Inflammatory Bowel Disease –
Diagnostic and Therapeutic Strategies

FALK SYMPOSIUM 154

Inflammatory Bowel Disease – Diagnostic and Therapeutic Strategies

Edited by

G. Adler
University Clinic Ulm
Ulm
Germany

C. Fiocchi
The Cleveland Clinic Foundation
Cleveland, Ohio
USA

L.B. Lazebnik
Institute of Gastroenterology
Moscow
Russia

G.I. Vorobiev
State Scientific Center of
Coloproctology
Moscow
Russia

Proceedings of the Falk Symposium 154 held in Moscow, Russia,
June 9–10, 2006

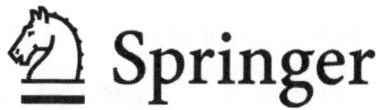

Library of Congress Cataloging-in-Publication Data is available.

ISBN-13 978-1-4020-6115-8

Published by Springer,
PO Box 17, 3300 AA Dordrecht, The Netherlands

Sold and distributed in North, Central and South America
by Springer,
101 Philip Drive, Norwell, MA 02061 USA

In all other countries, sold and distributed
by Springer,
PO Box 322, 3300 AH Dordrecht, The Netherlands

Printed on acid-free paper

Contents

SECTION II: MECHANISMS OF INFLAMMATORY BOWEL DISEASE: 2nd SESSION
Chair: GI Vorobiev, RB Sartor

SECTION III: MANAGEMENT OF INFLAMMATORY BOWEL DISEASE: 1st SESSION
Chair: AI Parfenov, WJ Sandborn

CONTENTS

SECTION IV: MANAGEMENT OF INFLAMMATORY BOWEL DISEASE: 2nd SESSION
Chair: YA Shelygin, SR Targan

List of principal contributors

EA Belousova
Moscow Regional Research
Clinical Institute
ul. Tschepkina 61/2-5
129110 Moscow
Russia

RS Blumberg
Harvard Medical School
Brigham and Women's Hospital
Division of Gastroenterology
75 Francis Street
Boston, MA 02115
USA

E Cario
University Hospital of Essen
Division of Gastroenterology and
  Hepatology
Institutsgruppe 1
Virchowstr. 171
D-45147 Essen
Germany

C Fiocchi
Department of Pathobiology
Lerner Research Institute
The Cleveland Clinic Foundation
9500 Euclid Avenue
Cleveland, Ohio 44195
USA

VY Golofeevsky
Military Medical Academy
Department of Hospital Therapy No.
  2
ul. Lebedeva 6
194044 St. Petersburg
Russia

H Herfarth
Division of Gastroenterology and
  Hepatology
University of North Carolina
4151 Bioinformatics Bldg
130 Mason Farm Road
Chapel Hill, NC 27599-7080
USA

DP Jewell
The Radcliffe Infirmary
Gastroenterology Unit
Nuffield Department of Medicine
Woodstock Road
Oxford, OX2 6HA
UK

IL Khalif
State Scientific Center of
  Coloproctology
Salyama Adil str. 2
123423 Moscow
Russia

NV Kostenko
Astrakhan Medical University
121, Bakinscay str.
414000 Astrakhan
Russia

LB Lazebnik
Center Research Institute of
  Gastroenterology
shosse Enthusiastov 86
111123 Moscow
Russia

JD Lewis
University of Pennsylvania
Center for Clinical Epidemiology and
  Biostatistics
7th Floor, Blockley Hall
423 Guardian Drive
Philadelphia, PA 19104-6021
USA

ID Loranskaya
Russian Medical Academy
Bol. Tishinskii per. 40-2-96
123557 Moscow
Russia

TT MacDonald
Barts and the London School of
  Medicine and Dentistry
Institute of Cell and Molecular
  Science
4 Newark Street
London, E1 2AT
UK

MF Neurath
Laboratory of Immunology
Department of Medicine
University of Mainz
Langenbeckstrasse 1
D-55101 Mainz
Germany

AS Peña
Department of Pathology
VU University Medical Center
PO Box 7057
NL-1007 MB Amsterdam
The Netherlands

C Prantera
Gastroenterology Unit
Azienda Ospedaliera
S. Camillo-Forlanini
Via Portuense, 292
I-00149 Rome
Italy

G Rogler
Department of Internal Medicine I
University of Regensburg
D-93042 Regensburg
Germany

WJ Sandborn
Inflammatory Bowel Disease Clinic
Division of Gastroenterology and
  Hepatology
Mayo Clinic
200 First Street SW
Rochester, MN 55905
USA

J-D Schulzke
Department of Gastroenterology,
  Infectious Diseases and
  Rheumatology
Medical Clinic I
Charité Campus Benjamin Franklin
D-12200 Berlin
Germany

GI Vorobiev
State Scientific Center of
  Coloproctology
Salyama Adil str. 2
123423 Moscow
Russia

M Zeitz
Medicine Clinic I
Department of Gastroenterology,
  Infectious Diseases and
  Rheumatology
Charité Campus Benjamin Franklin
Hindenburgdamm 30
D-12200 Berlin
Germany

List of chairpersons

LB Lazebnik
Center Research Institute of
 Gastroenterology
shosse Enthusiastov 86
111123 Moscow
Russia

AI Parfenov
Center Scientific Research
Institute of Gastroenterology
Entuziastov Shosse 86
111123 Moscow
Russia

WJ Sandborn
Inflammatory Bowel Disease Clinic
Division of Gastroenterology and
 Hepatology
Mayo Clinic
200 First Street SW
Rochester, MN 55905
USA

RB Sartor
University of North Carolina School
 of Medicine
Microbiology and Immunology
778 Burnett Womack Building
Chapel Hill, NC 27599-7080
USA

YA Shelygin
State Scientific Center of
 Coloproctology
Salyama Adil Str. 2
123423 Moscow
Russia

SR Targan
Cedars-Sinai Medical Center
Davis Research Center
#D-4063 (1865)
8700 Beverly Blvd
Los Angeles, CA 90048
USA

GI Vorobiev
State Scientific Center of
 Coloproctology
Salyama Adil Str. 2
123423 Moscow
Russia

M Zeitz
Medicine Clinic I
Department of Gastroenterology,
 Infectious Diseases and
 Rheumatology
Charite Campus Benjamin Franklin
Hindenburgdamm 30
D-12200 Berlin
Germany

Preface

This volume comprises the proceedings of the Falk Symposium No. 154 on 'Inflammatory bowel disease – diagnostic and therapeutic strategies'. The meeting was held in Moscow, Russia from June 9–10, 2006. The composition of the speakers represented a selected group of international experts from the United States of America, Russia and the rest of Europe. Of note, this meeting enjoyed the official co-sponsorship of the American Gastroenterological Association.

The major aim of the symposium was the presentation of the most recent progress in current understanding of IBD. State of the art lectures presented actual knowledge on the role of the immune system, the genetic factors, and the intestinal microflora in IBD. The second part of the meeting provided an evidence-based update on the current therapeutic options and discussed future perspectives for the management of IBD. In particular, emphasis was placed on various so-called 'biological' therapies that are opening a whole new therapeutic era.

The authors are grateful to Martin Falk and the Falk Foundation e.V., Freiburg for their generous support of the meeting and their excellent organization. Thanks to the generosity of the Falk Foundation, it was possible to bring together scientists and physicians from Europe, Russia, Asia and United States of America for fruitful discussion and exchange of ideas and experiences on IBD. We would like to thank Lancaster Publishing Services for their support in preparing this volume.

G. Adler, C. Fiocchi, G.I. Vorobiev, L.B. Lazebnik

Section I
Mechanisms of inflammatory bowel disease: 1st session

Chair: LB LAZEBNIK and M ZEITZ

1
State-of-the Art Lecture:
The multifactorial pathogenesis of inflammatory bowel disease

C. FIOCCHI

INTRODUCTION

Inflammation is the most common type of response the body mounts against the stimuli derived from the surrounding environment, and in the past several decades a worldwide surge in the frequency of chronic inflammatory diseases has been noted. Among them are inflammatory bowel diseases (IBD), whose clinical spectrum is represented primarily by Crohn's disease (CD) and ulcerative colitis (UC), although other forms of chronic gut inflammation also exist, including indeterminate, lymphocytic and collagenous colitis. In spite of remarkable progress made in the understanding of the cause and mechanisms of IBD[1-3], both CD and UC still represent major clinical challenges. One of the most serious limitations to the study of IBD is the practical fact that, by the time the patient manifests the first clinical symptoms, inflammation has already been present for a relatively long time and the gut almost invariably shows signs of chronic tissue damage. In reality the road to clinical disease starts at birth, when the future patient receives a set of genes from the parents that will determine his or her genetic susceptibility, and then continues with the exposure to conditioning environmental factors that may initiate subtle changes such as an increase in intestinal permeability or an immuno-regulatory imbalance leading to microscopic disease that will eventually evolve into macroscopic inflammation causing clinical symptoms[4]. The inflammatory injury in IBD tissue is eminently non-specific, mediated by the same substances involved in practically all other forms of acute or chronic inflammation, i.e. cytokines, growth factors, eicosanoids, neuropeptides, antibodies, reactive oxygen and nitrogen metabolites, and proteolytic enzymes. The factors that trigger the cascade of events that result in the exaggerated production of so many proinflammatory products are fairly well defined by now, and include genetic predisposition, the environment, the enteric commensal flora, and mucosal immune and non-immune cellular elements[1]. In this review each of these factors will be separately discussed,

3

aiming at highlighting the complexity of the multifactorial pathogenesis underlying both forms of IBD, and demonstrating how improved understanding of the role of each component has contributed to improve diagnosis and therapy of IBD patients.

ENVIRONMENTAL FACTORS

A remarkable feature of IBD is its evolution in time, particularly if one considers that this evolution has occurred incredibly quickly over a very short period of time[5,6]. Before the Second World War IBD was diagnosed almost exclusively in northern European countries and North America. From the 1950s to the 1970s both CD and UC began to be noticed in central and western Europe, Japan, Australia and South Africa, from the 1970s to the 1990s in the rest of Europe and South America, and in the last decade a surge of IBD in Asian countries has been documented[7]. A valid question related to this rapid increase in incidence is whether it is real or is simply due to a greater awareness by part of the medical community or improved diagnostic approaches. Studies have shown that this increase is indeed a true phenomenon, and no major differences in diagnostic capabilities are present in various countries with established or recently recognized IBD[8]. The progressive accumulation of IBD patients in clinics and hospitals is particularly noticeable in countries where CD and UC were considered practically nonexistent, i.e. Japan, Korea, China, and Malaysia[7], or even Puerto Rico[9].

Not only is IBD changing in incidence and prevalence during the last half-century, but the population being affected is also shifting to a progressively lower age group[10,11]. The percentage of children with IBD is increasing as a relative proportion of the entire IBD patient population, and at the same time the age of first diagnosis is dropping in the paediatric IBD patient population. Moreover, the new generations of these young CD and UC patients appear to have a different distribution among various racial groups and familial incidence when compared to older IBD patient populations. A recent study clearly demonstrates that the proportion of children with newly diagnosed IBD in the state of Wisconsin, USA, matches perfectly the relative proportions of the various ethnic groups (high Caucasian and low African-American, Hispanic, Asian, and other groups) in that state, and the vast majority of these paediatric patients do not have a family history, as traditionally observed only a few decades ago[12]. Taken together, these observations suggest an increasingly greater input of environmental over genetic factors in the appearance of IBD.

The rapid increase of CD and UC worldwide is not a unique phenomenon limited to IBD. For at least 50 years an increase in other autoimmune and chronic inflammatory diseases has been noted in parallel with IBD, as documented for asthma, type I diabetes and multiple sclerosis. What is even more intriguing is that such an increase has been accompanied by an equally well-documented decline in traditional infectious diseases, such as measles, rheumatic fever, hepatitis A and tuberculosis[13]. What is the cause-and-effect connection between these two events? What could explain the rise in chronic inflammatory and autoimmune diseases while infectious diseases tend to disappear? This must be investigated in the context of epidemiological evidence showing dramatic changes in the types of illnesses that afflict humanity and cause death during the past century. At the beginning of the 1900s tuberculosis, pneumonia, and diarrhoea – all infectious diseases – were responsible for 50% of all deaths in the United States of America, while at the end of the same century three-quarters of the same population was dying of heart disease and cancer[14]. Progress may be at the root of such striking changes in disease prevalence. Better housing, better nutrition, safer food and water, hygiene and sanitation, immunizations and the widespread use of antibiotics led to a decrease in disease transmission and host susceptibility, resulting in a drop in infectious diseases. At the same time, sheltered housing, clean food and water, selective nutrition, lack of parasites and new antigen exposure led to a restricted immune stimulation and an increase in host susceptibility, resulting in an increase in autoimmune/chronic inflammatory diseases[14]. These observations and conclusions constitute the basis for the 'hygiene hypothesis' that has been proposed to explain the rise, among other conditions, of IBD in the past few decades[15]. According to this hypothesis exposure to an increasingly 'clean' lifestyle with low microbial exposure would lead to a weak immune stimulation favouring Th2 responses that predispose to allergy and atopy, and perhaps explaining their increase worldwide. On the other hand, a 'dirty' lifestyle with high microbial exposure would lead to a strong Th1-mediated immune response conditioning the body to better defend itself against environmental insults later in life[16,17]. Though attractive, the hygiene hypothesis fails to explain why poor countries with low sanitation and a high incidence of parasites, that evoke a Th2 response, have a low incidence of allergic diseases, and countries with high hygiene and vaccination, that evoke a weak Th1 response, have a high incidence of typical Th1 conditions such as CD. Therefore, the existence of altered immunoregulatory networks with defective generation of suppressor cells or factors, such as interleukin (IL)-10 or transforming growth factor (TGF)-β has been postulated to complement the foundation of the hygiene hypothesis[18]. With specific reference to IBD, a multitude of environmental factors have been associated with IBD with either a predisposing or protective function, including smoking, diet, drugs, geography and social status, stress, microbes, intestinal permeability and appendectomy[19]. Of these, only smoking has been repeatedly shown to have a definitive association, being detrimental for CD but protective for UC[20].

GENETIC FACTORS

The existence of several members of the same family affected by IBD has been known for quite some time, either in the same generation or across generations, with an incidence of up to 30% of first-degree relatives having the disease, particularly in CD families[21]. This could be due to exposure to the same environmental factors or sharing the same genes. In reality all diseases are the result of combined environmental and genetic influences, and it is more a matter of how strong the influence of either one is, rather than whether a condition is due to one or the other[22]. To assess to what degree changes in the environment impact on disease appearance and phenotype is far more difficult than to establish whether a particular gene mutation brings about the manifestations of a particular illness. This has also been the case for CD and UC, and tremendous progress in the genetics of IBD has been achieved in little over 5 years after the discovery of the association of mutations of the *NOD2/CARD15* gene with stricturing small bowel CD[23,24]. These initial studies have provided not only more impetus for further genetic investigation, but also for better genotype–phenotype classifications of IBD patients and pharmacogenetics[25,26]. New genetic variations of the *OCTN* (IBD5) and *DLG5* genes have recently been reported, being associated with CD and IBD, respectively[27,28], and new linkages are now being continuously reported in various populations, such as polymorphism of toll receptor 9 (TLR-9) with CD[29], of ICAM-1 with CD[30], of TLR-4 with both CD and UC[31], and IL-10 with CD[32]. In regard to HLA, DRB1*1502 and DRB1*0103 are associated with UC in Jewish and non-Jewish populations[26]. At present there are at least 15 genetic loci with an association with IBD, seven being confirmed and replicated by several independent groups. There are numerous reports of single-nucleotide polymorphism (SNP) in IBD located in 40 different genes, and a preliminary report using an 'IBDchip' carrying 61 such SNP shows promise to predict clinical course and development of complications in IBD patients[33].

A perplexing aspect of genetic associations with IBD is their disparity according to the ethnicity of the population studied. An association with HLA-B5-DR2 was described more than 20 tears ago in Japanese patients with UC[34], but the most common *NOD2/CARD15* variants found in Western patients have not been detected in Japanese or Chinese patients with CD or UC[35,36]. The last observation was unexpected, but it opened the possibility that an assortment of gene mutations underlies the appearance of IBD in different populations, and some reports lend support to this possibility. Two studies from Japan describe an association of a polymorphism of the NRAMP1 gene with CD[37], and of IL-18 with UC patients[38]. It is unclear whether these findings represent genetic polymorphisms unique to Japanese subjects with IBD, or can be found in populations from other Asian nations, or even in IBD patients in other continents. Nevertheless, these findings underscore the value of pursuing genetic investigations in several and distinct IBD populations and searching for genes that may be able to distinguish genetically distinct subgroups of patients in different parts of the world, an observation that may provide new insights into IBD pathogenesis. The best example of how genetics can help to understand disease mechanisms is shown by the mutations of the *NOD2* gene found in Caucasian and Jewish populations. The product of *NOD2* is a cytosolic receptor found in antigen-presenting cells that recognizes muramyl dipeptide (MDP), a component of the bacterial cell wall commonly found in the gut[39,40]. This establishes a direct connection between the gut flora and the immune response to it, and it is reasonable to conceive that defective recognition of MDP by mutated NOD2 proteins may results in an abnormal immune response eventually resulting in CD[41,42].

MICROBIAL FACTORS

The idea that the gut flora was somehow linked to IBD pathogenesis has been proposed since the recognition of CD and UC as clinical entities, but only in the past few years has this concept been consolidated, due to discoveries in the field of IBD genetics, e.g. the association of *NOD2* mutations with ileal CD, and experimental and clinical evidence from animal models of IBD as well as humans[43]. An extremely rich enteric flora populates the gastrointestinal tract, with different types and concentrations of bacteria that augment progressively from the upper to the small and large bowel. Due to this complexity, and the practical reality that many microorganisms in the gut are not cultivable and therefore close to impossible to identify, evaluation of the composition of the gut flora in IBD presents many significant limitations. Nevertheless, when most reports are analysed as a whole, it appears that the flora of IBD patients differs from that of controls, is unstable and shows decreased diversity; in addition, some *E. coli* and *B. vulgatus* may play a detrimental role in disease pathogenesis[44]. The possibility that infectious agents are causing IBD has long been considered, but current evidence does not lend any solid support to this possibility[45]; and therefore putative pathogens as the cause of CD or UC will not be discussed here.

The enteric flora

This section will focus on the increasingly strong evidence that the gut commensal flora is the target of the pathogenic immune response in IBD. Since gut bacteria are essential to life, an equilibrium must exist between a massive amount of microorganisms (2×10^4) and the local immune system, resulting in the presence of an abundant number of immune cells in the mucosa that translates a state of 'physiological inflammation' necessary for protection against potentially harmful agents that may reach the intestinal lumen[46]. This immune equilibrium starts early in life when mucosal immune cells first recognize the various components of the normal flora and establish a state of tolerance to them and, under normal circumstances, this tolerance lasts a lifetime[47]. A number of cells and products are in place to recognize, sample and respond to intestinal bacteria.

Dendritic cells and Toll-like receptors

Mucosal dendritic cells are one of the first to enter in contact with gut bacteria[48], and several different subsets exist in the intestine and mesenteric lymph nodes[49]. Alterations of mucosal dendritic cells have recently been described in IBD[50], but it is still unclear whether they are primary or secondary to chronic gut inflammation. Dendritic cells recognize gut bacteria using a series of pattern recognition receptors, the best known being the Toll-like receptors (TLR), which are also expressed on various antigen-presenting cells (APC) and epithelial cells. Twelve TLR have been described so far, each homo- or heterodimer binding different bacterial products; they appear essential for recognition of commensal microflora and intestinal homeostasis[51], and are involved in signalling in the gut in health and disease[52]. Abnormalities of TLR expression have been described in IBD: TLR-3 is significantly down-regulated in intestinal epithelial cells in CD but not in UC, whereas TLR-4 is strongly up-regulated in both CD and UC[53]. In addition, several genetic polymorphisms of various TLR have been reported to be associated with IBD, including TLR-1, -2, -3, -4, and -6[54,55]. The true significance of these TLR alterations in the context of IBD pathogenesis is difficult to establish at the moment, and functional studies are needed. This is further complicated by the interaction of TLR with *NOD2*, as reported for the synergy normally existing between TLR-9 and *NOD2*, which appears to be lost in the presence of CD-associated *NOD2* mutations[56]. A commentary on this report suggests that altered *NOD2* signalling results in both enhanced T cell effector function and an impairment of regulatory T cell function[57].

Defensins

Another cellular system responsible for regulating the quantity of, and the interaction with, the lumenal flora is represented by the Paneth cells of the small intestinal crypts and their secreted products, primarily defensins[58,59]. Stimulation of Paneth cells by a variety of bacterial products results in multiple immune and non-immune functions that are important to the maintenance of intestinal homeostasis[59]. Of note, Paneth cells also produce abundant amounts of NOD2 protein, indicating synergism in antibacterial activity and bacterial recognition in the normal gut[60]. A series of recent reports indicate that a defect in defensins may exist in CD. Expression of human β-defensins (HBD) increases in the presence of gut inflammation, but this does not occur in CD for HBD-2 and -3[61]. Ileal expression of human α defensin 5 and 6 is impaired in active CD, and more so in patients with NOD2 mutations[62]. Finally, patients with CD of the ileum have a reduced antibacterial activity in their mucosal extracts in association with decreased α defensins independently of the degree of inflammation[63]. Based on these observations, the possibility that CD is a defensin deficiency syndrome has been suggested[64].

Animal models

Perhaps the best evidence that the gut flora plays a key role in IBD pathogenesis comes from animal models of IBD[65]. A large number of these have been created, and each has a different mechanism of induction and serves different experimental purposes. However, essentially all of them fail to develop gut inflammation when kept in a germ-free environment where the intestine is basically devoid of bacteria[66]; hence, the paradigm 'no bacteria, no colitis' has been proposed, and is presently widely accepted. This key observation allows the reconstitution of animals with single bacteria strains to assess their pathogenic potential, and distinct bacteria display different capabilities to induce gut inflammation[67–69]. Therefore, some crucial lessons have been learned from the evaluation of animal models of IBD: (1) completely different and independent factors (administration of exogenous agents, gene deletion, gene overexpression, and immune cell transfer) can cause IBD; (2) the genetic background of the animal influences the severity and location of inflammation; (3) colitis fails to develop in the absence of gut bacteria; (4) components of the normal gut flora are necessary to develop IBD.

Human studies

Evidence derived from human studies also lends considerable support to the notion of the importance of the flora in IBD pathogenesis. The number of bacteria associated with the inflamed mucosa is markedly greater in IBD than control subjects[70], and mucosal bacteria concentration is related to severity of gut inflammation[71]. In a particularly revealing clinical study it was shown that, in CD patients with small bowel disease, proximal diversion of the faecal stream after resection prevents disease recurrence, whereas exogenous infusion of lumenal contents in the distal stoma induces histological inflammatory changes within 1 week[72]. Another crucial report showed that mucosal lymphocytes of CD or UC patients with active disease proliferate when exposed to their own autologous aerobic and anaerobic flora, while those in patients with inactive disease do not, just as happens with lymphocytes from non-inflammatory control subjects[73]. This indicates that a state of immune tolerance to the gut flora is present in the normal mucosa (physiological inflammation), and tolerance is lost in IBD because the local immune system no longer recognizes the normal flora as self and mounts an inappropriate and persistent response against it (pathological inflammation). This being the case, it seems logical to conclude that modulation of the flora with antibiotics or probiotics may be therapeutically beneficial in IBD, and this appears to be the case. Alternatively, modulation of the mucosal immune response may also have beneficial effects, as will be discussed in the following section.

IMMUNE FACTORS

The intestinal immune system represents the effector arm of IBD pathogenesis, controlling the type and outcome of its response against aetiological agents. Even under physiological circumstances the intestinal immune response induces an inflammatory response, but this is tightly controlled in nature because tolerance to the potential offending agent is established. IBD patients, on the other hand, have lost or have a limited ability to develop tolerance, and pathological inflammation ensues and persists. The immunological consequences associated with this loss of tolerance or inability to regulate inflammation are numerous and varied, encompassing both the humoral and cell-mediated branch of immunity.

Humoral immunity

There is an exaggerated antibody production in IBD at both the systemic and mucosal level[74,75], more so in UC, where a marked increase in IgG production is observed, particularly of the IgG subclass I[76]. As a consequence, IBD patients display high titres of serum antibodies against a wide array of antigens present on colon epithelial cells, lymphocytes, cytoskeletal proteins, pancreatic proteins, cardiolipin, as well as dietary and bacterial antigens. Some of these antibodies are directed at autoantigens, as in the case of ECAC, human tropomyosin fraction 5 (hTM5) and neutrophils (pANCA)[77–79]. This raises the possibility that IBD could be an autoimmune condition, but little evidence supports the notion that truly pathogenic autoantibodies are present, although it is still possible that UC may have some component of autoimmunity. The studies by Das and collaborators have, over several years, generated enough data to partially support this possibility. Initially, a 40-kDa protein was isolated exclusively from the colon of UC but not CD patients, and an antibody developed against such protein recognized an epitope expressed by colonocytes[80], as well as all the other sites where the extraintestinal manifestations of IBD are frequently observed, such as the bile ducts, the skin, the eye and the joints[81]. The putative autoantigen was later identified as the structural protein hTM5 but, even though antibodies against the 40-kDa antigen were found to co-localize with complement components on UC colonocytes, suggesting the possibility of antibody-dependent, complement-mediated tissue damage[82], definitive proof of pathogenic autoimmunity in UC is still lacking.

IBD patients also have a multiplicity of antibacterial antibodies in the circulation. The range of bacteria that these antibodies react against is wide, but most of them probably represent a non-specific secondary phenomenon due to chronic inflammation. Some of the antibodies, however, appear to have some degree of specificity and may have the potential for differentiating CD from UC. Anti-*S. cerevisiae* antibodies (ASCA) are significantly more frequent in CD than UC[83,84]. The same may be the case for antibodies against I2[85], OmpC[86], and CBir1 flagellin[87]. Titres of these antibodies may also help in distinguishing clinical subgroups classified according to disease severity or complications.

Cell-mediated immunity

A large number of abnormalities of the cell-mediated immune system are found in IBD and, in general, they are considered more relevant to IBD pathogenesis. Only some of the most important will be reviewed here. Mucosal T cells from CD patients exhibit enhanced reactivity against a broad range of bacterial antigens, of both intestinal and non-intestinal origin[88]. The production of proinflammatory cytokines and chemokines is predictably high, as is the case for IL-1β, TNF-α, IL-6, IL-8 and many others[89–93]. Certainly more revealing are the patterns of immunoregulatory cytokines that allow better interpretation of whether and how the immune response is polarized in each form of IBD. These studies have been especially revealing of immunopathogenic events that are distinct for CD and UC. CD is a fairly typical Th1 response, with a predominant production of interferon (IFN)-γ, IL-12 and IL-18[94–96], whereas UC represents an atypical Th2-like condition with high production of IL-5 and IL-13 but low IL-4[97]. The functional capacity of mucosal T cells is also distinct between CD and UC. CD mucosal T cells proliferate and expand considerably more than UC cells[98,99], and are also more resistant to apoptosis[99,100]. The latter feature seems to be a basic characteristic of CD because induction of apoptosis of mucosal T cells by some biological agents, such as anti-TNF-α antibodies, seems essential to their therapeutic effects[101,102]. Another abnormality of the mucosal immune system that precludes down-regulation of inflammation in IBD is an excessive increase of SMAD7, a key signalling molecule that blocks phosphorylation of SMAD3 and prevents TGF-β from exerting its full suppressive and anti-inflammatory activity[103].

Innate immunity

All of the above cell-mediated abnormalities are related to adaptive immunity, where the T cell plays a central role, but they are all downstream of innate immunity events, where the initial response to inciting agents takes place. Evidence has recently emerged indicating that important defects of innate immunity may be present in IBD, CD in particular, and may actually lead to the above-mentioned alterations of adaptive immunity as secondary compensatory phenomena. CD patients carrying *NOD2* mutations exhibit severely impaired production of IL-1β and IL-8 by monocytes in response to MDP and TNF-α stimulation[104]. In addition, *NOD2* mutation-independent defects of innate immune responses have also been documented *in vivo* in CD patients. In response to acute injury there is a markedly decreased neutrophil accumulation and IL-8 production in the gut mucosa, but also impaired erythema, swelling and blood flow in response to *E. coli* injection in the patient's forearm[105]. Fascinatingly, both effects are absent in UC patients. These novel observations point to a systemic defect causing an inadequate acute innate immune response in CD, and suggest that abnormalities of both innate and adaptive immunity may be present in this condition, but whether and how the two might be interrelated remains to be established.

THERAPEUTIC IMPLICATIONS

In contrast to the early days of IBD therapy, where practically all drugs were used empirically based on a presumed or suspected anti-inflammatory activity, for close to two decades the treatment of CD and UC patients has evolved based on an increasingly evidence-based knowledge of the biological mechanisms and molecules involved in gut inflammation. This is a consequence of studies directed at unveiling the intricacies of mucosal immunity and the proinflammatory pathways of immune and non-immune cells. Just to cite a few, biologicals, probiotics, and leukapheresis are some examples of research-derived therapies. All these new and diverse approaches aim at the same ultimate goal, the improvement or elimination of gut inflammation, but each tries to achieve this beneficial effect by impacting on different components of IBD pathogenesis. Biologicals can be directed at blocking proinflammatory cytokines, receptors, cell adhesion molecules, signalling molecules, etc. or supplying extra amounts of natural suppressor molecules. Probiotics try to modulate the behaviour of the commensal gut flora so its recognition by the local immune system results in anti-inflammatory rather than proinflammatory effects. Leukapheresis physically removes cellular elements that execute or amplify inflammation. Although all represent major advances, none of them alone is likely to result in complete cure, an observation that underscores the complexity of the mechanisms of IBD, and the fact that most of the time we are trying to fix a problem that has been present for a long time, rather than attacking pathogenic steps at an earlier time point. The lesson here is that perhaps we should become more aggressive and intervene when the disease is of recent onset, as seen in paediatric IBD. Studies in animals models have shown that the pathogenic cytokines profile underlying gut inflammation shifts from one to another Th pattern during progression of disease[106], and the same may be true in humans. Early intervention with infliximab in children with the first attack of CD results in a much longer remission period as compared to children treated when the disease is chronic[107]. Therefore, in addition to learning how to intervene, we must also learn when to intervene during the evolution of the IBD process. Enough experience has proved that evolving knowledge based on solid experimental observations is the right path to discover more effective therapies, and at present the outlook has never been more promising for new breakthroughs in IBD pathogenesis and treatment[108].

In conclusion, the following points succinctly translate the main messages learned so far from an enormous amount of information gained on the pathogenesis of IBD:

- CD and UC share some epidemiological and clinical features, but represent distinct entities with different mechanisms of gut inflammation in each condition.

- Environmental changes, genetic predisposition, the enteric commensal flora, and the mucosal immune response are the key components of IBD pathogenesis.

- Loss of immune tolerance against the autologous enteric flora appears to be a central event in IBD pathogenesis, and modulation of the flora and/or the host's immune response against it seem essential to control gut inflammation.

- Current biological therapies are the direct result of an improved understanding of IBD pathogenesis, and further progress in this area will continue to generate new and better forms of therapy.

References

1. Fiocchi C. Inflammatory bowel disease: etiology and pathogenesis. Gastroenterology. 1998;115:182–205.
2. Podolsky DK. Inflammatory bowel disease. N Engl J Med. 2002;347:417–29.
3. MacDonald TT, Monteleone G. Immunity, inflammation, and allergy in the gut. Science. 2005;307:1920–5.
4. Cohen MB, Seidman E, Winter H et al. Controversies in pediatric inflammatory bowel disease. Inflamm Bowel Dis. 1998;4:203–27.
5. Ekbom A. Epidemiology of inflammatory bowel disease. In: Bistrian BR, Walker-Smith JA, editors. Inflammatory Bowel Diseases. Basel: Karger; 1999:7–21.

6. Loftus EV. Clinical epidemiology of inflammatory bowel disease: incidence, prevalence, and environmental influences. Gastroenterology. 2004;126:1504–17.
7. Ouyang Q, Tandon R, Goh K-L, Ooi CJ, Ogata H, Fiocchi C. The emergence of inflammatory bowel disease in the Asian Pacific region. Curr Opin Gastroenterol. 2005;21:408–13.
8. Lennard-Jones JE, Shivananda S. Clinical uniformity of inflammatory bowel disease at presentation and during the first year of disease in the north and south of Europe. Eur J Gastroenterol Hepatol. 1997;9:353–9.
9. Appleyard CB, Hernandez G, Rios-Bedoya CF. Basic epidemiology of inflammatory bowel disease in Puero Rico. Inflamm Bowel Dis. 2004;10:106–11.
10. Barton JR, Gillon S, Ferguson A. Incidence of inflammatory bowel disease in Scottish children between 1968 and 1983; marginal fall in ulcerative colitis, threefold increase in Crohn's disease. Gut. 1989;30:618–22.
11. Olafsdottir EJ, Fluge G, Haug K. Chronic inflammatory bowel disease in children in western Norway. J Pediatr Gastroenterol Nutr. 1989;8:454–8.
12. Kugathasan S, Judd RH, Hoffmann RG et al. Epidemiologic and clinical characteristics of children with newly diagnosed inflammatory bowel disease in Wisconsin: a statewide population-based study. J Pediatr. 2003;143:525–31.
13. Bach J-F. The effect of infections an susceptibility to autoimmune and allergic diseases. N Engl J Med. 2002;347:911–20.
14. Cohen ML. Changing patterns of infectious disease. Nature. 2000;406:762–7.
15. Feillet H, Bach J-F. Increased incidence of inflammatory bowel disease: the price of the decline of infectious burden? Curr Opin Gastroenterol. 2004;20:560–4.
16. Wills-Karp M, Santeliz J, Karp CL. The germless theory of allergic diseases: revisiting the hygiene hypothesis. Nature Rev. 2001;1:69–75.
17. Borchers AT, Keen CL, Gershwin ME. Hope for the hygiene hypothesis: when the dirt hits the fan. J Asthma. 2005;42:225–47.
18. Yazdanbakhsh M, Kremsner PG, van Ree R. Allergy, parasites, and the hygiene hypothesis. Science. 2002;296:490–4.
19. Danese S, Sans M, Fiocchi C. Inflammatory bowel disease: the role of environmental factors. Autoimmun Rev. 2004;3:390–400.
20. Birrenbach T, Bocker U. Inflammatory bowel disease and smoking. A review of epidemiology, pathophysiology, and therapeutic implications. Inflamm Bowel Dis. 2004;10:848–59.
21. Farmer RG, Michener WM. Association of inflammatory bowel disease in families. Front Gastrointest Res. 1986;11:17–26.
22. Chakravarti A, Little P. Nature, nurture and human disease. Nature. 2003;421:412–14.
23. Hugot J-P, Chamaiilard M, Zouali H et al. Association of NOD2 leucine-rich repeat variants with susceptibility to Crohn's disease. Nature. 2001;411:599–603.
24. Ogura Y, Bonen DK, Inohara N et al. A frameshift mutation in Nod2 associated with susceptibility to Crohn's disease. Nature. 2001;411:603–6.
25. Bonen DK, Cho JH. The genetics of inflammatory bowel disease. Gastroenterology. 2003;124:521–36.
26. Ahamd T, Tamboli CP, Jewell D, Colombel J-F. Clinical relevance of advances in genetics and pharmacogenetics. Gastroenterology. 2004;126:1533–49.
27. Peltekova VD, Wintle RF, Rubin LA et al. Functional variants of *OCTN* cation transporter genes are associated with Crohn's disease. Nat Genet. 2004;36:471–5.
28. Stoll M, Corneliussen B, Costello CM et al. Genetic variation in *DLG5* is associated with inflammatory bowel disease. Nat Genet. 2004;36:476–80.
29. Torok H-P, Glas J, Tonenchi L, Bruennler G. Crohn's disease is associated with a toll-like receptor-9 polymorphism. Gastroenterology. 2004;127:365–6.
30. Low JH, Williams FA, Yang X et al. Inflammatory bowel disease is linked to 19p13 and associated with ICAM-1. Inflamm Bowel Dis. 2004;10:173–81.
31. Franchimont D, Vermeire S, ElHousni H et al. Deficient host–bacteria interactions in inflammatory bowel disease? The toll-like receptor (TLR)-4 Asp299gly polymorphism is associated with Crohn's disease and ulcerative colitis. Gut. 2004;53:987–92.
32. Fernandez L, Martinez A, Mendoza JL et al. Interleukin-10 polymorphisms in Spanish patients with IBD. Inflamm Bowel Dis. 2005;11:739–43.

33. Sans M, Artieda M, Diego T et al. IBDchip: a new strategy to predict clinical course and development of complications in patients with inflammatory bowel disease (IBD). Gastroenterology. 2006;130:A-52 (Abstract).

34. Asakura H, Tsuchiya M, Aiso S et al. Association of the human lymphocyte-DR2 antigen with Japanese ulcerative colitis. Gastroenterology. 1982;82:413–18.

35. Inoue N, Tamura K, Kinouchi Y et al. Lack of common NOD2 variants in Japanese patients with Crohn's disease. Gastroenterology. 2002;123:86–91.

36. Leong RW, Armuzzi A, Ahmad T et al. NOD2/CARD15 gene polymorphisms and Crohn's disease in the Chinese population. Aliment Pharmacol Ther. 2003;17:1465–70.

37. Kojima Y, Kinouchi Y, Takahashi S, Negoro K, Hiwatashi N, Shimosegawa T. Inflammatory bowel disease is associated with a novel promoter polymorphism of natural resistance-associated macrophage protein 1 (NRAMP1) gene. Tiss Antigen. 2001;58:379–84.

38. Takagawa T, Tamura K, Takeda N et al. Association between IL-18 gene promoter polymorphisms and inflammatory bowel disease in a Japanese population. Inflamm Bowel Dis. 2005;11:1038–43.

39. Girardin SE, Boneca IG, Viala J et al. Nod2 is a general sensor of peptidoglycan through muramyl dipeptide (MDP) detection. J Biol Chem. 2003;278:8869–72.

40. Inohara N, Ogura Y, Fontalba A et al. Host recognition of bacterial muramyl dipeptide mediated through NOD2. J Biol Chem. 2003;278:5509–12.

41. Inohara N, Nunez G. Nods: intracellular proteins involved in inflammation and apoptosis. Nature Rev. 2003;3:371–82.

42. Eckmann L, Karin M. NOD2 and Crohn's disease: loss or gain of function? Immunity. 2005;22:661–7.

43. Fiocchi C. Microbial factors in the pathogenesis of IBD. Biosci Microflora. 2003;22:5–14.

44. Marteau P, Lepage P, Mangin I. Review article: Gut flora and inflammatory bowel disease. Aliment Pharmacol Ther. 2004;20(Suppl. 4):18–23.

45. Van Kruiningen HJ. Lack of support for a common etiology in Johne's disease of animals and Crohn's disease in humans. Inflamm Bowel Dis. 1999;5:183–91.

46. Fiocchi C. The normal intestinal mucosa: a state of 'controlled inflammation'. In: Targan SR, Shanahan F, editors. Inflammatory Bowel Disease: From Bench to Bedside, 2nd edn. Dordrecht: Kluwer, 2003:101–20.

47. Ogawa H, Fukushima K, Sasaki I, Matsuno S. Identification of genes involved in mucosal defense and inflammation associated with normal enteric bacteria. Am J Physiol. 2000;279: G492–9.

48. Rescigno M, Urbano M, Valzasina B et al. Dendritic cells express tight junction proteins and penetrate gut epithelial monolayers to sample bacteria. Nat Immunol. 2001;2:361–7.

49. Mowat AM. Anatomical basis of tolerance and immunity to intestinal antigens. Nat Rev Immunol. 2003;3:331–41.

50. Hart AL, Al-Hassi HO, Rigby RJ et al. Characteristics of intestinal dendritic cells in inflammatory bowel disease. Gastroenterology. 2005;129:50–65.

51. van Heel DA, Gosh S, Butler M et al. Muramyl dipeptide and toll-like receptor sensitivity in NOD2-associated Crohn's disease. Lancet. 2005;365:1794–6.

52. Abreu MT, Fukata M, Arditi M. TLR signaling in the gut in health and disease. J Immunol. 2005;174:4453–60.

53. Cario E, Podolsky DK. Differential alteration in intestinal epithelial cell expression of toll-like receptor 3 (TLR3) and TLR4 in inflammatory bowel disease. Infect Immun. 2000;68: 7010–17.

54. Oostenbrug LE, Drenth JPH, deJong DJ et al. Association between toll-like receptor 4 and inflammatory bowel disease. Inflamm Bowel Dis. 2005;11:567–75.

55. Pierik M, Joossens S, van Steen K et al. Toll-like receptor -1, -2, and -6 polymorphisms influence disease extension in inflammatory bowel disease. Inflamm Bowel Dis. 2006;12:1–8.

56. van Heel DA, Gosh S, Hunt KA et al. Synergy between TLR9 and NOD2 innate immune responses is lost in genetic Crohn's disease. Gut. 2005;54:1553–7.

57. Watanabe T, Kitani A, Strober W. NOD2 regulation of Toll-like receptor responses and the pathogenesis of Crohn's disease. Gut. 2005;54:1515–18.

58. Ouellette AJ. Mucosal immunity and inflammation. IV. Paneth cell antimicrobial peptides and the biology of the mucosal barrier. Am J Physiol. 1999;277:G257–61.

59. Selsted ME, Oullette AJ. Mammalian defensins in the antimicrobial immune response. Nat Immunol. 2005;6:551–7.

60. Ogura Y, Lala S, Xin W et al. Expression of NOD2 in Paneth cells: a possible link to Crohn's ileitis. Gut. 2003;52:1591–7.

61. Wehkamp J, Harder J, Weichenthal M et al. Inducible and constitutive ß-defensins are differentially expressed in Crohn's disease and ulcerative colitis. Inflamm Bowel Dis. 2003;9:215–23.

62. Wehkamp J, Harder J, Weichenthal M et al. NOD2(CARD15) mutations in Crohn's disease are associated with diminished mucosal α-defensin expression. Gut. 2004;53:1658–64.

63. Wehkamp J, Salzman NH, Porter E et al. Reduced Paneth cell α-defensins in ileal Crohn's disease. Proc Natl Acad Sci USA. 2005;102:18129–34.

64. Fellermann K, Wehkamp J, Herrlinger KR, Stange EF. Crohn's disease: a defensin deficiency syndrome? Eur J Gastroenterol Hepatol. 2003;15:627–34.

65. Strober W, Fuss IJ, Blumberg RS. The immunology of mucosal models of inflammation. Annu Rev Immunol. 2002;20:495–549.

66. Taurog JD, Richardson JA, Croft JT et al. The germfree state prevents development of gut and joint inflammatory disease in HLA-B27 transgenic rats. J Exp Med. 1994;180:2359–64.

67. Rath HC, Herfarth HH, Ikeda JS et al. Normal luminal bacteria, especially Bacteroides species, mediate chronic colitis, gastritis, and arthritis in HLA-B27/human β2 microglobulin transgenic rats. J Clin Invest. 1996;98:945–53.

68. Rath HC, Ikeda JS, Linde H-J, Scholmerich J, Wilson KH, Sartor RB. Varying cecal bacterial loads influences colitis and gastritis in HLA-B27 transgenic rats. Gastroenterology. 1999;116:310–19.

69. Rath HC, Wilson KH, Sartor RB. Differential induction of colitis and gastritis in HLA-B27 trangenic rats selectively colonized with Bacteroides vulgatus or Escherichia coli. Infect Immun. 1999;67:2969–74.

70. Schultsz C, Van den Berg FM, Kate FWT, Tytgat GNJ, Dankert J. The intestinal mucus layer from patients with inflammatory bowel disease harbors high numbers of bacteria compared with controls. Gastroenterology. 1999;117:1089–97.

71. Swidsinski A, Ladhoff A, Pernthaler A et al. Mucosal flora in inflammatory bowel disease. Gastroenterology. 2002;122:44–54.

72. D'Haens G, Geboes K, Peeters M, Baert F, Penninckx F, Rutgeerts P. Early lesions caused by infusion of intestinal contents in excluded ileum of Crohn's disease. Gastroenterology. 1998;114:262–7.

73. Duchmann R, Kaiser I, Hermann E, Mayet W, Ewe K, Meyer zum Buschenfelde K-H. Tolerance exists towards resident intestinal flora but it is broken in active inflammatory bowel disease (IBD). Clin Exp Immunol. 1995;102:448–55.

74. MacDermott RP, Nash GS, Bertovich MJ, Seiden MV, Bragdon MJ, Beale MG. Alterations of IgM, IgG, and IgA synthesis and secretion by peripheral blood and intestinal mononuclear cells from patients with ulcerative colitis and Crohn's disease. Gastroenterology. 1981;81:844–52.

75. MacDermott RP, Nash GS, Bertovich MJ et al. Altered patterns of secretion of monomeric IgA and IgA subclass 1 by intestinal mononuclear cells in inflammatory bowel disease. Gastroenterology. 1986;91:379–85.

76. Scott MG, Nahm MH, Macke K, Nash GS, Bertovich MJ, Macdermott RP. Spontaneous secretion of IgG subclasses by intestinal mononuclear cells: differences between ulcerative colitis, Crohn's disease, and controls. Clin Exp Immunol. 1986;66:209–15.

77. Roche JK, Fiocchi C, Youngman K. Sensitization to epithelial antigens in chronic mucosal inflammatory disease. Characterization of human intestinal mucosa-derived mononuclear cells reactive with purified epithelial cell-associated components in vitro. J Clin Invest. 1985;75:522–30.

78. Das KM, Dasgupta A, Mandal A, Geng X. Autoimmunity to cytoskeletal protein tropomyosin. A clue to the pathogenetic mechanisms for ulcerative colitis. J Immunol. 1993;150:2487–93.

79. Saxon A, Shanahan F, Landers C, Ganz T, Targan S. A distinct subset of anti-neutrophil cytoplasmic antibodies is associated with inflammatory bowel disease. J Allergy Clin Immunol. 1990;86:202–10.

80. Das KM, Sakamaki S, Vecchi M, Diamond B. The production and characterization of monoclonal antibodies to a human colonic antigen associated with ulcerative colitis:

cellular localization of the antigen by using the monoclonal antibody. J Immunol. 1987;139:77–84.

81. Das KM. Relationship of extraintestinal involvements in inflammatory bowel disease. New insights into autopimmune pathogenesis. Dig Dis Sci. 1999;44:1–13.

82. Takahashi F, Shah HS, Wise LS, Das KM. Circulating antibodies against human colonic extract enriched with a 40 kD protein in patients with ulcerative colitis. Gut. 1990;31:1016–20.

83. McKenzie H, Main J, Pennington CR, Parratt D. Antibody to selected strains of *Saccharomyces cerevisiae* (baker's and brewer's yeast) and *Candida albicans* in Crohn's disease. Gut. 1990;31:536–8.

84. Quinton JF, Sendid B, Reumaux D et al. Anti-*Saccharomyces cerevisiae* mannan antibodies combined with antineutrophil cytoplasmic autoantibodies in inflammatory bowel disease: prevalence and diagnostic role. Gut. 1998;42:788–91.

85. Dalwadi H, Wei B, Kronenberg M, Sutton CL, Braun J. The Crohn's disease-associated bacterial protein I2 is a novel enteric T cell superantigen. Immunity. 2001;15:149–58.

86. Mow WS, Vasiliauskas EA, Lin Y-C et al. Association of antibody responses to microbial antigens and complications of small bowel Crohn's disease. Gastroenterology. 2004;126:414–24.

87. Targan SR, Landers CJ, Yang H et al. Antibodies to CBir1 flagellin define a unique response that is associated independently with complicated Crohn's disease. Gastroenterology. 2005;128:2020–8.

88. Pirzer UC, Schurmann G, Post S, Betzler M, Meuer SC. Differential responsiveness to CD3-Ti vs CD2-dependent activation of human intestinal lymphocytes. Eur J Immunol. 1990;20:2339–42.

89. Youngman KR, Simon PL, West GA et al. Localization of intestinal interleukin 1 activity, protein and gene expression to lamina propria cells. Gastroenterology. 1993;104:749–58.

90. Braegger CP, Nicholls S, Murch SH, Stephens S, MacDonald TT. Tumour necrosis factor alpha in stool as a marker of intestinal inflammation. Lancet. 1992;339:89–91.

91. Mahida YR, Kurlak L, Gallagher A, Hawkey CJ. Circulating and tissue interleukin 6 (IL6) levels in inflammatory bowel disease. Gastroenterology. 1990;98:461 (Abstract).

92. Mahida YR, Ceska M, Effenberger F, Kurlak L, Lindley I, Hawkey CJ. Enhanced synthesis of neutrophil-activating peptide-I/interleukin-8 in active ulcerative colitis. Clin Sci. 1992; 82:273–5.

93. Reinecker H-C, Loh EY, Ringler DJ, Metha A, Rombeau JL, MacDermott RP. Monocyte-chemoattractant protein 1 gene expression in intestinal epithelial cells and inflammatory bowel disease mucosa. Gastroenterology. 1995;108:40–50.

94. Fais S, Capobianchi MR, Pallone F et al. Spontaneous release of interferon γ by intestinal lamina propria lymphocytes in Crohn's disease. Kinetics of *in vitro* response to interferon γ inducers. Gut. 1991;32:403–7.

95. Monteleone G, Biancone L, Marasco R et al. Interleukin 12 is expressed and actively released by Crohn's disease intestinal lamina propria mononuclear cells. Gastroenterology. 1997;112:1169–78.

96. Pizarro TP, Michie MH, Bentz M et al. IL-18, a novel immunoregulatory cytokine, is up-regulated in Crohn's disease: expression and localization in intestinal mucosal cells. J Immunol. 1999;162:6829–35.

97. Fuss IJ, Heller F, Boirivant M et al. Nonclassical CD1d-restricted NK T cells that produce IL-13 characterize an atypical Th2 response in ulcerative colitis. J Clin Invest. 2004;113: 1490–97.

98. Kugathasan S, Willis J, Dahms BB et al. Intrinsic hyperreactivity of mucosal T-cells to interleukin-2 in pediatric Crohn's disease. J Pediatr. 1998;133:675–81.

99. Sturm A, Leite AZ, Danese S et al. Divergent cell cycle kinetics underlie the distinct functional capacity of mucosal T-cells in Crohn's disease (CD) and ulcerative colitis (UC). Gut. 2004;53:1624–31.

100. Ina K, Itoh J, Fukushima K et al. Resistance of Crohn's disease T-cells to multiple apoptotic stimuli is associated with a Bcl-2/Bax mucosal imbalance. J Immunol. 1999; 163:1081–90.

101. Sturm A, Fiocchi C. Life and death in the gut: more killing, less Crohn's. Gut. 2002;50:148–9.

102. DiSabatino A, Ciccocioppo R, Cinque B et al. Defective mucosal T cell death is sustainably reverted by infliximab in a caspase dependent pathway in Crohn's disease. Gut. 2004;53:70–7.
103. Monteleone G, Kumberova A, Croft NM, McKenzie C, Steer HW, MacDonald TT. Blocking Smad7 restores TGF-α1 signaling in chronic inflammatory bowel disease disease. J Clin Invest. 2001;108:601–9.
104. Li J, Moran T, Swanson E et al. Regulation of IL-8 and IL-1ß expression in Crohn's disease associated with NOD2/CARD15 mutations. Hum Mol Genet. 2004;13:1715–25.
105. Marks DJB, Hardbord MWN, MacAllister R et al. Defective acute inflammation in Crohn's disease: a clinical investigation. Lancet. 2006;367:668–78.
106. Spencer DM, Veldman GM, Banerjee S, Willis J, Levine AD. Distinct inflammatory mechanisms mediate early versus late colitis in mice. Gastroenterology. 2002;122:94–105.
107. Kugathasan S, Werlin SL, Martinez A, Rivera MT, Heineken JB, Binion DG. Prolonged duration of response to infliximab in early but not late pediatric Crohn's disease. Am J Gastroenterol. 2000;95:3189–94.
108. Korzenik JR, Podolsky DK. Evolving knowledge and therapy of inflammatory bowel disease. Nat Rev Drug Discovery. 2006;5:197–209.

2
CD1d: at the cusp of innate and adaptive immunity in regulating mucosal inflammation

E. NIEUWENHUIS, A. KASER, S. DOUGAN, J. GLICKMAN,
T. MATSUMOTO, A. ONDERDONK and R. S. BLUMBERG

INTRODUCTION

The development of an immune response and consequently inflammation that is derived from immune-mediated mechanisms is initiated, perpetuated and ultimately controlled by the interaction between the two major arms of the immune system, innate immunity and adaptive (specific) immunity. Innate immunity represents an immediate, hard-wired response between structural components of microbes and pattern recognition receptors of the immune system. An example of this is the interaction between muramyl dipeptide (MDP) derived from Gram-positive and Gram-negative bacteria with NOD2/CARD15[1,2]. NOD2/CARD15 is expressed in both epithelial cells, including Paneth cells, and myeloid cells, including monocytes and macrophages[3]. Polymorphisms in NOD2/CARD15 are associated with increased risk for the development of Crohn's disease[1]. In contrast, adaptive or specific immunity is a slower immunological response that is obtained from the interaction between an antigen-presenting cell (APC) (dendritic cell, macrophage, B cell or intestinal epithelial cell) and a T cell that is associated with immunological memory. A classic paradigm for adaptive or specific immunity is the antigen-presentation pathway that is associated with the degradation of protein antigens into nominal peptides derived from a protein antigen wherein the peptide (9–16 amino acids) binds to proteins of the major histocompatibility complex (MHC)[4]. These human leukocyte-associated antigens (HLA) that are contained within the MHC locus on chromosome 6 interact with the T cell receptor (TCR) on a T cell leading to activation of T cell responses (Figure 1).

Innate and adaptive immune responses (Figure 2) are the molecular mechanisms by which T cells and APC interact and thus respond to antigens derived from microorganisms. Antigens differentially activate innate and adaptive immune mechanisms leading to activation of both the T cell and the APC which culminates in the secretion of cytokines by both cell types and the

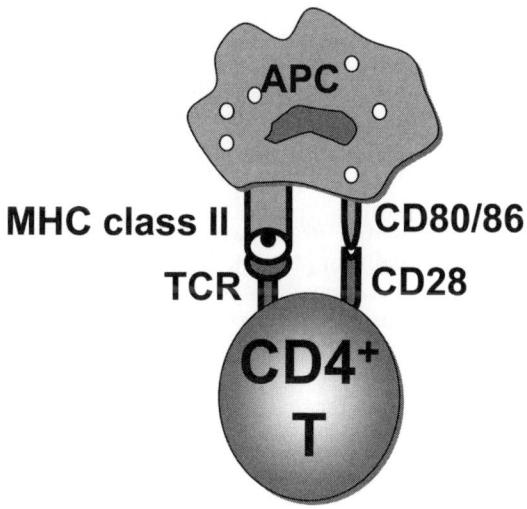

Figure 1 Antigen-presenting cell (APC) – T cell interaction: Signal 1, MHC class II–T cell receptor (TCR) interaction; signal 2 (costimulation), CD80/CD86–CD28 interaction

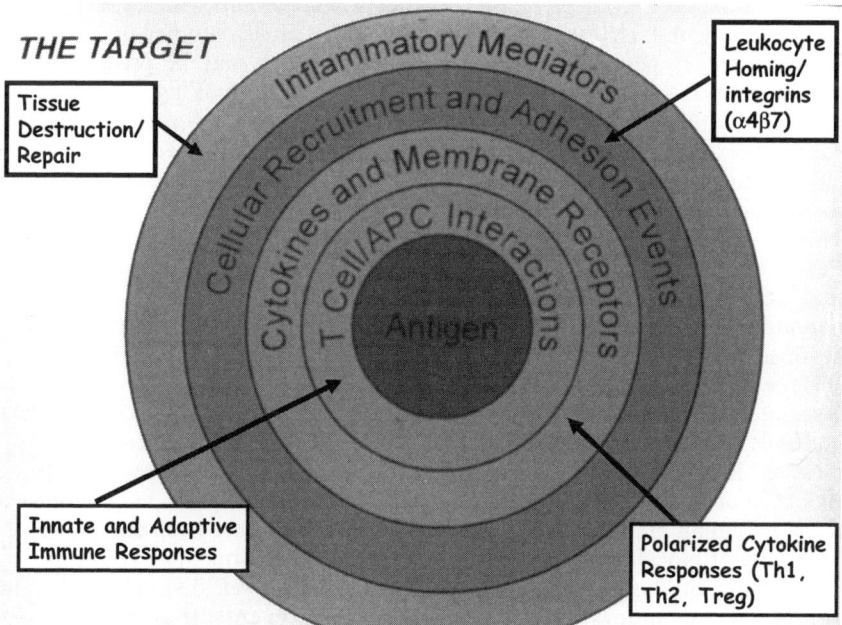

Figure 2 Layers of immune response that are the targets for therapies

up-regulation of membrane receptors. The cytokines produced by the T cell and APC will further affect endothelial cells, leading to the activation of local blood vessels and culminating in up-regulation of membrane receptors that increase adhesion and recruitment of many types of leukocytes into tissues. The leukocytes that are recruited through the activated endothelium play an important role in amplifying the immune response and are further activated by the local inflammatory milieu, resulting in the production of a wide range of inflammatory mediators.

Understanding the sequential events associated with the generation of inflammation is therapeutically important. By understanding the molecular events that lead to the generation of inflammation and tissue destruction (Figure 2), as would occur in inflammatory bowel disease (IBD), will help in the development of new therapeutic strategies to treat disease. There are two layers of potential therapeutic control: those that are directed against proinflammatory pathways or those that inhibit (or down-regulate) these aggressive pathways. For example, innate and adaptive immune responses lead to the production of proinflammatory cytokines such as T helper1 (Th1) promoting cytokines (tumour necrosis factor, interferon-γ, interleukin (IL)-12), Th2 cytokines (IL-4, IL-5, IL-13) and Th17 cytokines (IL-17, IL-23)[5]. It would therefore be predicted that antibody neutralization of these cytokines will lead to amelioration of intestinal inflammation. Indeed human clinical studies have now shown that blockade of IL-12, IL-23 and interferon-γ can cause amelioration of Crohn's disease, making it likely that Crohn's disease is mainly a Th1 and Th17-associated condition[6,7]. Clinical studies have not yet been extensively performed in ulcerative colitis but it may be predicted that blockade of IL-13 may also ameliorate this disease, making it likely that ulcerative colitis is mainly a Th2-associated disease[8,9]. Strong regulatory pathways exist in humans, that are mainly derived from the secretion of anti-inflammatory cytokines from T cells[10]. These so-called T regulatory (Treg) cells secrete high levels of anti-inflammatory cytokine such as IL-10 and TGF-β. These Treg cells are a major focus of research in the treatment of IBD. In a similar manner, blocking molecules on either endothelial cells or on leukocytes that are involved in their recruitment to the intestinal tissues is a major potential mechanism to treat these diseases. Indeed, leukocytes that are destined to migrate into intestinal tissues express molecules on their cell surface such as the mucosal-associated integrin (α4β7) or the mucosal-associated chemokine receptor (CCR9)[11]. In turn, endothelial cells express molecules on their cell surface such as the immunoglobulin supergene family member, MAdCAM1, that binds to the mucosal-associated addressin, α4β7[12]. Blockade of either α4β7, MAdCAM1 or CCR9, would be predicted to improve intestinal inflammation. Indeed, human clinical trials have been completed on the utility of blocking α4-associated proteins in the treatment of IBD through the success of therapeutics such as Tysabri[Tr] (see ref. 13). Therefore, in summary, by understanding the cascade of events that lead to the development of intestinal inflammation, tissue destruction and ultimately symptoms, drugs can be rationally developed, targeted and applied to the treatment of IBD.

CD1d AND CD1d-RESTRICTED T CELL PATHWAYS

Given the importance of innate and adaptive immunity in the development of inflammation in general, and IBD in particular, one molecule that has arisen as being of particular interest is CD1d. As will be seen in the discussion below, interest in CD1d occurs at multiple levels, but perhaps most interestingly is due to that fact that CD1d functions at the cusp between innate and adaptive immunity. The real interest perhaps in understanding proteins such as CD1d is that, by understanding the molecular immunology of this protein, and many others that regulate the aforementioned cascade of events associated with the development of inflammation, this will allow for the development of new classes of therapeutic agents. This discussion of CD1d is thus a template for other immunologically active molecules involved in the generation of intestinal inflammation.

CD1d is a MHC class I-related molecule[14]. As such, CD1d is structurally related to the HLA-A, B, and C proteins. CD1d thus consists of a heavy chain of approximately 45–48 kDa in non-covalent association with a light chain (β_2-microglobulin; 12 kDa). CD1d is expressed on APC. The APC include professional APC such as dendritic cells, macrophages and B cells and non-professional APC such as hepatocytes and intestinal epithelial cells (IEC). On the APC, CD1d displays small glycolipid antigens (Figure 3). These glycolipids are derived either from the host cell itself or from microbes[15]. A pharmacological agent that was developed, α-galactosylceramide (αGalCer), is a model glycolipid antigen[16]. CD1d bearing a glycolipid antigen such as αGalCer engages the T cell receptor (TCR) on a subset of T cells. These T cells are so-called natural killer T cells (NKT cells) that express both natural killer and T cell markers. A characteristic feature of these NKT cells is their expression of a characteristic TCR-α chain in non-covalent association with a polymorphic array of TCR-β chains. Most interestingly, NKT cells secrete a

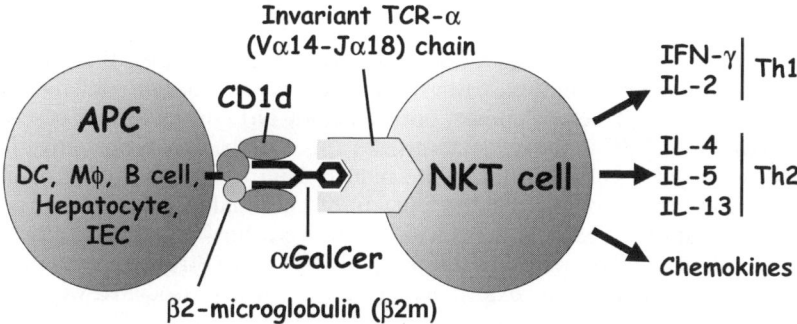

αGalCer (α-galactosylceramide): a model glycolipid antigen

Figure 3   CD1d-restricted pathways. DC, dendritic cell, Mφ, macrophage

large array of Th1, Th2, Th17 and other chemokines and cytokines. This engagement of NKT cells with CD1d bearing glycolipids on an APC occurs at the earliest phases of an immune response. One can therefore readily see how interesting it is to understand the biology in the context of mucosal immunology.

CD1d FUNCTION AT MUCOSAL SURFACES

The lumen of the human intestine contains a large quantity of microbial and dietary antigens. These antigens are largely excluded from the host by the properties of the epithelium, which forms a single cell layer that is generally impervious to the passage of large molecular weight molecules. Under normal circumstances, antigens derived from microbes and dietary sources are significantly excluded from the tissues underneath the epithelium, which contains a rich array of immune cells including lymphocytes, myeloid cells, natural killer cells and mast cells, among others[17]. Access of antigen to the immune system from the lumen is therefore restricted to those antigens which can be taken up directly by the epithelial cell and presented by the epithelial cell, those that can passage through the paracellular space between two different epithelial cells, those that can be transported across the epithelial cell or those that can be retrieved directly by dendritic cells which lie immediately beneath the epithelial barriers[18]. Therefore, it might be suggested that epithelial cells and dendritic cells are two of the first major subsets of cells to potentially process and present antigens derived from the intestinal lumen (Figure 4). Interestingly, both the IEC and DC functionally express CD1d on their cell surface[14,19]. When challenged by antigen, T lymphocytes in the lamina propria can be deviated to become either Th1 polarized cells secreting interferon-γ and TNF, which is important in the management of bacterial infections, for example. Alternatively, T cells in the lamina propria when challenged by antigen can be deviated to become Th2 cells that secrete IL-4, IL-5, IL-10 and IL-13, which is important to the pathogenesis of allergy and parasitic infestations, for example. Quite surprisingly, we have found that CD1d-restricted antigen-presentation pathways in mucosal tissues can regulate both types of polarized T cell responses; both Th2 and Th1. In the former case we have found that APC in the intestinal tissues appear to be capable of activating CD1d-restricted T cells (NKT cells) to induce them to secrete Th2 cytokines such as IL-13 that promote the development of intestinal inflammation that is similar to that observed in patients with ulcerative colitis[8,9,20]. Specifically, we have found, in collaboration with the group of Dr Warren Strober, that a model of human ulcerative colitis, oxazalone-induced colitis, is associated with very high concentrations of Th2 cytokines, and that this secretion of Th2 cytokines and mucosal inflammation is dependent on the expression of CD1d. Mice that are deficient in CD1d or mice in which CD1d is blocked with antibodies specific for this molecule do not develop colitis when exposed to oxazalone. Moreover, the functionally important and deleterious cytokine in this pathway is IL-13. Neutralization of IL-13 with an IL-13 decoy receptor also prevents the development of tissue inflammation in association with oxazalone exposure.

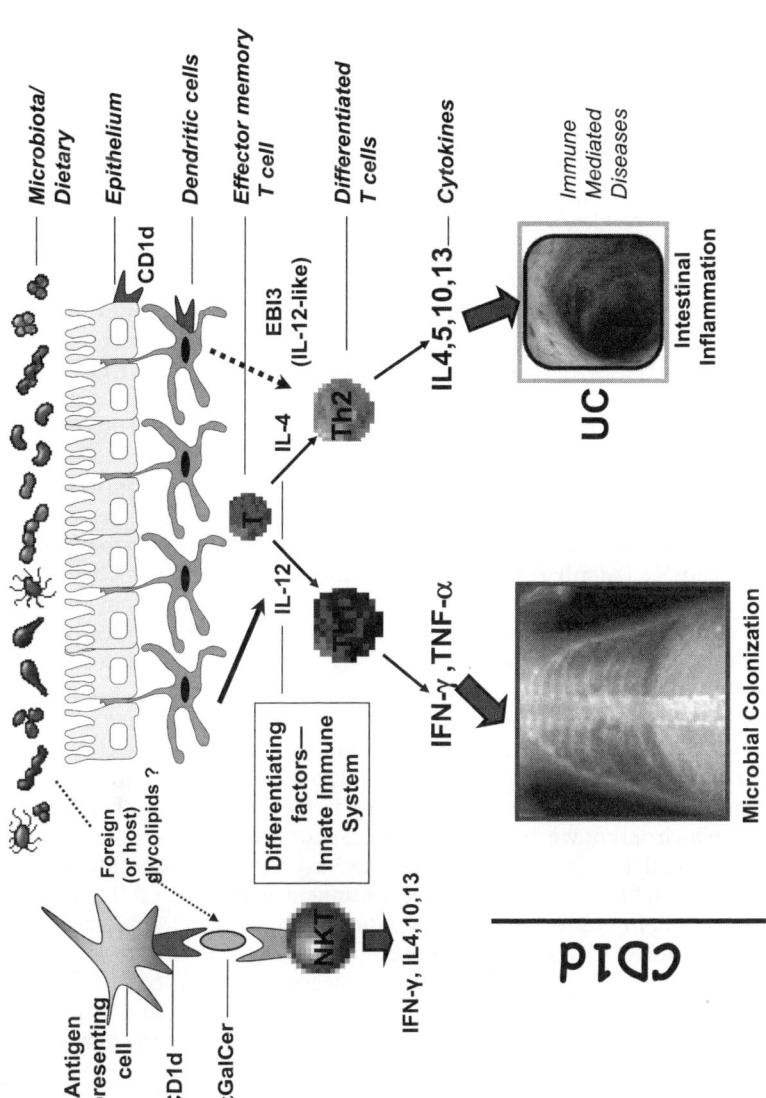

Figure 4 Immunoregulation at mucosal surfaces

23

This is probably related to the human condition because human patients with ulcerative colitis also exhibit increased Th2 cytokine secretion and specifically IL-13 secretion by lamina propria mononuclear cells when CD1d pathways are stimulated. This raises the possibility that targeting CD1d and NKT cell pathways, and the IL-13 cytokine in particular, may be an important future therapeutic target in the treatment of ulcerative colitis.

At the same time our group has identified an important role for CD1d and CD1d-restricted T cells in mediating an endogenous pathway of antimicrobial defence at the mucosal surfaces. This pathway is associated with excess Th1 cytokine secretion. We first made this observation in the mouse lung where we observed the ability of CD1d to regulate mucosal defence against a pathogenic bacterium, *Pseudomonas aeruginosa*[21]. Specifically, we observed that CD1d-deficient mice were highly susceptible to airway exposure with *Pseudomonas aeruginosa* and that such mice developed a very severe pneumonia. As a corrolary, activation of wild-type mice with αGalCer protected the mice from *Pseudomonas aeruginosa* pneumonia. This protection appeared to be due to the ability of CD1d-bearing APC and NKT cells to cause the secretion of chemokines such as MIP-2 that induced neutrophil recruitment and interferon-γ to induce macrophages to engulf and kill *Pseudomonas aeruginosa*.

Based upon these observations we sought to determine whether such a pathway of antimicrobial resistance that was orchestrated by CD1d was functional in intestinal mucosal surfaces. CD1d is expressed, as noted, on absorptive epithelial cells of the small and large intestine, as well as professional APC in the lamina propria, including both B lymphocytes and dendritic cells[14]. Paneth cells within intestinal crypts are responsible for antimicrobial secretion of so-called defensins, and also may express CD1d[22,23]. Given the importance of CD1d and CD1d-restricted T cells in the protection of the mucosal surfaces of the lung against bacterial infection, we examined the effects of CD1d in the regulation of mucosal colonization of the intestine with a pathogen (*Pseudomonas aeruginosa*), a presumptive pathogen (*Staphylococcus aureus*) or a normal commensal (*Escherichia coli*). In initial studies it was observed that wild-type mice exhibited decreased colonization of the intestine with *Pseudomonas aeruginosa* if the animal was treated with αGalCer, which is known to activate CD1d-restricted T cells *in vivo*. These studies suggest that CD1d pathways activate a programme of antimicrobial defence in the intestine. Therefore, we examined germ-free CD1d-deficient mice for their ability to manage colonization with a commensal bacterium, *E. coli*. When germ-free CD1d-deficient mice were monocolonized with *E. coli*, 10^9 colony-forming units of *E. coli* per gram of faeces was observed at 12 h after colonization, in contrast to wild-type mice which exhibited no detectable *E. coli* at that time point. Similar observations were made when germ-free CD1d-deficient mice were monocolonized with *S. aureus*. When germ-free mice were monocolonized with *E. coli* and the intestines examined 4 days after colonization, the major site within the intestine wherein bacterial over-colonization was detectable was within the jejunum. These studies suggested that CD1d was regulating an endogenous pathway of antimicrobial resistance that was most active in the small intestine. Since the small intestine is the major site for Paneth cell expression, and Paneth cells have been reported to express

CD1d and are the major cell type involved in antimicrobial defence, we examined Paneth cells in CD1d-deficient mice. These studies showed that Paneth cell structure was altered and that the Paneth cells exhibited diminished degranulation of their antimicrobial peptides upon colonization with *E. coli.* (unpublished observation). Taken together, these studies suggest that, in the absence of CD1d, Paneth cell function is abnormal. Interestingly Paneth cells may be dysfunctional in mice deficient of, and humans with polymorphisms in, NOD2/CARD15[3,24].

FUNCTION OF CD1d ON ABSORPTIVE EPITHELIAL CELLS

We have previously observed that CD1d is expressed by absorptive epithelial cells in both mouse and human epithelia[14]. The expression of CD1d on human epithelia has been easily detectable, in contrast to mouse epithelia, but a number of functional studies have indicated that CD1d is operative on both rodent and human IEC[14]. We have also observed that interferon-γ, which breaks the integrity of the epithelial barrier, is blocked by the paracrine secretion of IL-10 in response to CD1d ligation on the intestinal epithelial cell[25]. These studies have suggested that a CD1d-expressing IEC bearing phospholipids or glycolipids might be able to engage an NKT cell, resulting in

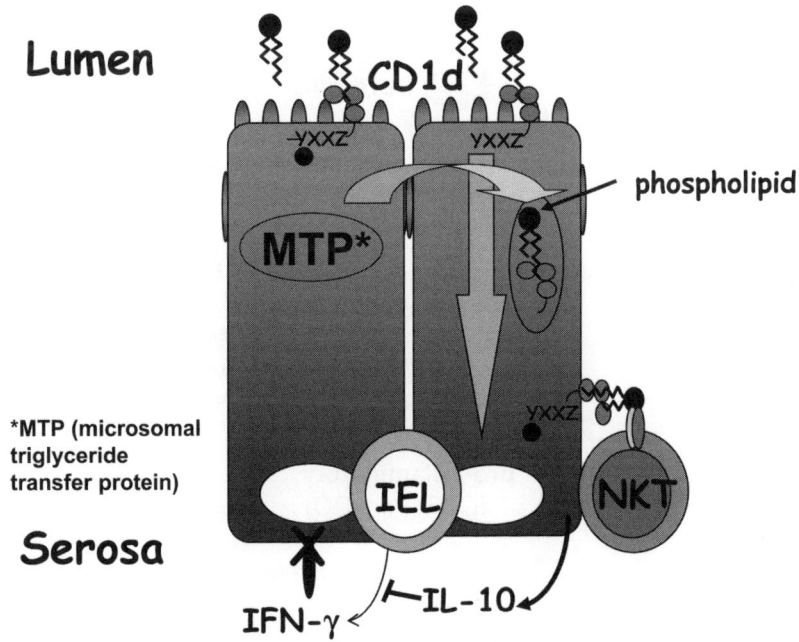

Figure 5 CD1d function in epithelium associated with barrier protection. Details as described in text. YXXZ, motif within CD1d cytoplasmic tail in single-letter amino acid code

the secretion of IL-10 by the epithelial cell itself (Figure 5). Such a pathway could theoretically provide an important means to protect the epithelial barrier from inflammatory destruction by cytokines such as interferon-γ. Indeed, preliminary studies suggest that this is the case. Epithelial cell lines when cultured with NKT cells result in the secretion of IL-10 from the epithelial cell and NKT lines. In contrast, co-culture of the same NKT cells with dendritic cells results in the secretion of IL-12, a proinflammatory cytokine (unpublished observation). These studies indicate that the relationship between NKT cells with different CD1d-bearing APC lead to markedly different cellular outcomes.

SUMMARY

We have shown that NKT cells that are restricted to respond to CD1d can regulate multiple different biological pathways in mucosal tissues by their interactions with discrete APC types (Figure 6). Such observations are important for unravelling the biology of mucosal tissues, but are also important for the development of therapeutics that can target mucosal inflammation at the earliest phases of the immune response. Specifically, we have observed that absorptive epithelial cells will respond to NKT cells via Cd1d with the secretion of IL-10, which promotes the strength of the epithelial barrier and prevents its destruction. In contrast, CD1d on a Paneth cell may

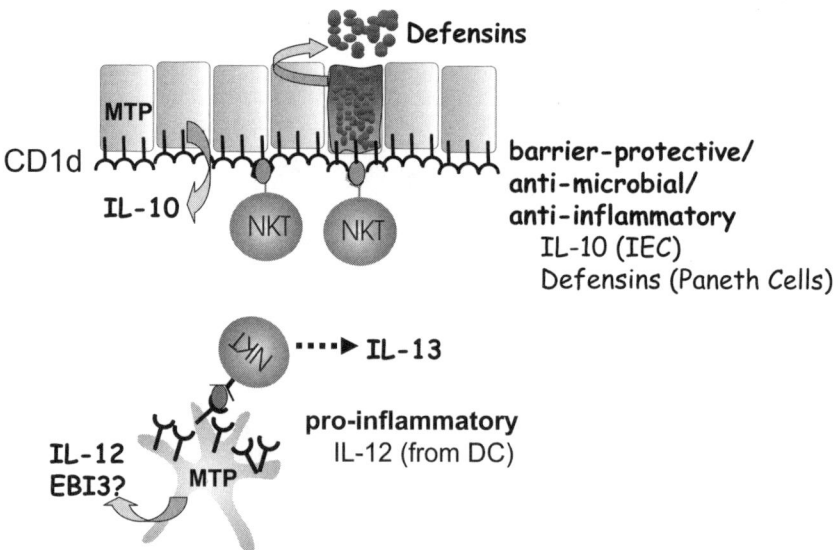

Figure 6   Summary of different functional outcomes related to specific APC–T cell interactions involving CD1d. EBI3, Epstein–Barr virus-induced gene 3 (IL-12 p40 homologue)

interact with NKT cells in a pathway that results in the regulation of Paneth cell function and the ability to secrete antimicrobial defensins. Such a pathway would be important in antimicrobial defence. In contrast, CD1d on dendritic cells in response to NKT cells induces the dendritic cell to secrete proinflammatory cytokines such as IL-12. Together, these studies show that the biological effects of CD1d–NKT cell interactions are likely to be quite heterogeneous. Therefore, is there any possibility for targeting CD1d-restricted pathways therapeutically if the cellular outcomes are so diverse? These studies teach us that targeting the end-products of the CD1d-restricted pathways may be one means to effect therapeutic opportunities from these observations. For example, blockade of IL-13 or directing IL-10 to the epithelial barrier more effectively might be beneficial. Alternatively, given observations that unique proteins such as microsomal triglyceride transfer protein (MTP) is highly active in the epithelium and involved in CD1d biology may make it possible to direct small molecules at this protein[26] (Figure 5). These and other approaches to develop the next generation of therapeutic agents that will target devastating diseases such as IBD are a major area of interest, and moreover, very feasible.

Acknowledgements

This work was supported by NIH Grants DK53056, DK44319, DK51362 and The Harvard Digestive Diseases Center.

References

1. Cho J. Genetic advances in inflammatory bowel disease. Curr Treat Options Gastroenterol. 2006;9:191–200.
2. Girardin SE, Boneca IG, Viala J et al. Nod2 is a general sensor of peptidoglycan through muramyl dipeptide (MDP) detection. J Biol Chem. 2003;278:8869–72.
3. Kobayashi KS, Chamaillard M, Ogura Y et al. Nod2-depndent regulation of innate and adaptive immunity in the intestinal tract. Inflamm Bowel Dis. 2005;11:860–1.
4. Villandangos JA, Schnorrer P, Wildon NS. Control of MHC class II antigen-presentation in dendritic cells: a balance between creative and destructive forces. Immunol Rev 2005;207:191–205.
5. Agnello D, Lankford CS, Bream J et al. Cytokines and transcription factors that T helper cell differentiation: new players and new insights. J Clin Immunol. 2003;23:147–61.
6. Mannon PJ, Fuss IJ, Mayer L et al. Anti-IL-12 Crohn's Disease Study Group. Anti-interleukin-12 antibody for active Crohn's disease. N Engl J Med. 2004;351:2045–8.
7. Hommes DW, Mikhajlova TL, Stoinov S et al. Fontolizumab, a humanized anti-interferon gamma antibody, demonstrates the safety and clinical activity in patients with moderate to severe Crohn's disease. Gut. 2006;55:1131–7.
8. Heller F, Fuss IJ, Nieuwenhuis EE, Blumberg RS, Strober W. Oxazolone colitis, a Th2 colitis model resembling ulcerative colitis, is mediated by IL-13 producing NK-T cells. Immunity. 2002;17:629–38.
9. Fuss IJ, Heller F, Boirivant M et al. Nonclassical Cd1d-restricted NK T cells that produce IL-13 characterize an atypical Th2 response in ulcerative colitis. J Clin Invest. 2004;113:1490–97.
10. Banham AH, Powrie FM, Suri-Payer E. FOXP3(+) regulatory T cells: current controversies and future perspectives. Eur J Immunol. 2006;36:2832–6.
11. Salmi M, Jalkanen S. Lymphocyte homing to the gut: attraction, adhesion, and commitment. Immunol Rev. 2005;206:100–13.
12. Adams DH, Eksteen B. Aberrant homing of mucosal T cells and extra-intestinal manifestations of inflammatory bowel disease. Nat Rev Immunol. 2006;6:244–51.

13. Sandborn WJ, Colombel JF, Enns R et al. International Efficacy of Natalizumab as Active Crohn's Therapy (ENACT-1) Trial Group; Evaluation of Natalizumab as Continuous Therapy (ENACT-2) Trial Group. Natalizumab induction and maintenance therapy for Crohn's disease. N Engl J Med. 2005;353:1912–25.

14. Dougan SK, Kaser A, Blumberg RS. CD1 Expression on antigen presenting cells. Curr Top Microbiol Immunol. 2007 (In press).

15. Kinjo Y, Turpin E, Wu D et al. Natural killer T cells recognize diacylglycerol antigens from pathogenic bacteria. Nat Immunol. 2006;7:978–86.

16. Kobayashi E, Motoki K, Uchida T, Fukushima H, Koezuka Y. KRN7000, a novel immunomodulator, and its antitumor activities. Oncol Res. 1995;7:529–34.

17. Ponda PP, Mayer L. Mucosal epithelium in health and disease. Curr Mol Med. 2005;5:549–56.

18. Yoshida M, Claypool SM, Wagner JS et al. Human neonatal Fc receptor mediates transport of IgG into luminal secretions for delivery of antigens to mucosal dendritic cells. Immunity. 2004;20:769–83.

19. van de Wal Y, Corazza N, Allez M et al. Delineation of a CD1d-restricted antigen presentation pathway associated with humans and mouse intestinal epithelial cells. Gastroenterology. 2003;124:1420–31.

20. Nieuwenhuis EE, Neurath MF, Corazza M et al. Disruption of T helper 2-immune responses in Epstein–Barr virus induced gene 3-deficient mice. Proc Natl Acad Sci USA. 2002;99:16951–6.

21. Nieuwenhuis EE, Matsumoto T, Exley M et al. Cd1d-dependent macrophage-mediated clearance of *Pseudomonas aeruginosa* from lung. Nat Med. 2002;8:588–93.

22. Wehkamp J, Stange EF. Paneth cells and the innate immune response. Curr Opin Gastroenterol. 2006;22:644–59.

23. Lacasse J, Martin LH. Detection of CD1 mRNA in Paneth cells of the mouse intestine by *in situ* hybridization. J Histochem Cytochem. 1992;40:1527–34.

24. Wehkamp J, Harder J, Weichenthal M et al. NOD2(CARD15) mutations in Crohn's disease are associated with diminished mucosal alpha-defensin expression. Gut. 2004;53:1658–64.

25. Colgan SP, Hershberg RM, Furuta GT, Blumberg RS. Ligation of intestinal epithelial CD1d induces bioactive IL-10: critical role of the cytoplasmic tail in autocrine signaling. Proc Natl Acad Sci USA. 1999;96:13938–43.

26. Brozovic S, Nagaishi T, Yoshida M et al. Cd1d function is regulated by microsomal triglyceride transfer protein. Nat Med. 2004;10:535–9.

3
Control of mucosal immune responses by transforming growth factor-β

T. T MACDONALD, A. DI SABATINO and G. MONTELEONE

INTRODUCTION

Inflammatory bowel diseases (IBD) affect about 150 000 people in the UK. The major costs to society are due to morbidity, with loss of individuals from the workforce, hospital inpatient and outpatient costs, and increasingly expensive new therapies. Crohn's disease (CD) continues to increase in incidence, with disease being seen more often in young individuals who will have to live with their disease for five or six decades. The IBD are also intractable, stigmatizing conditions associated with mutilating surgery and diarrhoea, and produce significant psychosocial morbidity. Current management rarely affects the natural history of these diseases and resection of diseased bowel is the consequence of the current inability to control these conditions.

It is beyond question that each of the major IBD, namely CD and ulcerative colitis (UC), is due to immunological hypersensitivity in the gut wall[1]. Though these diseases are quite different in terms of genetics and immunology, they share end-stage manifestations of tissue injury with elevated cytokines, free radicals, lipid mediators and matrix-degrading enzymes driving ulceration of the gut mucosa. In CD there is compelling evidence that disease is due to mis-recognition of the normal commensal bacterial flora as a pathogen. Thus while the body has invested in an extensive and highly active immune system to prevent gut infections, when immune activity is directed against the normal flora, chronic disease is the consequence.

Anti-cytokine therapy (such as infliximab) has led to a revolution in the treatment of IBD. A single infusion benefits 40% of patients in the short term, but long-term treatment maintains remission only in approximately 20% of those who initially responded[2]. This drop-off can be partly explained by the development of neutralizing antibodies against the chimeric antibody[3], and may be improved in clinical practice by immune suppression, humanized antibodies, phage-derived antibodies, and human monoclonal antibodies, but it is likely that none of these newer anti-TNF-α (tumour necrosis factor alpha)

29

antibodies will show significantly greater therapeutic efficacy than infliximab. Off anti-TNF-α therapy, patients rapidly relapse. Together with the significant risk of infection due to long-term TNF-α therapies[4], and their expense, there is an unmet need for novel approaches to heal the gut.

THE ROLE OF TGF-β IN THE CYTOKINE BALANCE IN IBD

The proinflammatory effector cytokines which cause inflammation in IBD gut exist alongside powerful anti-inflammatory cytokines such as interleukin 10 (IL-10) and transforming growth factor beta (TGF-β). The activity of the anti-inflammatory cytokines is inhibited for sound evolutionary reasons since it would not be beneficial to compromise anti-pathogen inflammatory responses in the gut until the agent is eliminated. In this context, excessive IL-10 in the inflamed mucosa cannot dampen immune responses because of elevated SOCS3 in inflammatory cells[5], and excess TGF-β cannot signal to inflammatory cells because of elevated intracellular Smad7 (Figure 1). In IBD, where the host has to modulate ongoing, chronic inflammation, improvement and even complete clinical remission can occur in placebo-treated patients[6], suggesting that the balance between immune-driven damage and the healing response is not so wide that it cannot be therapeutically manipulated.

We have been particularly interested in TGF-β, the most powerful endogenous inhibitor of gut inflammation, present at elevated concentrations in inflamed gut. Presence or absence of TGF-β is not an accurate reflection of the role of this cytokine in tissues. In the canonical signalling pathway, activated TGF-β receptors phosphorylate and activate the Smad2 and Smad3

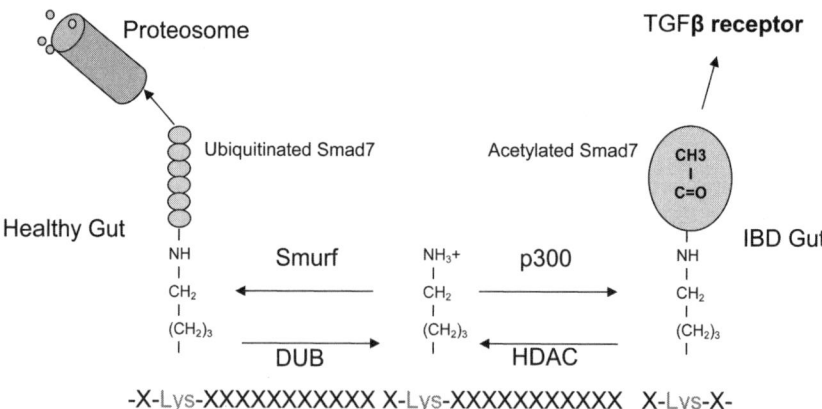

Figure 1 Diagrammatic illustration of how changes in Smad 7 acetylation and ubiquitination by ubiquitinating enzymes (Smurfs), deubiquitinating enzymes (DUB), p300, and histone deacteylation (HDAC) can determine whether Smad7 is degraded in the proteosome and is non-functional or can go to the membrane and block TGF-β signalling

transcription factors which form heterodimeric complexes with Smad4, enter the nucleus, and regulate the activity of target genes, either directly by binding to cognate DNA consensus sites or indirectly by interaction with other transcription factors[7]. Although there are three isoforms of TGF-β in humans, all signal through a common receptor.

When we studied Smad signalling in normal human gut mucosal tissues and cells[8] there was a basal level of phosphorylated Smad3 which was rapidly up-regulated by the addition of exogenous TGF-β_1. In contrast, samples from patients with active IBD exhibited reduced levels of endogenous phospho-Smad3 which was not enhanced by stimulation with exogenous TGF-β_1. Thus, in patients with IBD, there is a disruption of TGF-β_1 signalling despite the abundance of TGF-β1 in the inflamed gut.

THE ROLE OF Smad7

An inhibitory Smad, Smad7, blocks TGF-β_1 signalling[9]. This is partly due to the ability of Smad7 to physically interact with the activated TGF-β type I receptor to prevent the docking and phosphorylation of Smad2 and Smad3 to the TGF-β type I receptor[9]. We have shown that Smad7 protein is increased in IBD LPMC and TGF-β_1 cannot prevent proinflammatory cytokine production by IBD LPMC[8]. However, inhibition of Smad7 in lamina propria mononuclear cells (LPMC) and in explant tissues from patients with IBD using an antisense strategy restores both Smad3 phosphorylation and the ability of TGF-β_1 to inhibit cytokine production[8]. These studies also show that there is sufficient active TGF-β in inflamed gut to dampen inflammation. TGF-β_1 also completely prevents TNF-α-induced NF-κB activation in LPMC from normal individuals[10]. In samples from IBD patients, however, NF-κB activation proceeds unchecked and exogenous TGF-β_1 has no effect. If Smad7 is reduced with anti-sense, Smad3 activation is restored and NF-κB activation is immediately inhibited by endogenous TGF-β_1[10].

Upregulation of Smad7 is not a specific IBD-immune defect, as it is also over-expressed in *Helicobacter pylori*-associated gastritis[11]. We consider that the presence of Smad7 in different inflammatory conditions of the gut points to its importance.

If Smad7 is the crucial regulator of whether a cell can respond to TGF-β, then an obvious question is the control of the expression and localization of Smad7 in cells. Smad7 is induced in cell lines by the STAT1 pathway or by the NF-κB pathway[12]. TGF-β_1 itself can also increase Smad7[12]. In inflamed gut, especially CD, Stat1 and NF-κB activity are particularly prominent[10,13]. This would suggest that increased Smad7 is a downstream consequence of inflammation. However, taking a lead from elegant studies in cell lines[14,15], we have now shown that Smad7 regulation in IBD is complex but that this complexity has revealed a novel putative intervention strategy. In brief, Smad7 transcripts are abundant in healthy and IBD gut. Likewise the E3 ligases (Smurf 1 and 2) which export Smad7 from the nucleus to the cytoplasm are also abundant in healthy and diseased gut[16]. In health, however, Smad7 is rapidly ubiquitinated by Smurfs and degraded in the proteosome (Figure 1).

However, in IBD, Smad7 is resistant to ubiquitination because of acetylation at lysine residues. The molecule responsible for Smad7 acetylation is the transcriptional co-activator p300 which is markedly over-expressed in IBD. Knocking down p300 with siRNA in cells from IBD patients reduces Smad7 acetylation, increases its ubiquitination and, importantly, decreases Smad7 itself. Both ubiquitination and acetylation are counteracted by deubiquitinating enzymes and deacetylases. However, in IBD tissue there is no difference in the levels of deubiquitinating enzymes (Evans and MacDonald, unpublished data) and inhibition of deacetylating enzymes with trichostatin A did not increase Smad7 in IBD tissues[16].

Together, these data suggest that acetylation of Smad7 by p300 is the key determinant which maintains high levels of Smad7 inside the cell, rendering it unresponsive to TGF-β. Thus a rational approach to IBD therapy is to inhibit Smad7.

COULD Smad7 BE A NEW THERAPEUTIC TARGET IN IBD

We believe that there are now sufficient data to support the notion that modification of Smad7 acetylation may be therapeutic in humans. We have shown in Crohn's tissue that blocking Smad7 allows endogenous TGF-β to dampen TNF-α production[8]. We have also shown in mice that Smad7 antisense blocks trinitrobenzene sulphonic acid (TNBS) and oxazolone colitis by maintaining TGF-β responsiveness[17]. Protein acetylation is an important post-transcriptional modifier of many cellular functions and histone acetylation is important in gene expression, so it may be considered that blocking p300 acetyltransferase activity acetylation may have deleterious side-effects. However, inhibitors of histone de-acetylation have been used extensively in cancer patients[18].

Synthetic p300 inhibitors have been described[19,20]. The adenoviral protein E1A is a well-established inhibitor of p300 acetylation[21]. Natural products can also inhibit p300 acetylation; these include anacardic acid, an extract of cashew nut shells, with an IC50 in the μM range for its ability to inhibit p300 activity[22] and diferuloylmethane, the major ingredient of curcumin, which pharmacologically inhibits lymphocyte proliferation, is an antioxidant, inhibits NF-κB activity and is also a Ca-adenosine triphosphate pump inhibitor; but it is also a potent p300 inhibitor at low doses[23,24]. Based on its anti-inflammatory properties, previous studies have shown that it can inhibit TNBS colitis in mice by an unknown mechanism[25], and it has been shown in a small open-label study that oral curcumin capsules (up to 6 g/day) show benefit in ulcerative proctitis and CD[26]. We would suggest this activity is mediated through the effects of curcumin on Smad7 acetylation. It also shows no toxicity even at very high doses, and the limit on oral dosing appears to be the size of the capsules[27]. After feeding it can be detected in stools, showing that it reaches the distal colon, and peak serum levels of 2 μM can be achieved after feeding[28]. Although it is a food additive (E100) and the acceptable daily intake is 0.1 mg/kg largely based on animal studies, curcumin is widely available over the counter, and far higher doses have already been given to patients.

Overall, therefore, we consider that it would now be sensible to determine if it was possible to therapeutically modulate Smad7 to allow endogenous TGF-β to heal the diseased mucosa in IBD.

References

1. MacDonald TT, Montelone G. Immunity, inflammation and allergy in the gut. Science. 2005;307:1920–25.
2. Hanauer SB et al. Maintenance infliximab for Crohn's disease. Lancet. 2002;359:1541–9.
3. Baert F et al. Influence of immunogenicity on the long-term efficy of infliximab in Crohn's disease. N Engl J Med. 2003;348:277–8.
4. Keane J et al. TB associated with infliximab, a TNF-neutralizing agent. N Engl J Med. 2001;345:1098–104.
5. Lovato P et al. Constitutive STAT3 activation in intestinal T cells from patients with Crohn's disease. J Biol Chem. 2003;278:16777–81.
6. Targan SR et al. A short-term study of chimeric monoclonal antibody cA2 to TNFalpha for Crohn's disease. N Engl J Med. 1997;337:1029–35.
7. Dennler S et al. Direct binding of Smad3 and Smad4 to critical TGF-β-inducible elements in the promoter of human plasminogen activator inhibitor-type 1 gene. EMBO J. 1998;17: 3091.
8. Montelone G et al. Blocking Smad7 restores TGFß1 signalling in chronic inflammatory bowel disease. J Clin Invest. 2001;108:601–8.
9. Montelone G et al. Smad7 in TGFß-mediated negative regulation of gut inflammation. Trends Immunol. 2004;25:513–17.
10. Monteleone G et al. A failure of TGFß1 negative regulation maintains sustained NF-κB activation in gut inflammation. J Biol Chem. 2004;279:3925–32.
11. Monteleone I et al. Defective TGFß1 signalling associates with high Smad7 in the gastric mucosa of patients with *H. pylori* infection. Gastroenterology. 2004;26:674–82.
12. ten Dijke P, Hill CS. New insights into TGF-ß-Smad signaling. Trends Biochem Sci. 2004; 29:265–73.
13. Schreiber S et al. Activation of STAT 1 in human chronic IBD. Gut. 2002;51:379–85.
14. Gronroos E. Control of Smad7 stability by competition between acetylation and ubiquitination. Mol Cell. 2002;10:483–93.
15. Simonsson M et al. The balance between acetylation and deacetylation controls Smad7 stability. J Biol Chem. 2005;280:21797–803.
16. Monteleone G et al. Post-transcriptional regulation of Smad7 in the gut of patients with inflammatory bowel disease. Gastroenterology. 2005;129:1420–9.
17. Boirivant M et al. Targeted inhibition of Smad7 with a specific antisense oligonucleotide facilitates TGF-ß1-mediated suppression of mucosal inflammation. Gastroenterology. 2006;131:1786–98.
18. Kelly WK, Marks PA. Drug insight: histone deacetylase inhibitors – development of the new targeted anticancer agent suberoylanilide hydroxamic acid. Nat Clin Pract Oncol. 2005;2:150–7.
19. Nishihara A et al. E1A inhibits TGF-β signaling through binding to Smad proteins. J Biol Chem. 1999;274:28716–23.
20. Cebrat M et al. Synthesis and analysis of potential prodrugs of coenzyme A analogues for the inhibition of the histone acetyltransferase p300. Bioorg Med Chem. 2003;11:3307–13.
21. Balasubramanyam K et al. Small molecule modulators of histone acetyltransferase p300. J Biol Chem. 2003;278:19134–40.
22. Rahman I et al. Redox modulation of chromatin remodelling : impact on histone acetylation and deacetylation, NF-KB and pro-inflammatory gene expression. Biochem Pharmacol. 2004;68:1255–67.
23. Egan ME et al. Curcumin, a major constituent of turmeric, corrects cystic fibrosis defects. Science. 2004;304:600–2.
24. Balasubramanyam K et al. Curcumin, a novel p300/CREB-binding protein-specific inhibitor of acetyltransferase, represses the acetylation of histone/nonhistone proteins and

histone acetyltransferase-dependent chromatin transcription. J Biol Chem. 2004;279: 51163–71.

25. Sugimoto S et al. Curcumin prevents and ameliorates TNBS colitis in mice. Gastroenterology. 2002;123:1912–22.
26. Holt PRR et al. Curcumin therapy in IBD: a pilot study. Dig Dis Sci. 2005;50:11:2191–93.
27. Benford D. Curcumin. WHO Food Additives Series 52, 2004.
28. Cheng Al et al. Phase 1 clinical trial of curcumin, a chemopreventative agent, in patients with high-risk or pre-malignant lesions. Aniticancer Res. 2001;21:2895–900.

4
Immunoregulation: Crohn's disease versus ulcerative colitis

F. HELLER and M. ZEITZ

INTRODUCTION

Since Burrill Bernhard Crohn's first description of ileitis terminalis as a separate disease entity in contrast to colitis ulcerosa in 1932 much has been learned about the differences and similarities between M. Crohn (CD) and colitis ulcerosa (UC)[1-3]. The common feature in inflammatory bowel disease (IBD) is that of a chronic recurring inflammation of intestine. The inflammation is induced by the mucosa-associated immune system (MALT). Now there is ample evidence that the stimuli for the immune system are luminal antigens from the bacterial flora. Genetic and environmental factors influence the reaction of the immune system to these antigens. Several genetic loci have been described that contribute to IBD susceptibility in humans as well as in animal models[4].

IMMUNOREGULATION IN THE MUCOSAL IMMMUNE SYSTEM

The immune reaction of the MALT is orchestrated by differentiated CD4$^+$ T cells (Figure 1). These T cells can differentiate into phenotypes with specialized functional properties that induce specific immune responses. One such pathway of inflammation is mediated by T helper 1 (Th1) T cells. Naive T cells differentiate into cells with this phenotype under the influence of interleukin-12 (IL-12) produced by antigen-presenting-cells (APC). After binding of IL-12 to its surface receptor the transcription factor STAT-4 is phosphorylated. Phosphorylated STAT proteins dimerize and than translocate to the nucleus, where they bind to and transactivate genes containing the gamma-activated sequence (GAS). Differentiated Th1 cells also express T-bet, a transcription factor that induces IFN-γ production and the expression of IL-12 receptors on the cell surface. Thereby the inflammatory response to activation of such differentiated cells is directed by the transcription factors that became active during the priming of the naive T cell. Th1 differentiated T cells produce IL-2, IFN-γ and TNF-α, and are thereby important regulators of cell-mediated

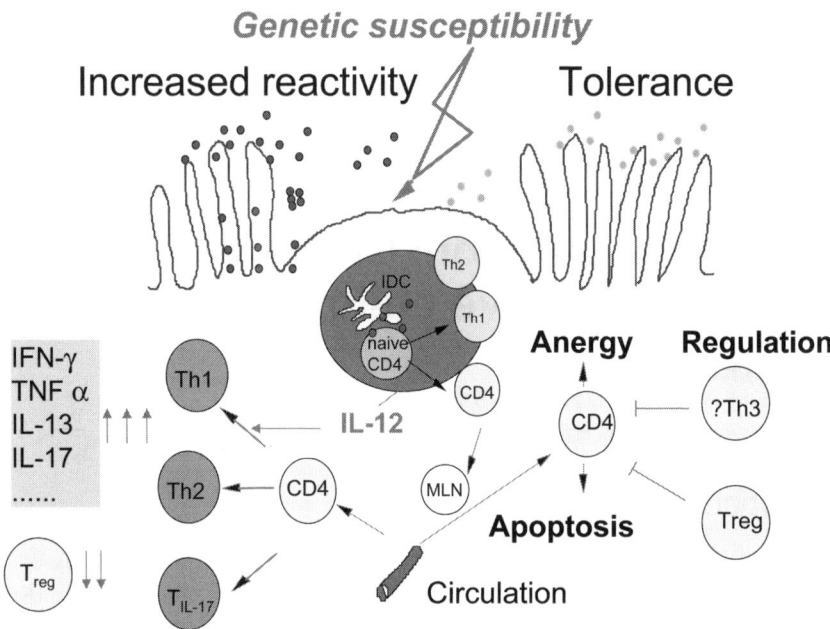

Figure 1 Immune reactions in the mucosal immune system are orchestrated by differentiated CD4[+] T cells; these can have inflammatory or regulatory properties

immune responses. If the priming of naive CD4[+] T cells occurs under the influence of IL-4 the transcription factors STAT-6, GATA-3, NFAT and c-MAF are activated. Such T cells develop a Th2 phenotype and, upon activation, produce IL-4, IL-5, IL-10 and IL-13[5]. In contrast to these inflammatory subsets of T helper cells some cells adopt a regulatory phenotype and specifically inhibit immune reactions in their close proximity. While some of these regulatory T cells have been primed during thymic development it is possible that a subset of regulatory cells can also be generated in the periphery in response to non-self antigens. Depending on the animal model in which these cells have been defined they have been named Th3 cells or Tr1 cells. Th3 cells exert their function with the suppressive cytokines TGF-β, some of it membrane-bound on the surface[6]. Tr1 cells can differentiate from naive T cells and are characterized by IL-10 production[7].

Since the gastrointestinal mucosa is under the constant challenge of microbial and dietary foreign antigens the MALT requires a balanced activation of these T helper subsets. The inappropriate activation of one subset or the inappropriate formation of a subset can destabilize the mucosal homeostasis and ultimately lead to a destructive unwanted inflammation (Figure 2).

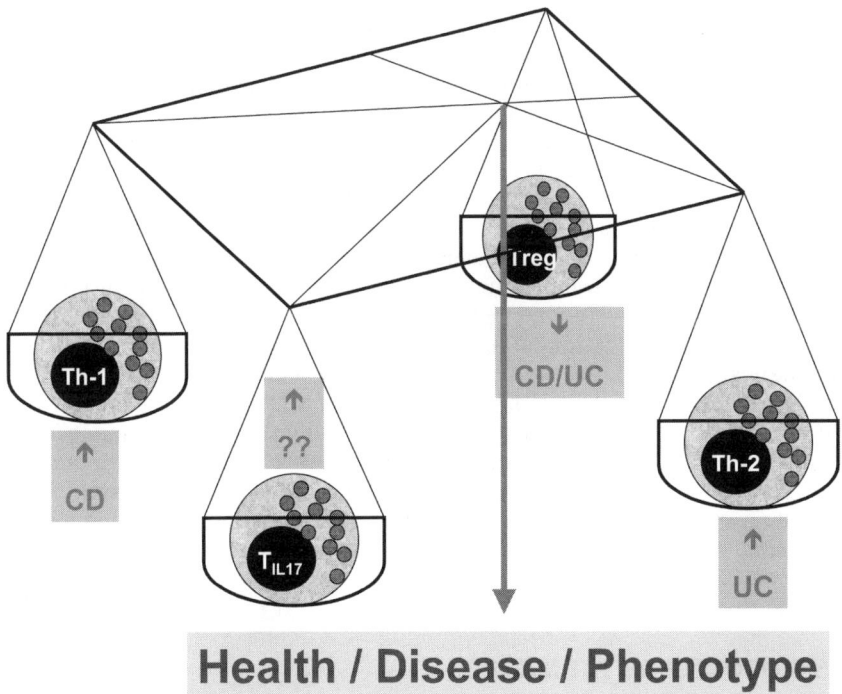

Figure 2 Mucosal homeostasis requires a balanced state of activation of the mucosal T-helper subsets. Activation or suppression of separate subsets can lead to inflammation

IMMUNOREGULATION IN IBD

While the clinical pictures of Crohn's disease (CD) and ulcerative colitis (UC) share some similarities, analysis of the involved Th subsets indicates the activation of very different types of Th subsets. The T cells infiltrating the lamina propria in CD exhibit a Th1 phenotype and the increased production of IL-12 by APC can be demonstrated. In UC, on the contrary, the number of T cells with a Th1 phenotype and the production of Th1 cytokines are decreased. Analysis of the inflammatory pathways in UC has been difficult to interpret since IL-4, the marker cytokine of Th2 inflammation, was not produced in large quantities in human samples and even in oxazalone colitis, an animal model of UC, was only initially and mildly detectable[8]. Recently we found that the inflammatory T cells in UC and in the mouse model oxazalone colitis produce large quantities of IL-13. The disease in the animal model could be cured by treatment with an IL-13-neutralizing antibody. When analysing cytokine production from T cells we found that the lamina propria was infiltrated with NKT cells. Such cells bear markers of conventional T cells and NK cells. These cells have been shown to react to glycolipids, unlike conventional T cells which respond to peptides. The antigen is presented to

37

NKT cells by CD1d on APC, while peptide antigens are inserted into MHC-II and bind to the T cell receptor[9]. When human samples were stimulated with CD1d and α-galactosylceramide, a prototype glycolipid that stimulates the majority of NKT cells, the inflammatory cells responded with the production of IL-13, while blockade of CD1d by antibodies abrogated the disease in the animal model and inhibited production of IL-13 from human UC samples[10].

While these findings demonstrate the result of the imbalance of mucosal homeostasis, a destructive Th1 or Th2 inflammation, it is still unclear which pathway leads to the initial imbalance of the mucosal immune system. As alluded to above, these inflammatory responses can result from insufficient suppression or function of regulatory cells, but also from enhanced proliferation or activation of inflammatory subsets. Therefore Maul and colleagues analysed the number of CD4[+] T cells bearing markers of regulatory cells: FOXP3 and high expression of CD25. In these studies CD patients in an acute phase of the disease had slightly increased numbers of regulatory cells in the lamina propria. When these were compared with samples from patients with acute diverticulitis the IBD patients had significantly fewer regulatory cells. These findings suggest that intestinal inflammation induces an expansion of regulatory cells, and this expansion is insufficient in IBD to counterbalance the inflammatory response[11].

OSTEOPONTIN AS Th1 MARKER

Osteopontin is a glycoprotein secreted by intestinal epithelial cells, macrophages, dendritic cells and B cells. It contains the characteristic RGD sequence seen in extracellular matrix proteins and shares receptor binding on cells with extracellular matrix proteins, including αv and β1 integrins. It also binds to CD44. Osteopontin increases the adhesion of activated T cells and is a T cell chemoattractant, but importantly it supports Th1 responses and inhibits Th2 responses[12,13]. Therefore Wittig and colleagues studied the production of osteopontin in IBD patients. Preliminary results show that osteopontin was detectable in significantly higher concentrations in serum of patients with active CD compared to patients without active disease or patients with UC. The concentration of osteopontin correlates with disease activity as measured by the CDAI. In biopsy samples from IBD patients osteopontin concentration is detectable in high amounts in active CD but not in control samples, and only in small amounts in samples from UC patients. An important cellular source seem to be dendritic cells, since these cells produce the highest amount of osteopontin when stimulated *in vitro* compared to monocytes, peripheral blood mononuclear cells (PBMC) or total lamina propria cells (LPMC).

PROTEASOME FUNCTION IN IBD

Proteasomes are multisubunit multicatalytic proteases that are responsible for the majority of non-lysosomal protein degradation within eukaryotic cells, and have a central role in the generation of peptides presented by MHC class I molecules as well as in the degradation of intracellular proteins[14]. The proteolytic properties of proteasomes depend on their constitution of different subunits, which have specific catalytic activities. The constitution of the proteasomes is influenced by inflammatory cytokines, the most prominent cytokine in this context being IFN-γ. Under the influence of IFN-γ proteasomes convert to immuno-proteasomes with altered cleavage sites in proteolysis[15]. Steinhoff and colleagues studied the constitution of proteasomes and their enzymatic activity from patients with IBD. One striking finding in these studies was the observation that proteasomes from CD patients exhibit an increased chymotrypsin-like activity and reduced caspase-like activity. Proteasomes from UC patients, on the contrary, had an increased caspase-like activity but reduced chymotrypsin-like activity. Corresponding to that the proteasomes of CD patients consisted of an increased fraction of β1i subunits and decreased fraction of β1 units compared to controls and UC patients. Steinhoff and colleagues very nicely demonstrated the functional consequence of these changes[16]. The proteasome enhances NF-κB activation, a transcription factor promoting Th1 activity in T cells. Early in the pathway leading to NF-κB activation p65 (rel) needs to dissociate from p105. The decoy protein p105 is degraded by proteasomes, thereby an enhanced activity of these proteasomes in CD leads to an increase in active p65. The next step in the activation cascade is the nuclear translocation of p65 dimerized with p50 (NF-κB), which is prevented by IκB, but since IκB is again degraded by proteasomes the transcriptional activity of NF-κB is enhanced. It was concluded from these studies that CD proteasomes contribute significantly to the overwhelming Th1 activity in the mucosa.

THE IL-23/IL-17 AXIS IN INFLAMMATION

Recently Harrington and colleagues reported another important cytokine and most likely new subtype of inflammatory cells important in intestinal inflammation[17]. Under the influence of IL-23 an inflammatory T-cell subset is activated, that is clearly distinct from Th1 or Th2 cells. These IL-17-producing CD4[+] T cells were dubbed Th17 or Th$_{IL-17}$ cells. IL-17, a proinflammatory cytokine predominantly produced by activated T cells, enhances T-cell priming and stimulates fibroblasts, endothelial cells, macrophages, and epithelial cells to produce multiple proinflammatory mediators, including IL-1, IL-6, TNF-α, NOS-2, metalloproteases, and chemokines, resulting in the induction of inflammation. IL-17 expression is increased in patients with a variety of allergic and autoimmune diseases, such as rheumatoid arthritis, multiple sclerosis, IBD, and asthma, suggesting the contribution of IL-17 to the induction and/or development of such diseases. Yen and colleagues demonstrated, in a mouse model of intestinal inflammation, that IL-23 and IL-17 are important key figures in the inflammatory process apart from IL-12. These studies indicate that T cells differentiated under the influence of IL-23 drive an intestinal inflammation in mice that resembles human CD[18].

CONCLUSION

T cells in the mucosal immune system specialize during their process of differentiation into distinct T-helper subsets. The Th1 and Th2 subsets have an inflammatory activity while Th3 cells exhibit a regulatory function. It is essential for mucosal homeostasis that these subsets maintain a balanced state of activation. Recent work adds important insights into mucosal inflammation. A newly described inflammatory subset of T-helper cells is induced by IL-23 and is characterized by the production of IL-17 that plays an important role in intestinal inflammation distinct from Th1 cells. In UC the inflammation is induced by CD1d restricted NKT cells, which produce IL-13 as their main pathogenic feature. In CD osteopontin promotes the activation of Th1 cells and its production correlates with disease activity. The regulatory cells found in the mucosa can be further specified by their high expression of CD25 and FOXP3. These cells increase in number during inflammation, but not as much as in other intestinal inflammations, such as diverticulitis, which might explain their inability to control inflammation in IBD. Proteasomes degrade intracellular self and non-self proteins. Their constitution and activity is influenced by inflammatory cytokines. In CD they cleave proteins, preventing the excessive activation of NF-κB, thereby leading to enhanced activation of this inflammatory transcription factor.

References

1. Crohn BB, Ginzburg L, Oppenheimer GD. Regional ileitis; a pathologic and clinical entity. Am J Med. 1952;13:583–90.
2. Crohn BB. Segmental (granulomatous) disease of the colon. Isr J Med Sci. 1968;4:146–8.
3. Crohn BB, Ginzburg L, Oppenheimer GD. Landmark article Oct 15, 1932. Regional ileitis. A pathological and clinical entity. By Burril B. Crohn, Leon Ginzburg, and Gordon D. Oppenheimer. J Am Med Assoc. 1984;251:73–9.
4. Bouma G, Strober W. The immunological and genetic basis of inflammatory bowel disease. Nat Rev Immunol. 2003;3:521–33.
5. Kuo CT, Leiden JM. Transcriptional regulation of T lymphocyte development and function. Annu Rev Immunol. 1999;17:149–87.
6. Nakamura K, Kitani A, Strober W. Cell contact-dependent immunosuppression by CD4 (+)CD25(+) regulatory T cells is mediated by cell surface-bound transforming growth factor beta. J Exp Med. 2001;194:629–44.
7. Groux H OGA, Bigler M, Rouleau M, Antonenko S, de Vries JE, Roncarolo MG. A CD4+ T-cell subset inhibits antigen-specific T-cell responses and prevents colitis. Nature. 1997; 389:737–42.
8. Fuss IJ, Neurath M, Boirivant M et al. Disparate CD4+ lamina propria (LP) lymphokine secretion profiles in inflammatory bowel disease. Crohn's disease LP cells manifest increased secretion of IFN-gamma, whereas ulcerative colitis LP cells manifest increased secretion of IL-5. J Immunol. 1996;157:1261–70.
9. Heller F, Fuss IJ, Nieuwenhuis EE, Blumberg RS, Strober W. Oxazolone colitis, a Th2 colitis model resembling ulcerative colitis, is mediated by IL-13-producing NK-T cells. Immunity. 2002;17:629–38.
10. Fuss IJ, Heller F, Boirivant M et al. Nonclassical CD1d-restricted NK T cells that produce IL-13 characterize an atypical Th2 response in ulcerative colitis. J Clin Invest. 2004;113: 1490–7.
11. Maul J, Loddenkemper C, Mundt P et al. Peripheral and intestinal regulatory CD4+ CD25 (high) T cells in inflammatory bowel disease. Gastroenterology. 2005;128:1868–78.
12. O'Regan AW, Nau GJ, Chupp GL, Berman JS. Osteopontin (Eta-1) in cell-mediated immunity: teaching an old dog new tricks. Immunol Today. 2000;21:475–8.

13. Sato T, Nakai T, Tamura N et al. Osteopontin/Eta-1 upregulated in Crohn's disease regulates the Th1 immune response. Gut. 2005;54:1254–62.
14. Coux O, Tanaka K, Goldberg AL. Structure and functions of the 20S and 26S proteasomes. Annu Rev Biochem. 1996;65:801–47.
15. Gaczynska M, Rock KL, Goldberg AL. Gamma-interferon and expression of MHC genes regulate peptide hydrolysis by proteasomes. Nature. 1993;365:264–7.
16. Visekruna A, Joeris T, Seidel D et al. Proteasome-mediated degradation of IkappaBalpha and processing of p105 in Crohn disease and ulcerative colitis. J Clin Invest. 2006;116: 3195–203.
17. Harrington LE, Hatton RD, Mangan PR et al. Interleukin 17-producing CD4[+] effector T cells develop via a lineage distinct from the T helper type 1 and 2 lineages. Nat Immunol. 2005;6:1123–32.
18. Yen D, Cheung J, Scheerens H et al. IL-23 is essential for T cell-mediated colitis and promotes inflammation via IL-17 and IL-6. J Clin Invest. 2006;116:1310–16.

5
Role of Toll-like receptors in inflammatory bowel diseases

E. CARIO and D. K. PODOLSKY

The intestinal epithelium constitutes an anatomical as well as immunological barrier that forms a bipolar interface between the diverse populations of lumenal microbes and immune cells of the underlying lamina propria. The intestinal epithelial barrier must exert a highly defined process of discrimination – excluding potential host-threatening agents from microbial species while allowing host-beneficial substances (e.g. nutrients) to permeate. Mucosal imbalance within this complex network of cell and microbial interactions appears to play a key role in the pathogenesis of inflammatory bowel diseases (IBD). To counteract potential harmful effects of lumenal toxins and to protect barrier homeostasis, intestinal epithelial cells (IEC) produce several defensive factors, including trefoil peptides, mucins[1] and defensins[2]. However, these host-protective defence mechanisms are severely dysregulated in colitis[3,4]. Host–microbial interactions may also be impaired in colitis by intestinal epithelial products such as chitinase 3-like-1[5] which facilitates bacterial adhesion and invasion perpetuating acute intestinal inflammation.

The intestinal mucosa must rapidly recognize lumenal pathogens to initiate appropriate immune responses, but maintain hyporesponsiveness to omnipresent harmless commensals. Toll-like receptors (TLR) comprise a class of pattern-recognition receptors that specifically discriminate between 'self' and microbial 'non-self' based on the recognition of broadly conserved molecular patterns[6]. TLR play a key role in microbial recognition, control of adaptive immune responses and induction of antimicrobial effector pathways, leading to efficient elimination of most host-threatening pathogens. Eleven mammalian TLR have been identified which share three structural features: an extracellular ligand-binding domain with leucine-rich repeats, a short transmembrane region and a cytoplasmic Toll/IL-1 receptor domain similar to that of the interleukin-1 receptor family and essential for initiation of downstream signalling cascades. TLR are inducibly or constitutively expressed in varying combinations throughout the whole gastrointestinal tract by many different cell types, including epithelial cells[7], monocytes/macrophages[8] or myofibroblasts[9].

Various so-called pathogen-associated molecular patterns (PAMP) selectively activate different TLR, i.e. each TLR binds specific 'molecular signatures' present on diverse commensals or pathogens; e.g. TLR2 – lipopeptide; TLR4 – lipopolysaccharide (LPS); TLR5 – flagellin and TLR9 – CpG DNA. Subcellular compartmentalization of TLR appears to be one critical determinant controlling immune responsiveness[10]. Individual TLR differentially activate distinct, but partially overlapping, signalling events via diverse cofactors and adaptor proteins mediating specific immune responses. To date at least five different adaptor proteins have been identified in humans: MyD88, Mal/TIRAP, TRIF/TICAM-1, TRAM/Tirp/TICAM-2 and SARM. Downstream, different signalling modules and partially interacting complexes result in the activation of several transcription factors, including NF-κB, AP-1, Elk-1, CREB, STAT. These result in the subsequent transcriptional activation of unique and common genes encoding pro- and anti-inflammatory cytokines and chemokines as well as the induction of costimulatory molecules which control the activation of antigen-specific and non-specific adaptive immune responses by lamina propria cells[11]. Several proteins which negatively modulate immune responses by interference with the TLR-signalling complex have recently been identified. These include PI3K-Akt[12], Tollip[13,14], PPARγ[15], SIGIRR (or TIR8)[16,17] and A20[18] in the healthy intestine. These proteins may block exaggerated inflammatory responses to omnipresent harmless commensals and their products. The functional activity of individual TLR is affected by a variety of additional mechanisms. For example, TLR4 ultimately requires the co-receptor MD-2 for optimal LPS recognition and signalling. Functional trypsin appears to impair epithelial LPS recognition and responsiveness by proteolysis of MD-2[19].

Accumulating evidence underscores the important role that basal activation of TLR plays in innate host defence in the healthy intestinal mucosa, maintaining mucosal as well as commensal homeostasis. Commensals not only suppress[20,21] but also actively induce expression of a variety of host genes that participate in important physiological functions, including barrier protection and defence strategies[22]. Recent observations imply that the continuous recognition of selective commensals by TLR under steady-state conditions is essential in mucosal protection against exogenous injury[23]. Moreover, TLR2 can directly confer intestinal epithelial barrier function[24]. TLR-mediated signals may also regulate the gatekeeping functions of the follicle-associated epithelium to promote antigen capture by dendritic cells in organized mucosal lymphoid tissues[25]. Finally, TLR-signalling pathways may be critically involved in commensal-induced production of antimicrobial peptides, such as defensins[26] and BPI[27], to help prevent pathogenic bacteria from crossing the mucosal barrier. Interestingly, epithelial BPI co-localizes with TLR4 upon LPS stimulation, although the mechanism of interaction remains to be defined[28]. The full spectrum of host-beneficial signalling pathways activated by commensal-derived TLR ligands which may balance responsiveness and survival and confer integrity of the healthy, intestinal mucosa needs to be delineated in depth.

The pathogenesis of chronic recurrent intestinal inflammation in IBD is thought to involve broken epithelial barrier function and the resident microflora as triggers with subsequent aberrant stimulation of the underlying mucosal immune system in genetically susceptible individuals[29]. 'Healthy' intestinal mucosa expresses relatively little TLR2 or TLR4 protein *in vivo*[30]. However, TLR4/MD-2 expression is significantly increased in IEC and lamina propria mononuclear cells (LPMNC) throughout the lower gastrointestinal tract in association with acute IBD[19,30,31]. LPS may then be internalized by IEC[10,32] and elicit immune responses and trigger downstream events, most notably NF-κB activation resulting in the transcriptional activation of genes encoding cytokines and chemokines[7,14,19,33]. Active inflammation in IBD may thus be triggered by broken host tolerance to omnipresent LPS due to altered pattern recognition through dysregulation of TLR4/MD-2 signalling complex. Th1 cytokines, such as IFN-γ and TNF-α, strongly up-regulate TLR4 expression in IEC, possibly acting in an autocrine loop which may lead to perpetuation of intestinal inflammation by altering TLR4 responsiveness to commensals[33,34]. In contrast, Th2 cytokines efficiently suppress TLR4 expression[35].

The most common variant of TLR4 (D299G polymorphism) has been associated with IBD in selected populations[36], but the functional phenotypic significance remains unresolved in IBD. Several studies have recently demonstrated that TLR4-deficient mice are more susceptible to dextran sodium sulfate (DSS) colitis[23,37–39], although this appears to be variable, perhaps reflecting genetic heterogeneity in mice used for these studies[40]. Toxic effects on colonic epithelium with loss of commensal-mediated cytoprotection of the intestinal epithelial barrier due to TLR4-/MyD88 dysfunction and subsequent bacterial translocation[38] have been suggested as possible mechanisms by which DSS induces increased morbidity and mortality in TLR4/MyD88-deficient mice. Indeed, intestinal epithelial permeability has been found to be severely altered in the absence of MyD88[41]. Furthermore, activated macrophages promote proliferation and survival of colonic epithelial progenitors, and this may be severely impaired following injury in the absence of MyD88[42].

The functional effects of altered TLR signalling may depend on the temporal relationship to the initial insult. While basal TLR4 activation may be protective against acute injury through its beneficial effects in the intestinal epithelium, following damage TLR4/MyD88 signalling may promote chronic intestinal inflammation through its proinflammatory effects on the underlying lamina propria. Thus, while the studies referenced above suggested a protective role for TLR4 against the priming insult, a recent study demonstrated that the absence of TLR4 in STAT3-deficient mice dramatically reduced intestinal inflammation. The latter findings suggest that commensal-mediated TLR4 dysfunction of mucosal T cells contributes to the development of intestinal inflammation through the TH1-pathway[43]. This hypothesis is supported by the recent observation that blocking TLR4 with a specific antagonist inhibited development of Th1-mediated colitis in MDR1α-deficient mice. Lipid A-mimetics which specifically block binding of LPS to the TLR4/MD-2 complex, are currently under clinical investigation as possible novel therapeutics for the treatment of IBD[44–46].

Flagellins, the ligands of TLR5, have been found to be the dominant antigens in sera from colitic C3H/HeJBir mice, and also from subsets of IBD patients[47–49]. In addition, flagellin-specific CD4+ T cells induce severe colitis when adoptively transferred into immunodeficient SCID mice[48], implying aberrant TLR5 (and/or other TLR)-mediated T regulatory immune responses in colitis. Intracolonic administration of *Salmonella* flagellin perpetuates inflammatory responses in DSS colitis[50]. Interestingly, a recent study suggests that individuals carrying a TLR5 polymorphism which could result in a dominant-negative receptor exhibit significantly lower levels of flagellin-specific IgG and IgA and might be protected from developing CD[51]. Intracolonic EHEC H7 flagellin directly up-regulates the expression of epithelial cell proinflammatory chemokines in healthy mucosa[52], while *Salmonella* flagellin has no such effect[50]. Thus, it appears that cells may be able to discriminate among flagellin ligands. Further studies are needed to dissect the complex interplay of environmental and microbial factors, serotypic differences as well as distinct host pattern-recognition molecules with functional variations in distinct cell types (and also organs) that may modify disease expression and the relationships between these variables and IBD phenotypes in the genetically susceptible host.

Further characterization of the physiological and pathophysiological mechanisms within this network of possible cell–cell, ligand–ligand and PRR–PRR signalling interactions could lead to promising novel approaches that exploit TLR pathways as a means to induce salutary immune responses for treatment of IBD. Prophylactic application of selective TLR ligands may enhance commensal-mediated tissue-protective processes in order to prevent acute flares of inflammatory activity in IBD patients. Conversely, if an acute inflammatory episode has been initiated, some of the proinflammatory effects could be abrogated by blocking uncontrolled signal transduction by specific TLR inhibitors.

References

1. Kindon H, Pothoulakis C, Thim L, Lynch-Devaney K, Podolsky DK. Trefoil peptide protection of intestinal epithelial barrier function: cooperative interaction with mucin glycoprotein. Gastroenterology. 1995;109:516–23.
2. Wehkamp J, Fellermann K, Herrlinger KR, Bevins CL, Stange EF. Mechanisms of disease: defensins in gastrointestinal diseases. Nat Clin Pract Gastroenterol Hepatol. 2005;2:406–15.
3. Mashimo H, Wu DC, Podolsky DK, Fishman MC. Impaired defense of intestinal mucosa in mice lacking intestinal trefoil factor. Science. 1996;274:262–5.
4. Wehkamp J, Salzman NH, Porter E et al. Reduced Paneth cell alpha-defensins in ileal Crohn's disease. Proc Natl Acad Sci USA. 2005;102:18129–34.
5. Mizoguchi E. Chitinase 3-like-1 exacerbates intestinal inflammation by enhancing bacterial adhesion and invasion in colonic epithelial cells. Gastroenterology. 2006;130:398–411.
6. Janeway CA Jr, Goodnow CC, Medzhitov R. Danger – pathogen on the premises! Immunological tolerance. Curr Biol. 1996;6:519–22.
7. Cario E, Rosenberg IM, Brandwein SL, Beck PL, Reinecker HC, Podolsky DK. Lipopolysaccharide activates distinct signaling pathways in intestinal epithelial cell lines expressing Toll-like receptors. J Immunol. 2000;164:966–72.
8. Smith PD, Smythies LE, Mosteller-Barnum M et al. Intestinal macrophages lack CD14 and CD89 and consequently are down-regulated for LPS- and IgA-mediated activities. J Immunol. 2001;167:2651–6.
9. Otte JM, Rosenberg IM, Podolsky DK. Intestinal myofibroblasts in innate immune responses of the intestine. Gastroenterology. 2003;124:1866–78.

10. Cario E, Brown D, McKee M, Lynch-Devaney K, Gerken G, Podolsky DK. Commensal-associated molecular patterns induce selective toll-like receptor-trafficking from apical membrane to cytoplasmic compartments in polarized intestinal epithelium. Am J Pathol. 2002;160:165–73.
11. Cario E. Bacterial interactions with cells of the intestinal mucosa: Toll-like receptors and NOD2. Gut. 2005;54:1182–93.
12. Cario E, Akira S, Gerken G, Podolsky DK. Toll-like receptor 2-induced activation of the PI3K-Akt-pathway limits immune responsiveness and promotes survival of intestinal epithelial cells via MyD88. Gastroenterology. 2005;128:A4.
13. Melmed G, Thomas LS, Lee N et al. Human intestinal epithelial cells are broadly unresponsive to Toll-like receptor 2-dependent bacterial ligands: implications for host–microbial interactions in the gut. J Immunol. 2003;170:1406–15.
14. Otte JM, Cario E, Podolsky DK. Mechanisms of cross hyporesponsiveness to Toll-like receptor bacterial ligands in intestinal epithelial cells. Gastroenterology. 2004;126:1054–70.
15. Dubuquoy L, Jansson EA, Deeb S et al. Impaired expression of peroxisome proliferator-activated receptor gamma in ulcerative colitis. Gastroenterology. 2003;124:1265–76.
16. Garlanda C, Riva F, Polentarutti N et al. Intestinal inflammation in mice deficient in Tir8, an inhibitory member of the IL-1 receptor family. Proc Natl Acad Sci USA. 2004;101:3522–6.
17. Qin J, Qian Y, Yao J, Grace C, Li X. SIGIRR inhibits interleukin-1 receptor- and toll-like receptor 4-mediated signaling through different mechanisms. J Biol Chem. 2005;280:25233–41.
18. Boone DL, Turer EE, Lee EG et al. The ubiquitin-modifying enzyme A20 is required for termination of Toll-like receptor responses. Nat Immunol. 2004;5:1052–60.
19. Cario E, Golenbock DT, Visintin A, Runzi M, Gerken G, Podolsky DK. Trypsin-sensitive modulation of intestinal epithelial MD-2 as mechanism of lipopolysaccharide tolerance. J Immunol. 2006;176:4258–66.
20. Neish AS, Gewirtz AT, Zeng H et al. Prokaryotic regulation of epithelial responses by inhibition of IκB-α ubiquitination. Science. 2000;289:1560–3.
21. Kelly D, Campbell JI, King TP et al. Commensal anaerobic gut bacteria attenuate inflammation by regulating nuclear-cytoplasmic shuttling of PPAR-gamma and RelA. Nat Immunol. 2004;5:104–12.
22. Hooper LV, Gordon JI. Commensal host–bacterial relationships in the gut. Science. 2001; 292:1115–18.
23. Rakoff-Nahoum S, Paglino J, Eslami-Varzaneh F, Edberg S, Medzhitov R. Recognition of commensal microflora by toll-like receptors is required for intestinal homeostasis. Cell. 2004;118:229–41.
24. Cario E, Gerken G, Podolsky DK. Toll-like receptor 2 enhances ZO-1-associated intestinal epithelial barrier integrity via protein kinase C. Gastroenterology. 2004;127:224–38.
25. Chabot S, Wagner JS, Farrant S, Neutra MR. TLRs regulate the gatekeeping functions of the intestinal follicle-associated epithelium. J Immunol. 2006;176:4275–83.
26. Vora P, Youdim A, Thomas LS et al. Beta-defensin-2 expression is regulated by TLR signaling in intestinal epithelial cells. J Immunol. 2004;173:5398–405.
27. Canny G, Levy O, Furuta GT et al. Lipid mediator-induced expression of bactericidal/permeability-increasing protein (BPI) in human mucosal epithelia. Proc Natl Acad Sci USA. 2002;99:3902–7.
28. Canny G, Cario E, Lennartsson A et al. Functional and biochemical characterization of epithelial bactericidal/permeability-increasing protein. Am J Physiol Gastrointest Liver Physiol. 2006;290:G557–67.
29. Podolsky DK. Inflammatory bowel disease. N Engl J Med. 2002;347:417–29.
30. Cario E, Podolsky DK. Differential alteration in intestinal epithelial cell expression of toll-like receptor 3 (TLR3) and TLR4 in inflammatory bowel disease. Infect Immun. 2000;68: 7010–17.
31. Hart AL, Al-Hassi HO, Rigby RJ et al. Characteristics of intestinal dendritic cells in inflammatory bowel diseases. Gastroenterology. 2005;129:50–65.
32. Neal MD, Leaphart C, Levy R et al. Enterocyte TLR4 mediates phagocytosis and translocation of bacteria across the intestinal barrier. J Immunol. 2006;176:3070–9.
33. Suzuki M, Hisamatsu T, Podolsky DK. Gamma interferon augments the intracellular pathway for lipopolysaccharide (LPS) recognition in human intestinal epithelial cells

through coordinated up-regulation of LPS uptake and expression of the intracellular Toll-like receptor 4-MD-2 complex. Infect Immun. 2003;71:3503–11.

34. Abreu MT, Arnold ET, Thomas LS et al. TLR4 and MD-2 expression is regulated by immune-mediated signals in human intestinal epithelial cells. J Biol Chem. 2002;277: 20431–7.

35. Mueller T, Terada T, Rosenberg IM, Shibolet O, Podolsky DK. Th2 cytokines down-regulate TLR expression and function in human intestinal epithelial cells. J Immunol. 2006;176:5805–14.

36. Franchimont D, Vermeire S, El Housni H et al. Deficient host-bacteria interactions in inflammatory bowel disease? The toll-like receptor (TLR)-4 Asp299gly polymorphism is associated with Crohn's disease and ulcerative colitis. Gut. 2004;53:987–92.

37. Rachmilewitz D, Katakura K, Karmeli F et al. Toll-like receptor 9 signaling mediates the anti-inflammatory effects of probiotics in murine experimental colitis. Gastroenterology. 2004;126:520–8.

38. Fukata M, Michelsen KS, Eri R et al. Toll-like receptor-4 is required for intestinal response to epithelial injury and limiting bacterial translocation in a murine model of acute colitis. Am J Physiol Gastrointest Liver Physiol. 2005;288:G1055–65.

39. Ohkawara T, Takeda H, Nishihira J et al. Macrophage migration inhibitory factor contributes to the development of acute dextran sulphate sodium-induced colitis in Toll-like receptor 4 knockout mice. Clin Exp Immunol. 2005;141:412–21.

40. Mahler M, Bristol IJ, Leiter EH et al. Differential susceptibility of inbred mouse strains to dextran sulfate sodium-induced colitis. Am J Physiol. 1998;274:G544–51.

41. Thomas KE, Sapone A, Fasano A, Vogel SN. Gliadin stimulation of murine macrophage inflammatory gene expression and intestinal permeability are MyD88-dependent: role of the innate immune response in celiac disease. J Immunol. 2006;176:2512–21.

42. Pull SL, Doherty JM, Mills JC, Gordon JI, Stappenbeck TS. Activated macrophages are an adaptive element of the colonic epithelial progenitor niche necessary for regenerative responses to injury. Proc Natl Acad Sci USA. 2005;102:99–104.

43. Kobayashi M, Kweon MN, Kuwata H et al. Toll-like receptor-dependent production of IL-12p40 causes chronic enterocolitis in myeloid cell-specific Stat3-deficient mice. J Clin Invest. 2003;111:1297–308.

44. Christ WJ, Asano O, Robidoux AL et al. E5531, a pure endotoxin antagonist of high potency. Science. 1995;268:80–3.

45. Mullarkey M, Rose JR, Bristol J et al. Inhibition of endotoxin response by e5564, a novel Toll-like receptor 4-directed endotoxin antagonist. J Pharmacol Exp Ther. 2003;304:1093–102.

46. Fort MM, Mozaffarian A, Stover AG et al. A synthetic TLR4 antagonist has anti-inflammatory effects in two murine models of inflammatory bowel disease. J Immunol. 2005;174:6416–23.

47. Targan SR, Landers CJ, Yang H et al. Antibodies to CBir1 flagellin define a unique response that is associated independently with complicated Crohn's disease. Gastroenterology. 2005;128:2020–8.

48. Lodes MJ, Cong Y, Elson CO et al. Bacterial flagellin is a dominant antigen in Crohn disease. J Clin Invest. 2004;113:1296–306.

49. Sitaraman SV, Klapproth JM, Moore DA 3rd et al. Elevated flagellin-specific immunoglobulins in Crohn's disease. Am J Physiol Gastrointest Liver Physiol. 2005;288: G403–6.

50. Rhee SH, Im E, Riegler M, Kokkotou E, O'Brien M, Pothoulakis C. Pathophysiological role of Toll-like receptor 5 engagement by bacterial flagellin in colonic inflammation. Proc Natl Acad Sci USA. 2005;102:13610–15.

51. Gewirtz AT, Vijay-Kumar M, Brant SR, Duerr RH, Nicolae DL, Cho JH. Dominant-negative TLR5 polymorphism reduces adaptive immune response to flagellin and negatively associates with Crohn's disease. Am J Physiol Gastrointest Liver Physiol. 2006;290:G1157–63.

52. Miyamoto Y, Iimura M, Kaper JB, Torres AG, Kagnoff MF. Role of Shiga toxin versus H7 flagellin in enterohaemorrhagic *Escherichia coli* signalling of human colon epithelium *in vivo*. Cell Microbiol. 2006;8:869–79.

6
Animal models in inflammatory bowel disease

R. ATREYA, M. WALDNER and M. F. NEURATH

INTRODUCTION

Inflammatory bowel disease (IBD) comprises Crohn's disease (CD) and ulcerative colitis (UC), which are defined as relapsing inflammations of unknown cause that can affect the entire gastrointestinal tract. Both disease entities are characterized by distinct clinical and pathological attributes[1]. While UC primarily involves the colonic mucosa and submucosa, and is marked by continuous inflammation of the large intestine, CD is characterized by transmural, segmental inflammation that for the most part involves the distal ileum and colon, but can also potentially affect any part of the gastrointestinal tract[2]. Although the precise aetiology of IBD still remains unclear, considerable progress has been made in the past few years with regard to the identification of pivotal pathogenic mechanisms. There is accumulating evidence that genetic predisposition, environmental factors, infectious agents, impairment of local tolerance and mucosal imbalance with ongoing activation of the intestinal immune system contribute to the perpetuation of the inflammatory cascade[3].

While patient-oriented investigations and subsequent *in-vitro* studies have contributed to the growing insight regarding pathological mucosal immune responses, most progress has been derived from the development of various experimental animal models of chronic intestinal inflammation. Although these models are not able to mimic all multidimensional aspects visible in IBD, such as the spontaneous, relapsing course of disease or specific extraintestinal manifestations, they provide irreplaceable assistance in the study of specific pathophysiological events. They enable the study of early pathological events before disease onset, the identification of genes that determine susceptibility and of bacterial antigens involved in disease pathogenesis, and the examination of immunological processes and interactions of central immune cell populations during the course of the disease. The results obtained led to the development of novel therapeutic strategies that can be tested in appropriate animal models resulting in possible therapeutic alternatives for IBD patients[4-6].

Animal models of IBD can be divided into four main categories: models of spontaneous colitis consisting of mutant mouse strains; inducible colitis models (chemical, and immunological); adoptive transfer models in immunocompromised host animals and genetically engineered models (knockout and transgenic)[6].

The following paragraphs provide an overview of a variety of established experimental models of chronic intestinal inflammation, elucidating current general mechanisms that are believed to be involved in chronic mucosal inflammation, as well as emerging therapeutic alternatives that are derived from these models.

MODELS OF SPONTANEOUS COLITIS

Spontaneous models of chronic intestinal inflammation comprise animals with a predisposition to develop signs of mucosal inflammation without any genetic or immunological manipulation and therefore may have an advantage in mimicking the complexity of human disease as compared to other experimental models. One of the first models to be described is the cottontop tamarin, which is a special inbred primate that suffers from UC-like mucosal inflammation and subsequent colon cancer[8]. This inflammatory process is probably caused by environmental factors, genetic factors (due to only a single MHC class I locus[9]) and bacterial antigens[10]. With regard to mice, two models of spontaneous colitis have been described and are presented in the following paragraphs. Due to the somewhat remarkable similarity of these experimental models to IBD there is great promise for further identification of genetic susceptibility factors studies regarding the interaction of the intestinal microflora with the mucosal immune system.

C3H/HeJBir mice

C3H/HeJBir mice, generated by selective breeding of C3H/HeJ mice, are a substrain of mice that reproducibly and spontaneously develop signs of colitis involving the ileocaecal region and extending into the right side of the colon in the third week of life. The transmural inflammation occurs in young mice and tends to resolve with age, usually without any signs of recurrence, and is characterized by a Th1-type cell response[11]. Cell transfer studies showed that activated C3H/HeJBir CD4[+] T cells reactive to bacterial antigens induced colitis upon transfer into severe combined immunodeficiency (SCID) mice, demonstrating the pathogenic importance of antigens of the enteric bacterial flora[12]. Further studies identified specific microbial antigens (bacterial flagellins) in the commensal flora, which activate the pathogenic T cells[13]. Moreover a colitis susceptibility gene locus that seems to regulate CD4[+] T-cell response to these bacterial antigens was also detected[14].

SAMP/Yit mice

One of the most recently developed spontaneous IBD mouse model consists of the SAMP/Yit mice, which have been derived by selective breeding of AKR mice. This inbred strain spontaneously develops a chronic terminal ileitis with discontinuous, transmural inflammatory lesions, bearing a remarkable resemblance to CD[15]. One may adoptively transfer the chronic ileitis by CD4+ T cells into SCID mice[16]. A subsequently generated SAMP/YitFc substrain expressed even more clinical features reminiscent of CD. Among other characteristics a subgroup of mice developed perianal ailments with corresponding ulceration and fistulas, representing the first time such occurrence in any experimental model of IBD[17]. Further studies revealed that this Th1 mediated inflammation, which occurs in mice as early as 10 weeks of age, could be ameliorated by inhibition of the cytokine TNF-α, which led to an induction of apoptosis in lamina propria mononuclear cells[18]. The administration of broad-spectrum antibiotics led to the suppression of the intestinal Th1 cytokine production and down-regulation of activated T cells, indicating the important pathogenic role of the intestinal flora[19]. Their pivotal role was also emphasized by the fact that SAMP/YitFc mice, which were raised under strictly aseptic conditions, showed no signs of intestinal inflammation as compared to mice housed under standard conditions[15]. Another study showed that combined blockade of adhesion molecules, such as the intracellular adhesion molecule (ICAM)-1 and vascular cell adhesion molecule (VCAM)-1, suppressed the acute inflammatory process in the SAMP/Yit mice transfer model[20]. As spontaneous models of IBD are a valuable asset for the study of genes responsible for disease susceptibility, it recently became possible to localize the genes promoting the inflammation-associated epithelial damage in these mice[21]. Vidrich et al. used SAMP/YitFc mice to reveal that alterations in the normal pattern of epithelial differentiation prior to intestinal inflammation may be an initiating factor in this experimental model, leading to activation of pathogenic T cells reactive to bacterial antigens[22,23].

INDUCIBLE COLITIS MODELS

The group of inducible colitis models are overall the most widely used experimental IBD animal models, as the simplicity of the induction process and the immediate mucosal inflammation are unparalleled[24]. The induction of chronic or transient intestinal inflammation in experimental colitis models is instigated in various different ways leading to acute damage of the epithelial barrier. The most common experimental models rely on the administration of an exogenous chemical agent or the involvement of a secondary immune component[23]. One of the first animal models to be presented was the immune complex colitis model in rabbits[25]. A modified version, in which the transient mucosal inflammation was induced by instillation of a formaldehyde solution into the distal colon followed by systemic administration of immune complexes, enabled the detailed study of proinflammatory sequences in acute colitis, as the profile of inflammatory mediators exhibit a strong resemblance to

IBD[7,26]. Another rather simple model of experimental IBD is acetic acid-induced colitis, in which mucosal inflammation can be induced by luminal administration of acetic acid in a dose-dependent fashion[27]. This easily inducible model is useful for evaluating early events of inflammation and ensuing mechanisms of mucosal healing, but due to the lack of chronification its value is also limited. A model with some similarity to CD is generated by the treatment of rats with indomethacin, which leads to extensive chronic ulcerations in the small bowel in genetically susceptible animals. Subsequent studies emphasized the protective role of prostacyclins regarding the initial epithelial injury in indomethacin-induced colitis[28]. Further models include carageenan colitis, in which continuous administration of degraded carrageenan polymers in the drinking water of guinea-pigs initially causes caecal inflammation, which then extends to the left side of the colon[29]. Data obtained from this model revealed the importance of specific anaerobic bacteria of the endogenous flora for the development of mucosal ulcerations[30]. Peptidoglycan-polysaccharide (PG-PS) colitis consists of intramural injection of the bacterial cell wall component PG-PS, which leads to the induction of granulomatous transmural enterocolitis and sometimes even extraintestinal manifestations, depending on the genetic background of the rats used[31]. This model provided insights regarding the importance of cell wall components of resident enteric bacteria in the induction of the inflammatory process in a susceptible host when exposed to the mucosal immune system. Among the class of inducible colitis models dextran sulphate sodium colitis (DSS) and hapten-based colitis models, employing either trinitrobenzene sulphonic acid (TNBS) or oxazolone, are the most commonly used models, and will therefore be discussed in more detail.

DSS colitis

The addition of DSS polymers to the drinking water of rodents induces haematochezia, neutrophil infiltration and lesions in the distal colon inducing a consistent level of colitis. Both acute and chronic models of DSS colitis are described[32]. Remarkably DSS can also evoke colitis in SCID mice, suggesting that T cells are not required for development of mucosal inflammation, indicating that acute colitis is induced by innate immunity but not acquired immunity in this setting[33]. This is also visible by the initial activation of macrophages and the consecutive production of proinflammatory cytokines, which then lead to the activation of intestinal lymphocytes resulting in chronic colitis[34]. The importance of genetic factors in models of mucosal inflammation has also been shown in relation to DSS colitis, as different mouse strains comprise different susceptibilities to disease[35]. This model has also proved to be quite beneficial in the testing of new therapeutic strategies such as anti-TNF-α antibodies[36] or antibodies to various cell adhesion molecules[37,38]. Finally pretreatment of mice with DSS colitis with azoxymethane led to the development of invasive colorectal adenocarcinomas at the site of the most severe colitic injury[39]. Therefore this model is predestined for further examination of colorectal carcinogenesis in mucosal inflammation.

TNBS colitis

One of the most intensively studied models of mucosal inflammation is the TNBS colitis. This hapten-induced colitis is induced by luminal instillation of TNBS in ethanol in susceptible rodent strains. This immunologically mediated colitis model is based on the ethanol-mediated disruption of the mucosal barrier and the hapten-induced delayed-type hypersensitivity immune response. TNBS-induced colitis is associated with a transmural granulomatous inflammation limited to the colon as a result of an interleukin (IL)-12 driven, Th1-mediated cytokine response resembling CD. Consequently administration of anti-IL-12 antibodies resulted in disease prevention or complete disappearance of already-existing inflammatory lesions[40]. The rapid therapeutic effect is due to Fas-mediated T-cell apoptosis in the lamina propria[41]. In addition disease could also be prevented by application of anti-CD40L, indicating a role of CD40L–CD40 interaction in Th1-mediated inflammation[42]. Another major lesson learned from the TNBS model of colitis is the importance of regulatory mechanisms in the mucosal immune system. The mechanism of oral tolerance was displayed by oral administration of TNP-haptenated colonic protein that led to the prevention of colitis induced by intestinal TNBS application, due to the induction of regulatory cells producing transforming growth factor beta (TGF-β)[43] and IL-10[44]. The therapeutic implications of these data are visible in the successful administration of intranasal TGF-β plasmids leading to amelioration of TNBS colitis through induction of TGF-β production by T cells and macrophages[45]. The TNBS colitis model convinces in its potential for the investigation of alterations in cytokine profiles in gut inflammation and the development and testing of new therapeutic strategies.

Oxazolone colitis

The rectal administration of the haptenating agent oxazolone in ethanol causes a severe mucosal inflammation in treated SJL/J mice, that affects the distal half of the colon. Histopathological studies reveal a reduction of epithelial cells, goblet cells and accompanying bowel wall oedema. Overall these characteristics are reminiscent of UC rather than CD. Consistently, lamina propria cells in oxazolone colitis exhibited increased production of the Th2 cytokines IL-4 and IL-5, but normal or reduced levels of the Th1 cytokine IFN-γ, which strongly resembles the cytokine profile of UC. The pathogenic role of the Th2 response is emphasized by the fact that anti-IL-4 antibody treatment ameliorates disease, whereas anti-IL-12 application worsens it. Further studies revealed a high TGF-β production in this model, which is more elevated in the non-inflamed proximal colon than in the inflamed regions of the distal colon, indicating an anti-inflammatory role of TGF-β in disease pathogenesis, a notion further supported by the fact that anti-TGF-β antibody treatment led to exacerbation of disease[46]. This colitis model is therefore valuable for further investigations of downstream inflammatory cytokines involved in disease pathogenesis.

ADOPTIVE TRANSFER MODELS IN IMMUNOCOMPROMISED HOST

Adoptive transfer models consist of an adoptive transfer of specific cell types or bone marrow precursor cells into immunocompromised hosts, resulting in profound mucosal inflammation. The reconstitution of the immunodeficient animals with subsets of specific cells enables the functional assessment of these cells in disease pathogenesis. One mouse model that exhibits severe small intestinal inflammation is induced by adoptive transfer of heatshock protein (hsp) 60-specific CD8[+] T-cell clones preactivated by bacterial hsp60 into SCID mice. The inflammatory reactions were MHC class I-dependent and featured a functional role of TNF-α, as intestinal lesions were decreased in mice lacking the TNF-α receptor. This colitis model denotes that specific T cells with defined antigen specificity are able to cause severe intestinal inflammation. Furthermore it is one of the few models in which signs of mucosal inflammation are also found under germ-free conditions[47]. Another colitis model consists of the bone marrow reconstituted Tgε26 mouse. Mice with the Tgε26 defect bear an abnormal structure of the thymus, leading to intrathymic T cell and natural killer cell death. The transplantation of T-cell-depleted bone marrow is able to rescue the fetal mice[48]. Adoptive transfer studies of Tgε26 mice which are reconstituted with wild-type bone marrow depleted from T cells show that these mice develop a Th1-mediated colitis. These data suggest abnormal T-cell development in the bone marrow as a major factor of colitis induction in this model[23]. These models, together with a consecutively presented CD45RB[high] transfer model, have further defined the pivotal pathogenic role of regulatory T-cell populations and inflammatory cytokines in IBD.

CD45RB[high] SCID-transfer colitis

The CD45RB[high] transfer model is one of the most widely used models of mucosal inflammation. The transfer of CD4[+]CD45RB[high] T cells from immunocompetent mice to SCID or recombination activating gene (RAG) deficient mice leads to a severe Th1-mediated colitis with transmural inflammation[49,50]. The importance of the microbial flora for disease pathogenesis was proved in studies showing that the transfer of cells to SCID mice raised under germ-free conditions led to reduced levels of inflammation[51]. One of the most interesting features of this model is that transfer of CD4[+] T cells or CD4[+]CD45RB[low] T-cell subsets along with the CD4[+]CD45RB[high] T cells does not result in mucosal inflammation. It could be shown that the protective effect mediated by the CD4[+]CD45RB[low] T cells was due to the production of the regulatory cytokine TGF-β[52]. Moreover further studies elucidated that CD25[+] T cells were the essential regulatory cells among the CD4[+]CD45RB[low] cells[53], producing elevated TGF-β levels when stimulated[54]. In further studies IL-10 could also be identified as a main regulatory cytokine in SCID-transfer colitis, as CD4[+]CD45RB[high] T cells from IL-10 transgenic mice do not induce colitis after transfer[55]. Correspondingly the CD4[+]CD45RB[low] T cells derived from IL-10-deficient mice were not able to prevent the induction of colitis when transferred with CD4[+]CD45RB[high] T cells[56]. Moreover the regulatory class of Tr1 cells that mainly produce IL-10 were able to suppress the onset of mucosal inflammation when cotransferred with CD4+CD45RB[high] T cells into SCID mice[57]. Recent data have shown that adoptive transfer of CD4+CD25- T cells also results in colitis resembling IBD with a rapid onset and limited variability between individuals[58]. Analogous to other experimental models of colitis, the severity of the SCID-transfer colitis is significantly diminished when the recipient SCID mice are bred under germ-free conditions[59].

The SCID-transfer model has helped tremendously to further define the role of regulatory T-cell populations in mediating the inflammatory process, and elucidates the importance of the balance between effector and regulatory cell populations for the maintainance of mucosal homeostasis. Furthermore it is highly suitable for pharmacological testing of new interventional strategies.

GENETICALLY ENGINEERED MODELS

Genetically engineered models form the largest group of experimental models of IBD and, due to advances in recombinant DNA technologies, are the group that has recently been expanding the most. The generation of animals with a single deletion of a target gene (knockout animals) or increased expression of a particular gene (transgenic animals) has enabled the study of candidate genes in IBD and specific immunoregulatory pathways involved in disease pathogenesis[60]. These models clearly show that many different immune defects can lead to quite similar IBD phenotypes. With the availability of increasing numbers of genetically engineered models it seems possible to unravel the multiple pathways involved in the regulation of mucosal inflammation.

Transgenic models

One of the first reported transgenic colitis model are rats transgenic for human HLA B27 and β_2-microglobulin which develop a spontaneous inflammation of the stomach, ileum and the entire colon, as well as inflammation of the joints[61]. Various studies have revealed a coherence between different bacteria of the resident microbial flora and inflammation of the gut[62]. IL-7 transgenic mice expressed signs of chronic colitis caused by infiltrating CD4+ T cells. Interestingly, high levels of IL-7 were found in the acute phase in the inflamed regions of the mucosa while IL-7 was decreased in the chronic phase[63]. A further model that once more emphasizes the importance of the intestinal epithelial barrier for mucosal homeostasis is the transgenic mice mode for dominant negative N-cadherin. The altered intestinal intercellular adhesion leads to the induction of mucosal inflammation[64]. As some of the previously described models have already shown the importance of the regulatory cytokine TGF-β in IBD, a more detailed interaction of defects in TGF-β signalling and mucosal inflammation could be examined with transgenic dominant-negative TGF-β receptor (TGF-β RII) mice. This model showed that alterations in TGF-β signalling in intestinal T cells[65], as well as in epithelial cells[66] led to inflammation of the gut. Another model that genetically intervenes in the molecular pathways involved in IBD pathogenesis is the signal transducer and activator of transcription-4 (STAT-4) transgenic mouse. These mice have an increased disposition towards an IL-12-driven Th1 response after CD4$^+$ T-cell activation which leads to chronic transmural colitis. Interestingly T cells from these mice primed with autologous bacterial antigen *in vitro* and then adoptively transferred to SCID mice are able to induce colitis[67].

Gene knockout models

IL-2-deficient mice

Mice with IL-2 deficiency exhibit multiorgan disease which is then followed by the development of a Th1-driven transmural colitis. As in many other models, IL-2$^{-/-}$ mice do not develop colitis under germ-free conditions[68]. Further studies examining the cause of colitis in IL-2 deficiency concluded that an inadequate TGF-β regulatory response to the activation of intestinal T cells against components of the luminal bacterial flora is responsible for mucosal inflammation[69].

IL-10-deficient mice

IL-10-deficient mice spontaneously develop chronic enterocolitis marked by epithelial cell hyperplasia and massive infiltration of lymphocytes and activated macrophages. In the acute phase the disease is marked by a Th1 cytokine profile and can be treated by anti-IL-12 antibodies[70]. Germ-free bred IL-10-deficient mice do not develop colitis, indicating that antigens in the mucosal microflora are pivotal for initiation of intestinal inflammation[71]. Furthermore IL-10-deficient mice exhibit an increased intestinal permeability leading to an increased exposure of mucosal antigens towards the mucosal immune system, thus leading to the ensuing inflammatory reaction[72]. The absent immunoregulatory effect of IL-10 in this model is underscored by above-mentioned studies that show that CD4$^+$CD45RB^{low} T cells from IL-10-deficient mice are not able to prevent colitis in the SCID transfer model[56]. Finally not only IL-10 deficiency leads to colitis but so also do defects in IL-10 signalling. This is visible in CRF2-4 knockouts that exhibit a deficiency for the CRF-2 receptor that is elemental for IL-10 signal transduction, leading to signs of chronic intestinal inflammation[73].

STAT-3 knockout mice

STAT-3 in macrophages is an important transcription factor mediating the signal transduction pathways of IL-10 and IL-6. Mice with specific inhibition of the STAT-3 gene in macrophages and neutrophils develop a Th1-mediated enterocolitis producing elevated amounts of proinflammatory cytokines (TNF-α, IFN-γ, IL-6) when stimulated with lipopolysaccharide (LPS). As the suppressive effects of IL-10 on inflammatory cytokine production from macrophages and neutrophils are completely abolished, the dominance of these cytokines leads to the development of chronic intestinal inflammation[74]. These data are consistent with the concept of heightened exposure to microbial flora with subsequent stimulation of the mucosal immune system being the decisive factor in the initiation of mucosal inflammation.

TCR-α chain knockout mice

Chronic colitis also develops in gene-targeted mice deficient for the TCR-αchain. The colitis in these mice is characterized by histological lesions that are rather characteristic for UC, e.g. the presence of distorted crypts and a rather superficial inflammation of the gut. Moreover colitis in this model is associated with a Th2-type cytokine profile, with a dominance of IL-4. Consistent with these data further experiments show a beneficial therapeutic effect of anti-IL-4 antibodies in this model and TCR-α/IL-4 double knockout mice similarly exhibit fewer signs of inflammation[75]. Another point derived from this model is the role of B cells in the pathogenesis of mucosal inflammation. Double mutant TCR-α chain-deficient and μIg-deficient mice, which have no B cells, develop more severe colitis than single mutant TCR-α chain-deficient mice[76]. This observation may be explained by data that suggest that B cells may produce regulatory cytokines such as IL-10 and thus may play a role in controlling mucosal homeostasis[23].

NF-κBp50 mice

Nuclear factor (NF)-κB is a transcription factor known to be critically involved in promoter regulation of various proinflammatory cytokines, and thus takes up an important role in IBD pathogenesis. Recent data have also elucidated that, in contrast to the p65 subunit, the p50 subunit of NF-κB also possesses inhibitory activity[23]. In a series of adoptive transfer experiments using RAG-$2^{-/-}$ or $p50^{-/-}p65^{+/-}$Rag-$2^{-/-}$ mice as hosts for $p50^{-/-}p65^{+/-}$ lymphocyte populations, it could be shown that *Helicobacter hepaticus*-induced colitis in $p50^{-/-}p65^{+/-}$Rag-$2^{-/-}$ mice could not be suppressed by $p50^{-/-}p65^{+/-}$ splenocytes. Colitis in these animals is marked by elevated macrophage production of the inflammatory cytokine IL-12p40 and administration of an anti-IL-12p40 antibody prevented disease. These results suggest that inhibition of *H. hepaticus*-induced IL-12p40 expression by NF-κB subunits is crucial in preventing intestinal inflammation in response to bacterial antigens[77].

TNFΔARE mice

The targeted gene deletion of AU-rich elements (ARE) in the 3′-untranslated region of TNF-α mRNA leads to increased production of the cytokine TNF-α. The augmented expression of the proinflammatory cytokine TNF-α leads to severe mucosal inflammation in the TNFΔARE mouse model. The transmural inflammation is predominantly located in the terminal ileum and is accompanied by signs of polyarthritis. This model of colitis emphasizes the pathogenic role of TNF-α and suggests that defective function of ARE may be involved in the development of CD in a subset of patients[78].

PATHOGENIC MECHANISMS OF MUCOSAL INFLAMMATION

Despite the steadily increasing number of varying experimental models for IBD, they all have some basic pathogenic principles in common that have improved our understanding of the mechanisms involved in the process leading to chronic mucosal inflammation. The lessons derived from these models led to a pathogenic concept that is based on genetic susceptibility causing alterations of the epithelial barrier. Subsequently, the intestinal mucosal immune system is exposed to enteric bacterial antigens from the commensal flora, leading to an uncontrolled activation of the intestinal immune system. This ultimately leads to gastrointestinal inflammation and perpetuation of disease[3].

Genetic susceptibility

Multiple studies have shown that genetic factors have an influence in various models of mucosal inflammation. This relation is visible in the DSS or TNBS colitis model, in which the induction of colitis depends on the genetic background of the mouse strains used[5,35]. Moreover, genetic analysis of susceptibility to DSS colitis in C3H/HEJ mice led to the identification of several quantitative trait loci[79]. In IBD the identification of the *NOD-2* gene has correspondingly pointed out the significance of genetic susceptibility for development of disease[80]. Recent data have even identified the peroxisome proliferator-activated receptor-gamma as a susceptibility gene in SAMP1/YitFc mice, as well as in human CD[81].

The bacterial flora

Various studies with experimental models for IBD have demonstrated that the incidence of colitis in the vast majority of the models depends on the presence of the microbial flora indicating that gut inflammation is driven by resident bacterial antigens. The disturbance of the epithelial barrier, as in transgenic mice for dominant negative N-cadherin[64], probably leads to increased exposure of the mucosal immune system towards the enteric antigens. Furthermore the administration of antibiotics has led to abrogation of disease in SAMP/YitFc mice[19]. However, not all components of the microbial flora have the capacity to induce inflammation, as selective colonialization experiments have revealed. In C3/HeJBir mice bacterial flagellins[13], and in IL-10-deficient mice *H. hepaticus*[82] have been identified as major contributors of disease pathogenesis. On the other hand specific bacterial species are even able to prevent the onset of mucosal inflammation[83]. The pathogenic importance of the enteric flora in human disease has been documented in diverse studies[84,85].

Alterations of the epithelial barrier

Animal models which possess a defect in epithelial barrier protein, such as the transgenic mice for dominant negative N-cadherin[64], or in mice lacking the trefoil factor[86], develop severe signs of gut inflammation due to the increased exposure of the mucosal immune system towards the enteric flora. A disturbance of the epithelial structure with heightened intestinal permeability has also been visible in CD[87], as well as in UC[88].

The mucosal immune system

The different mouse models all indicate that uncontrolled CD4[+] T-cell activation is the central pathogenic mechanism involved in the initiation and regulation of the inflammatory process. The involvement of CD4[+] T cells in disease pathogenesis has most elegantly been shown in the adoptive transfer model. These activated CD4[+] T cells, through Th1 or Th2 polarized immune response, induce the intestinal inflammation in the animal models. Due to the changed grade of activation in these cells, there is an abnormal cytokine production pattern, The IL-12-driven Th1 cytokine response is present in most of the experimental models. The mucosa of patients with established CD is also characterized by CD4[+] T cells with a Th1 phenotype, marked by the production of IFN-γ[89]. Fittingly the histological aspect of transmural inflammation in these models is consistent with human CD. In contrast to these findings, oxazolone-induced colitis and the colitis in TCR-α-deficient mice are mediated by Th2 cell response, characterized by excessive IL-4 production. Similarly the mucosa in patients with UC may be dominated by CD4[+] lymphocytes with an altered Th2 phenotype, characterized by the production of IL-5, but not IL-4[89]. The above-mentioned colitis models also indicate the crucial role of the regulatory cytokines IL-10 and TGF-β in maintaining mucosal homeostasis upon activation. The functional absence of these cytokines in the related mouse models led to intestinal inflammation[65,66,70]. In the SCID transfer model the counter-regulation of CD4[+]CD45RB[high] T cells through CD25[+] T cells (t_r1) is also dependent on TGF-β[53].

TREATMENT OF MUCOSAL INFLAMMATION

Studies in animal models of intestinal inflammation have not only allowed significant progress in the understanding of the pathogenic mechanisms involved in disease pathogenesis but have also highlighted potential immune targets that form the basis for novel therapeutic strategies. Analogous to the successful administration of anti-TNF-α antibodies in the SCID model of colitis[90], and the DSS-induced colitis91 the anti-TNF-α antibody has proved its therapeutic efficacy in various human trials, and is well established in the treatment of CD[92,93] and UC[94]. The therapeutic rationale herein seems to be the rapid and augmented induction of intestinal T-lymphocyte apoptosis[95]. The attractive therapeutic approach of inhibiting major proinflammatory cytokines is also implemented in the administration of a neutralizing anti-IL-12 antibody in TNBS-induced colitis where it led to the induction of apoptosis of intestinal CD4[+] T cells and to consecutive abrogation of mucosal inflammation[40,41]. A recent study report showed that treatment with a monoclonal antibody against IL-12 also induced clinical response and remission in patients with CD[96]. Another potential target of forthcoming therapies is the proinflammatory cytokine IL-6, which conveys an increased apoptotic resistance of intestinal CD4[+] T cells through its soluble receptor (sIL-6R)[97]. The administration of a neutralizing antibody against the sIL-6R had a therapeutic effect in the SCID transfer and TNBS model, as well as in IL-10-deficient mice. This blockade of the IL-6 signalling pathway was recently carried out in a clinical trial with a humanized anti-IL-6R monoclonal antibody for active CD. This preliminary study showed an overall therapeutic benefit[98]. However, other therapeutic approaches that have shown encouraging effects in experimental models have only been marginally effective in human disease. Therefore, a careful evaluation is necessary regarding therapeutic conclusions from animal models; nevertheless the above results give hope for the development of new therapeutic strategies that are based on sound pathophysiological rationales derived from experimental models of inflammatory bowel diseases.

References

1. Podolsky DK. Inflammatory bowel disease. N Engl J Med. 1991;325:928–37.
2. Duchmann R, Zeitz M. Crohn's disease. In: Ogra PL, Mestecky J, Lamm M, Strober W, Bienenstock J, McGhee JR, editors. Mucosal Immunology, 2nd edn. San Diego: Academic Press, 1999:1055–80.
3. Podolsky DK. Inflammatory bowel disease. N Engl J Med. 2002;347:417–29.
4. Elson CO, Sartor RB, Tennyson GS, Riddell RH. Experimental models of inflammatory bowel disease. Gastroenterology. 1995;109:1344–67.
5. Pizarro TT, Arseneau KO, Bamias G, Cominelli F. Mouse models for the study of Crohn's disease. Trends Mol Med. 2002;9:218–22.
6. Wirtz S, Neurath MF. Animal models of intestinal inflammation: new insights into the molecular pathogenesis and immunotherapy of inflammatory bowel disease. Int J Colorectal Dis. 2000;15:144–60.
7. Strober S, Fuss IJ, Blumberg RS. The immunology of mucosal models of inflammation. Annu Rev Immunology. 2002;20:495–549.
8. Madara JL, Podolsky DK, King NW, Sehgal PK, Moore R, Winter HS. Characterization of spontaneous colitis in cotton-top tamarins (Saguinus oedipus) and its response to sulfasalazine. Gastroenterology. 1985;88:13–19.
9. Watkins DI, Chen ZW, Hughes AL, Evans MG, Tedder TF, Letvin NL. Evolution of the MHC class I genes of a New World primate from ancestral homologues of human non-classical genes. Nature. 1990;346:60–3.
10. Mansfield KG, Lin KC, Xia D et al. Enteropathogenic Escherichia coli and ulcerative colitis in cotton-top tamarins (Saguinus oedipus). Infect Dis. 2001;184:803–7.
11. Sundberg JP, Elson CO, Bedigian H, Birkenmeier EH. Spontaneous, heritable colitis in a new substrain of C3H/HeJ mice. Gastroenterology. 1994;107:1726–35.
12. Cong Y, Brandwein SL, McCabe RP et al. CD4+ T cells reactive to enteric bacterial antigens in spontaneously coliticC3H/HeJBir mice: increased T helper cell type 1 response and ability to transfer disease. J Exp Med. 1998;187:855–64.
13. Lodes MJ, Cong Y, Elson CO et al. Bacterial flagellin is a dominant antigen in Crohn disease. J Clin Invest. 2004;113:1296–306.
14. Beckwith J, Cong Y, Sundberg JP, Elson CO, Leiter EH. Cdcs1, a major colitogenic locus in mice, regulates innate and adaptive immune response to enteric bacterial antigens. Gastroenterology. 2005;129:1473–84.
15. Matsumoto S, Okabe Y, Setoyama H et al. Inflammatory bowel disease-like enteritis and caecitis in a senescence accelerated mouse P1/Yit strain. Gut. 1998;43:71–8.
16. Kosiewicz MM, Nast CC, Krishnan A et al. Th1-type responses mediate spontaneous ileitis in a novel murine model of Crohn's disease. J Clin Invest. 2001;107:695–702.
17. Rivera-Nieves J, Bamias G, Vidrich A et al. Emergence of perianal fistulizing disease in the SAMP1/YitFc mouse, a spontaneous model of chronic ileitis. Gastroenterology. 2003;124: 972–82.

18. Marini M, Bamias G, Rivera-Nieves J et al. TNF-alpha neutralization ameliorates the severity of murine Crohn's-like ileitis by abrogation of intestinal epithelial cell apoptosis. Proc Natl Acad Sci USA. 2003;100:8366–71.

19. Bamias G, Marini M, Moskaluk CA et al. Down-regulation of intestinal lymphocyte activation and Th1 cytokine production by antibiotic therapy in a murine model of Crohn's disease. Immunology. 2002;169:5308–14.

20. Burns RC, Rivera-Nieves J, Moskaluk CA, Matsumoto S, Cominelli F, Ley K. Antibody blockade of ICAM-1 and VCAM-1 ameliorates inflammation in the SAMP-1/Yit adoptive transfer model of Crohn's disease in mice. Gastroenterology. 2001;121:1428–36.

21. Kozaiwa K, Sugawara K, Smith MF Jr et al. Identification of a quantitative trait locus for ileitis in a spontaneous mouse model of Crohn's disease: SAMP1/YitFc. Gastroenterology. 2003;125:477–90.

22. Vidrich A, Buzan JM, Barnes S et al. Altered epithelial cell lineage allocation and global expansion of the crypt epithelial stem cell population are associated with ileitis in SAMP1/YitFc mice. Am J Pathol. 2005;166:1055–67.

23. Elson CO, Cong Y, McCracken VJ, Dimmitt RA, Lorenz RG, Weaver CT. Experimental models of inflammatory bowel disease reveal innate, adaptive, and regulatory mechanisms of host dialogue with the microbiota. Immunol Rev. 2005;206:260–76.

24. Hoffmann JC, Pawlowski NN, Kuhl AA, Hohne W, Zeitz M. Animal models of inflammatory bowel disease: an overview. Pathobiology. 2003;70:121–30.

25. Kirsner JB. Experimental 'colitis' with particular reference to hypersensitivity reactions in the colon. Gastroenterology. 1961;40:307–12.

26. Mee AS, McLaughlin JE, Hodgson HJ, Jewell DP. Chronic immune colitis in rabbits. Gut. 1979;20:1–5.

27. MacPherson BR, Pfeiffer CJ. Experimental production of diffuse colitis in rats. Digestion. 1978;17:135–50.

28. Yamada T, Sartor RB, Marshall S, Specian RD, Grisham MB. Mucosal injury and inflammation in a model of chronic granulomatous colitis in rats. Gastroenterology. 1993;104:759–71.

29. Onderdonk AB. The carrageenan model for experimental ulcerative colitis. Prog Clin Biol Res. 1985;186:237–45.

30. Breeling JL, Onderdonk AB, Cisneros RL, Kasper DL. *Bacteroides vulgatus* outer membrane antigens associated with carrageenan-induced colitis in guinea pigs. Infect Immun. 1988;56:1754–9.

31. Sartor RB, Cromartie WJ, Powell DW, Schwab JH. Granulomatous enterocolitis induced in rats by purified bacterial cell wall fragments. Gastroenterology. 1985;89:587–95.

32. Okayasu I, Hatakeyama S, Yamada M, Ohkusa T, Inagaki Y, Nakaya R. A novel method in the induction of reliable experimental acute and chronic ulcerative colitis in mice. Gastroenterology. 1990;98:694–702.

33. Dieleman LA, Ridwan BU, Tennyson GS, Beagley KW, Bucy RP, Elson CO. Dextran sulfate sodium-induced colitis occurs in severe combined immunodeficient mice. Gastroenterology. 1994;107:1643–52.

34. Dieleman LA, Palmen MJ, Akol H et al. Chronic experimental colitis induced by dextran sulphate sodium (DSS) is characterized by Th1 and Th2 cytokines. Clin Exp Immunol. 1998;114:385–91.

35. Mahler M, Bristol IJ, Leiter EH et al. Differential susceptibility of inbred mouse strains to dextran sulphate sodium-induced colitis. Am J Physiol. 1998;274:G544–51.

36. Hartmann G, Bidlingmaier C, Siegmund B et al. Specific type IV phosphodiesterase inhibitor rolipram mitigates experimental colitis in mice. Pharmacol Exp Ther. 2000;292:22–30.

37. Soriano A, Salas A, Salas A et al. VCAM-1, but not ICAM-1 or MAdCAM-1, immunoblockade ameliorates DSS-induced colitis in mice. Lab Invest. 2000;80:1541–51.

38. Kato S, Hokari R, Matsuzaki K et al. Amelioration of murine experimental colitis by inhibition of mucosal addressin cell adhesion molecule-1. Pharmacol Exp Ther. 2000;295:183–9.

39. Okayasu I, Ohkusa T, Kajiura K, Kanno J, Sakamoto S. Promotion of colorectal neoplasia in experimental murine ulcerative colitis. Gut. 1996;39:87–92.

40. Neurath MF, Fuss I, Kelsall BL, Stuber E, Strober W. Antibodies to interleukin 12 abrogate established experimental colitis in mice. J Exp Med. 1995;182:1281–90.

41. Fuss IJ, Marth T, Neurath MF, Pearlstein GR, Jain A, Strober W. Anti-interleukin 12 treatment regulates apoptosis of Th1 T cells in experimental colitis in mice. Gastroenterology. 1999;117:1078–88.

42. Stuber E, Strober W, Neurath M. Blocking the CD40L-CD40 interaction *in vivo* specifically prevents the priming of T helper 1 cells through the inhibition of interleukin 12 secretion. J Exp Med. 1996;183:693–8.

43. Neurath MF, Fuss I, Kelsall BL, Presky DH, Waegell W, Strober W. Experimental granulomatous colitis in mice is abrogated by induction of TGF-beta-mediated oral tolerance. J Exp Med. 1996;183:2605–16.

44. Fuss IJ, Boirivant M, Lacy B, Strober W. The interrelated roles of TGF-beta and IL-10 in the regulation of experimental colitis. Immunology. 2002;168:900–8.

45. Kitani A, Fuss IJ, Nakamura K, Schwartz OM, Usui T, Strober W. Treatment of experimental (trinitrobenzene sulfonic acid) colitis by intranasal administration of transforming growth factor (TGF)-beta1 plasmid: TGF-beta1-mediated suppression of T helper cell type 1 response occurs by interleukin (IL)-10 induction and IL-12 receptor beta2 chain downregulation. Exp Med. 2000;192:41–52.

46. Boirivant M, Fuss IJ, Chu A, Strober W. Oxazolone colitis: a murine model of T helper cell type 2 colitis treatable with antibodies to interleukin 4. J Exp Med. 1998;188:1929–39.

47. Steinhoff U, Brinkmann V, Klemm U et al. Autoimmune intestinal pathology induced by hsp60-specific CD8 T cells. Immunity. 1999;11:349–58.

48. Hollander GA, Simpson SJ, Mizoguchi E et al. Severe colitis in mice with aberrant thymic selection. Immunity. 1995;3:27–38.

49. Leach MW, Bean AG, Mauze S, Coffman RL, Powrie F. Inflammatory bowel disease in C. B-17 scid mice reconstituted with the CD45Rbhigh subset of CD4+ T cells. Am J Pathol. 1996;148:1503–15.

50. Powrie F, Leach MW, Mauze S, Menon S, Caddle LB, Coffman RL. Inhibition of Th1 responses prevents inflammatory bowel disease in scid mice reconstituted with CD45 Rbhi CD4+ T cells. Immunity. 1994;1:553–62.

51. Aranda R, Sydora BC, McAllister PL et al. Analysis of intestinal lymphocytes in mouse colitis mediated by transfer of CD4+, CD45RBhigh T cells to SCID recipients. Immunology. 1997;158:3464–73.

52. Powrie F, Carlino J, Leach MW, Mauze S, Coffman RL. A critical role for transforming growth factor-beta but not interleukin 4 in the suppression of T helper type 1-mediated colitis by CD45RB(low) CD4+ T cells. J Exp Med. 1996;183:2669–74.

53. Read S, Malmstrom V, Powrie F. Cytotoxic T lymphocyte-associated antigen 4 plays an essential role in the function of CD25(+)CD4(+) regulatory cells that control intestinal inflammation. Exp Med. 2000;192:295–302.

54. Nakamura K, Kitani A, Strober W. Cell contact-dependent immunosuppression by CD4 (+)CD25(+) regulatory T cells is mediated by cell surface-bound transforming growth factor beta. J Exp Med. 2001;194:629–44.

55. Hagenbaugh A, Sharma S, Dubinett SM et al. Altered immune responses in interleukin 10 transgenic mice. Exp Med. 1997;16:2101–10.

56. Asseman C, Mauze S, Leach MW, Coffman RL, Powrie FJ. An essential role for interleukin 10 in the function of regulatory T cells that inhibit intestinal inflammation. Exp Med. 1999; 190:995–1004.

57. Groux H, O'Garra A, Bigler M et al. A CD4+ T-cell subset inhibits antigen-specific T-cell responses and prevents colitis. Nature. 1997;389:737–42.

58. Kjellev S, Lundsgaard D, Poulsen SS, Markholst H. Reconstitution of Scid mice with CD4 +CD25- T cells leads to rapid colitis: an improved model for pharmacologic testing. Int Immunopharmacol. 2006;6:1341–54.

59. Aranda R, Sydora BC, McAllister PL et al. Analysis of intestinal lymphocytes in mouse colitis mediated by transfer of CD4+, CD45RBhigh T cells to SCID recipients. J Immunol. 1997;158:3464–73.

60. Singh B, Powrie F, Mortensen NJ. Immune therapy in inflammatory bowel disease and models of colitis. Br J Surg. 2001;88:1558–69.

61. Hammer RE, Maika SD, Richardson JA, Tang JP, Taurog JD. Spontaneous inflammatory disease in transgenic rats expressing HLA-B27 and human beta 2m: an animal model of HLA-B27-associated human disorders. Cell. 1990;63:1099–112.

62. Rath HC, Ikeda JS, Linde HJ, Scholmerich J, Wilson KH, Sartor RB. Varying cecal bacterial loads influences colitis and gastritis in HLA-B27 transgenic rats. Gastroenterology. 1999;116:310–19.

63. Watanabe M, Watanabe N, Iwao Y et al. The serum factor from patients with ulcerative colitis that induces T cell proliferation in the mouse thymus is interleukin-7. J Clin Immunol. 1997;17:282–92.

64. Hermiston ML, Gordon JI. Inflammatory bowel disease and adenomas in mice expressing a dominant negative N-cadherin. Science. 1995;270:1203–7.

65. Gorelik L, Flavell RA. Abrogation of TGFbeta signaling in T cells leads to spontaneous T cell differentiation and autoimmune disease. Immunity. 2000;12:171–81.

66. Hahm KB, Im YH, Parks TW et al. Loss of transforming growth factor beta signalling in the intestine contributes to tissue injury in inflammatory bowel disease. Gut. 2001;49:164–5.

67. Wirtz S, Finotto S, Kanzler S et al. Cutting edge: chronic intestinal inflammation in STAT-4 transgenic mice: characterization of disease and adoptive transfer by TNF- plus IFN-gamma-producing CD4+ T cells that respond to bacterial antigens. J Immunol. 1999;162:1884–8.

68. Sadlack B, Merz H, Schorle H, Schimpl A, Feller AC, Horak I. Ulcerative colitis-like disease in mice with a disrupted interleukin-2 gene. Cell. 1993;75:253–61.

69. Ludviksson BR, Ehrhardt RO, Strober W.J. TGF-beta production regulates the development of the 2,4,6-trinitrophenol-conjugated keyhole limpet hemocyanin-induced colonic inflammation in IL-2-deficient mice. Immunology. 1997;159:3622–8.

70. Kuhn R, Lohler J, Rennick D, Rajewsky K, Muller W. Interleukin-10-deficient mice develop chronic enterocolitis. Cell. 1993;75:263–74.

71. Sellon RK, Tonkonogy S, Schultz M et al. Resident enteric bacteria are necessary for development of spontaneous colitis and immune system activation in interleukin-10-deficient mice. Infect Immun. 1998;66:5224–31.

72. Madsen KL, Malfair D, Gray D, Doyle JS, Jewell LD, Fedorak RN. Interleukin-10 gene-deficient mice develop a primary intestinal permeability defect in response to enteric microflora. Inflamm Bowel Dis. 1999;5:262–70.

73. Spencer SD, Di Marco F, Hooley J et al. The orphan receptor CRF2-4 is an essential subunit of the interleukin 10 receptor. Exp Med. 1998;187:571–8.

74. Takeda K, Clausen BE, Kaisho T et al. Enhanced Th1 activity and development of chronic enterocolitis in mice devoid of Stat3 in macrophages and neutrophils. Immunity. 1999;10:39–49.

75. Mizoguchi A, Mizoguchi E, Bhan AK. The critical role of interleukin 4 but not interferon gamma in the pathogenesis of colitis in T-cell receptor alpha mutant mice. Gastroenterology. 1999;116:320–6.

76. Mizoguchi A, Mizoguchi E, Smith RN, Preffer FI, Bhan AK. Suppressive role of B cells in chronic colitis of T cell receptor alpha mutant mice. J Exp Med. 1997;186:1749–56.

77. Tomczak MF, Erdman SE, Poutahidis T et al. NF-kappa B is required within the innate immune system to inhibit microflora-induced colitis and expression of IL-12 p40. Immunology. 2003;171:1484–92.

78. Kontoyiannis D, Pasparakis M, Pizarro TT, Cominelli F, Kollias G. Impaired on/off regulation of TNF biosynthesis in mice lacking TNF AU-rich elements: implications for joint and gut-associated immunopathologies. Immunity. 1999;10:387–98.

79. Mahler M, Bristol IJ, Sundberg JP et al. Genetic analysis of susceptibility to dextran sulfate sodium-induced colitis in mice. Genomics. 1999;55:147–56.

80. Hugot JP, Chamaillard M, Zouali H et al. Association of NOD2 leucine-rich repeat variants with susceptibility to Crohn's disease. Nature. 2001;411:599–603.

81. Sugawara K, Olson TS, Moskaluk CA et al. Linkage to peroxisome proliferator-activated receptor-gamma in SAMP1/YitFc mice and in human Crohn's disease. Gastroenterology. 2005;128:351–60.

82. Kullberg MC, Ward JM, Gorelick PL et al. *Helicobacter hepaticus* triggers colitis in specific-pathogen-free interleukin-10 (IL-10)-deficient mice through an IL-12- and gamma interferon-dependent mechanism. Infect Immun. 1998;66:5157–66.

83. Madsen KL, Doyle JS, Jewell LD, Tavernini MM, Fedorak RN. *Lactobacillus* species prevents colitis in interleukin 10 gene-deficient mice. Gastroenterology. 1999;116:1107–14.

84. Sartor RB. Postoperative reccurence of Crohn's disease: the enemy is within the fecal stream. Gastroenterology. 1998;114:398–400.
85. D'Haens GR, Geboes K, Peeters M, Baert F, Penninckx F, Rutgeerts P. Early lesions of recurrent Crohn's disease caused by the infusion of intestinal contents in excluded colon. Gastroenterology. 1998;104:262–8.
86. Mashimo H, Wu DC, Podolsky DK, Fishman MC. Impaired defense of intestinal mucosa in mice lacking intestinal trefoil factor. Science. 1996;274:262–5.
87. Katz KD, Hollander D, Vadheim CM et al. Intestinal permeability in patients with Crohn's disease and their healthy relatives. Gastroenterology. 1989;97:927–31.
88. Schmitz H, Barmeyer C, Fromm M et al. Altered tight junction structure contributes to the impaired epithelial barrier function in ulcerative colitis. Gastroenterology. 1999;116:301–9.
89. Fuss IJ, Neurath M, Boirivant M et al. Disparate CD4+ lamina propria (LP) lymphokine secretion profiles in inflammatory bowel disease. Crohn's disease LP cells manifest increased secretion of IFN-gamma, whereas ulcerative colitis LP cells manifest increased secretion of IL-5. Immunology. 1996;157:1261–70.
90. Powrie F, Leach MW, Mauze S, Menon S, Caddle LB, Coffman RL. Inhibition of Th1 responses prevents inflammatory bowel disease in scid mice reconstituted with CD45RBhi CD4+ T cells. Immunity. 1994;1:553–62.
91. Murthy S, Cooper HS, Yoshitake H, Meyer C, Meyer CJ, Murthy NS. Combination therapy of pentoxifylline and TNFalpha monoclonal antibody in dextran sulphate-induced mouse colitis. Aliment Pharmacol Ther. 1999;13:251–60.
92. Targan SR, Hanauer SB, van Deventer SJ et al. A short-term study of chimeric monoclonal antibody cA2 to tumor necrosis factor alpha for Crohn's disease. Crohn's Disease cA2 Study Group. N Engl J Med. 1997;337:1029–35.
93. Rutgeerts P, D'Haens G, Targan S et al. Efficacy and safety of retreatment with anti-tumor necrosis factor antibody (infliximab) to maintain remission in Crohn's disease. Gastroenterology. 1999;117:761–9.
94. Rutgeerts P, Sandborn WJ, Feagan BG et al. Infliximab for induction and maintenance therapy for ulcerative colitis. N Engl J Med. 2005;353:2462–76.
95. Van den Brande JM, Braat H, van den Brink GR et al. Infliximab but not etanercept induces apoptosis in lamina propria T-lymphocytes from patients with Crohn's disease. Gastroenterology. 2003;124:1774–85.
96. Mannon PJ, Fuss IJ, Mayer L et al., anti-IL-12 Crohn's Disease Study Group. Anti-Interleukin-12 antibody for active Crohn's disease. N Engl J Med. 2005;351:2069–79.
97. Atreya R, Mudter J, Finotto S et al. Blockade of interleukin 6 trans signaling suppresses T-cell resistance against apoptosis in chronic intestinal inflammation: evidence in Crohn disease and experimental colitis in vivo. Nat Med. 2000;6:583–8.
98. Ito H, Takazoe M, Fukuda Y et al. A pilot randomized trial of a human anti-interleukin-6 receptor monoclonal antibody in active Crohn's disease. Gastroenterology. 2004;126:989–96.

7
Epidemiology of inflammatory bowel disease in Russia

E. A. BELOUSOVA ON BEHALF OF RUSSIAN IBD STUDY GROUP

INTRODUCTION

Epidemiological investigations of the inflammatory bowel diseases (IBD) have a long history. In most European countries, USA, Canada, and other countries they have been carried out for the past few decades. Such studies in Europe have been performed since the mid-1940s. This allowed us to follow up the dynamics of incidence of ulcerative colitis (UC) and Crohn's disease (CD), to reveal the trend of their spread and to estimate the possible association between development of the disease and factors predisposing to it.

PREVALENCE AND INCIDENCE OF IBD IN THE WORLD

The pevalence of UC in different countries fluctuates within 21–268 cases per 100 000 population and of CD from 9 to 199 cases per 100 000. The incidence of UC was shown to be 5–15 patients and that of CD 5–10 patients per 100 000 population per year[1-3].

Systematic studies in various countries disclosed common world trends of IBD epidemiology such as geographical, demographic, socioeconomic, and temporal.

Geographic trends

The existence of a north–south gradient of IBD prevalence and of incidence with higher rates in northern Europe and North America was confirmed in studies from the USA[4,5], Manitoba in Canada[6], Europe[7-13] and in the European Cooperative Study of Inflammatory Bowel Disease including 20 European centres[14] (Table 1). An interesting point of view was presented by A. Ekbom; in his opinion, in the near future, the north–south gradient will be evened out and turned in a west–east direction: to Eastern Europe, the former Soviet Union, the Far East, and Asia[15]. Low means of CD prevalence and incidence were found in Japan[16].

Table 1 Prevalence and incidence of IBD in various countries (per 100 000 population)

Country	Ulcerative colitis		Crohn's disease	
	Prevalence	Incidence	Prevalence	Incidence
Sweden, Orebro[8,9]	234	11.1	146	6.7
Denmark, Copenhagen[2,10,14]	161	9.8	54	7.3
Norway, Oslo[14]		15.6		7.9
England, North Tees[11]	268	22.2	156	7.4
USA, Minnesota[4,5]	229	8.3	133	6.9
Canada, Manitoba[6]	170	14.3	199	14.6
Italy, Palermo[14]		11.0		6.6
Italy, Florence[14]		8.7		3.3
North Portugal, Braga[12]		4.3		2.8
Portugal, Almada[14]		2.6		1.6
Spain, Galicia, Vigo[13]		5.8		4.4
Spain[14]		9.8		5.2
Japan[16]			5.9	0.5

Demographic trends

Demographic trends concern the age of disease onset and frequency of UC and CD in male and female patients. According to the majority of epidemiological studies the predominant peak of UC and CD incidence occurs in the age group 20–40 years. In some countries a second peak of UC incidence was found after 60 years[1,3].

The frequency of UC was found to be equal in patients of both sexes, but CD incidence in females was higher than in males, and formed a female/male ratio of 1.3[4–7,9].

Socioeconomic trends

UC and CD were found to be more common in highly developed industrial counties than in predominantly agricultural or less developed countries[3]. The incidence of UC and CD is higher in urban as compared with rural inhabitants[4,7,17].

Temporal trends

Different trends in the incidence of CD and UC have been observed over the past 40 years; the incidence dramatically increased in some countries (Denmark, Canada) or reached a plateau in others[5–8,10].

AIM OF THIS INVESTIGATION

Our aim was to study the epidemiology of IBD in Russia, to compare the data obtained with the same epidemiological parameters from other countries, and to assess the correspondence between the epidemiological situation in Russia and world trends.

METHODS

IBD in Russia is an extremely serious problem, as in the rest of the world. Owing to the importance of the problem, a Russian IBD Study Group was established in 2002 under the aegis of the Russian Association of Coloproctology. This group included gastroenterologists, coloproctologists, and practical physicians who were interested in IBD from all over the country. One of the global objectives of this group was to assess the epidemiological situation in various regions of Russia. Investigators from regional IBD study groups carried out epidemiological studies. Investigators from the Moscow region group conducted and coordinated this study, due to their experience in this field.

Five main regions of Russia were included in the study: Moscow region (Moscow excluded), Krasnoyarsky region (chief city Krasnoyarsk), city of Novosibirsk, Nizhni Novgorod region (chief city Nizhni Novgorod), Rostov region (chief city Rostov-on-Don) (Figure 1, Table 2).

The following parameters were studied:

1. Prevalence – the number of IBD cases per 100 000 population in a particular territory at the given moment.

2. Incidence – the number of new IBD cases per 100 000 population in a particular territory per year.

3. Mortality – the number of lethal IBD cases per 100 000 population per year.

4. Female/male ratio in UC and CD.

5. Urban/rural ratio in both diseases.

6. Age of disease onset.

7. Frequency of complications and surgery

CHARACTERISTICS OF THE STUDY AND SOURCES OF INFORMATION

This was a population-based study with enrollment of all UC and CD patients revealed in all medical organizations (hospitals and outpatient clinics) in every examined region. At the beginning of the study all physicians and all hospital staff of the regions were informed about the goal of the study. The information was received through medical documentation, medical statistical reports from Health Care Committees, and by examination of new patients by investigators. The study was retrospective and/or prospective concerning different periods of time. The common protocol elaborated by investigators of the Moscow Regional Research Clinical Institute was used to unify the study. The diagnosis of UC was confirmed by endoscopy and histology, the diagnosis of CD was made by endoscopy and/or X-rays, and sometimes by histology. The study was performed among an adult population (age more than 18 years).

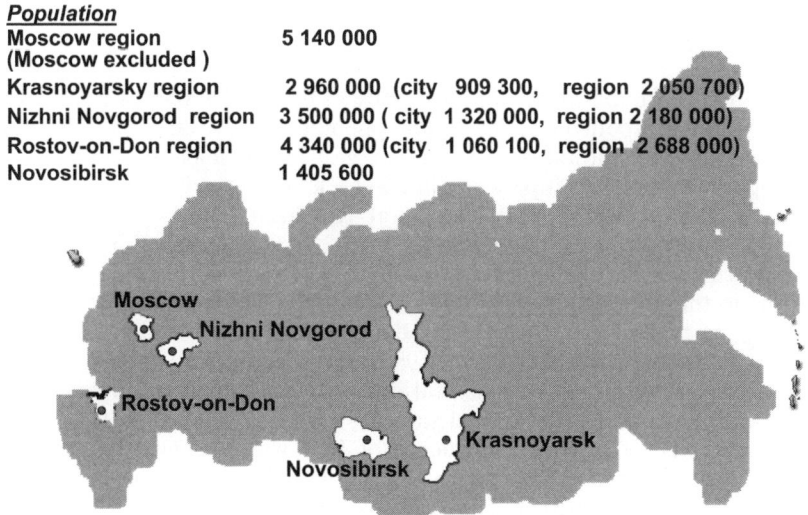

Population
Moscow region (Moscow excluded)	**5 140 000**
Krasnoyarsky region	**2 960 000 (city 909 300, region 2 050 700)**
Nizhni Novgorod region	**3 500 000 (city 1 320 000, region 2 180 000)**
Rostov-on-Don region	**4 340 000 (city 1 060 100, region 2 688 000)**
Novosibirsk	**1 405 600**

Figure 1   Russian regions examined in the epidemiological study

Table 2   Epidemiological study of IBD in Russia

Region	Geographical location	Period of study	Population	Number of IBD patients
Moscow region (Moscow excluded)	Centre of eastern part of Russia	1981–2005	5 140 000	UC 1453 CD 416
Krasnoyarsky region	Eastern Siberia	2000–2005	2 960 000	UC 292 CD 69
City of Novosibirsk	Eastern Siberia	2003–2005	1 405 600	UC 308 CD 131
Nizhni Novgorod region	Centre of eastern part of Russia	2005	3 500 000	UC 410 CD 121
Rostov-on-Don region	South	2004–2005	4 340 000	UC 578 CD 145
Total				UC 3041 CD 932

CHARACTERISTIC OF REGIONS

The Moscow region

This is an area around Moscow in the centre of the eastern part of Russia with a population of about 6 915 000 (adult population 5 140 000). It is both an industrial and agricultural region, consisting of 75 municipalities with central municipal hospital and outpatient clinic in each. The principal medical centre of the region is the Moscow Regional Research Clinical Institute. As mentioned previously, all physicians from the medical regional organizations were informed of the goal of the study, which resulted in admittance of all IBD patients to the principal medical centre where they were primarily diagnosed, regularly or periodically treated or followed up. In the Moscow region the study was both retrospective (1981–1993) and prospective (1994–2005). The retrospective study dealt with medical documentation from all inpatient and outpatient clinics and with medical statistics from the Moscow region. In the prospective study the current incidence of IBD was evaluated and all IBD patients from municipal hospitals and principal centre were taken into consideration. We created a database involving the period 1981–2005 and including 1869 IBD patients (1453 UC and 416 CD)[18,19].

The Krasnoyarsky region

This is the largest territory of eastern Siberia, extending for about 2200 km from south to north, straight to the Arctic Ocean, and covering three geographical zones: mountains, taiga, and tundra. The southern, industrial part, of the region is the most inhabited. The total population is about 2 960 000 (adult population 2 368 000). The main city of the region is Krasnoyarsk with 909 340 inhabitants.

The study in the Krasnoyarsky region was both retrospective, including the period 2000–2003, and prospective, 2004–2005. All IBD patients from all areas of the region were treated and followed up in three largest hospitals of Krasnoyarsk, and the medical documentation was analysed. The database included 292 UC and 69 CD patients[20].

The Novosibirsky region

The Novosibirsky region (main city Novosibirsk) is in eastern Siberia, approximately 800 km from the Krasnoyarsky region to the east. The prospective epidemiological study during 2003–2005 was carried out only in Novosibirsk (1 405 600 population); the surrounding territories were excluded. Only IBD patients who live in Novosibirsk and who are treated in city hospitals were enrolled in the study. Over a period of three years 308 UC patients and 131 CD patients were found.

The Nizhni Novgorod region

This is in the centre of the eastern part of Russia. Machine-building and other industries as well as agriculture are practised. The main city of the region is Nizhni Novgorod, a commercial port and one of the largest industrial cities in central Russia. The total population of the region is 3 500 000 (adult population about 2 800 000). The population of Nizhni Novgorod is 1 320 000 (adult population about 1 056 000). The retrospective–prospective study was carried out in 2005. IBD patients from Nizhni Novgorod were treated in city hospitals and university clinics, patients from the surrounding areas were treated, as usual, in the largest regional hospital. Using medical documentation, medical reports from the Health Care Committee, and results of examination of new patients, a database was created for 410 UC and 121 CD patients.

The Rostov-on-Don region

This region, with a population of 4 340 000, is the southern area where industry and agriculture are practised in approximately equal proportions. The main city of the region is Rostov-on-Don – the largest industrial city and commercial river port in the south of Russia. The adult population of Rostov-on-Don is 1 060 100. The study included retrospective and prospective steps within the period 2004–2005; 578 UC patients and 145 CD patients were enrolled in the database[21].

RESULTS

As a result of the studies it was established that the prevalence of UC in three of the five regions studied (Krasnoyarsky region, Nizhni Novgorod region, and Rostov region) were very much the same and fluctuated within an interval of 12.6–$14.6/10^5$ population. The prevalence in the chief industrial cities is 2.5–6.5-fold higher than in surrounding territories. The sole exception is the Moscow region, where UC prevalence is $28.3/10^5$ inhabitants, which is more than 2-fold higher than in other regions (Figure 2). Almost the same trend in the regions mentioned is noted for CD, but the prevalence of the latter is 3.5–4.2-fold higher than that of UC (Figure 3). In our opinion this fact can be explained by the proximity to Moscow and the influence of the megalopolis on the lifestyle of the regional population. Compared with the present data from the majority of countries the prevalence of UC and CD in Russia is 3–8-fold lower (Table 1), but similar to early epidemiological findings obtained in Italy[22], Spain[23], Portugal[24,25] and Norway[26], as well as to the prevalence and incidence in Japan[16] (Table 3).

The prevalence of UC and CD between females and males was studied in four of the five regions examined. UC prevalence was equal (female/male ratio = 1.0) in both Moscow and Krasnoyarsky regions. In the Rostov region UC prevalence among females was somewhat lower (f/m ratio = 0.8), but in Novosibirsk it was higher (f/m ratio = 1.4) (Figure 4). More clear-cut regularity was revealed in CD in all regions, with a higher prevalence among females (f/m ratio = 1.2–1.7) (Figure 4).

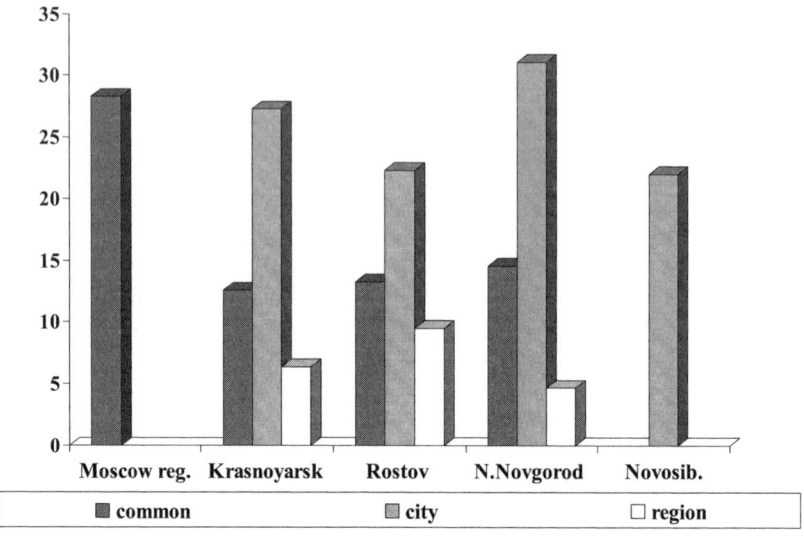

Figure 2   Prevalence of UC in different regions of Russia (per 100 000 population)

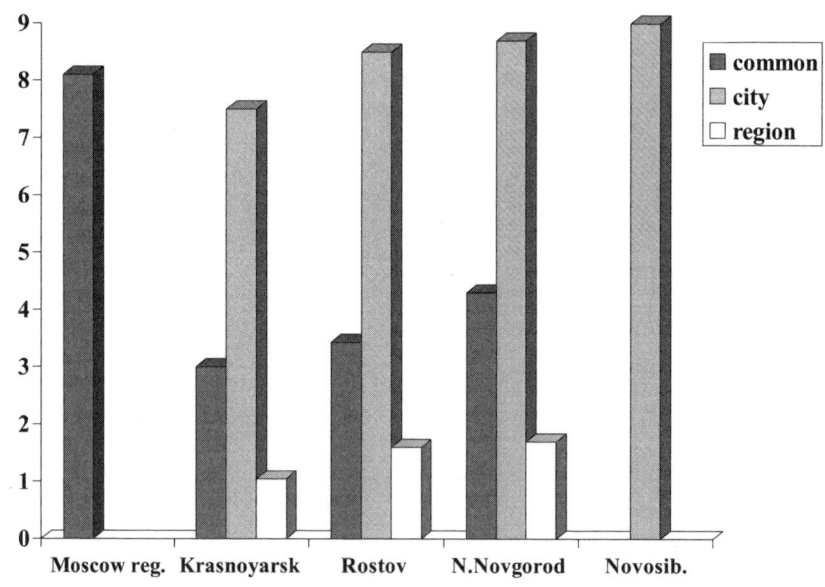

Figure 3   Prevalence of CD in different regions of Russia (per 100 000 population)

Table 3 Comparison between prevalence and incidence of IBD in Russia and in other countries (per 100 000 population)

Region	Years of study	UC Prevalence	UC Incidence	CD Prevalence	CD Incidence
Moscow region[18,19]	1981–1992		0.6–1.2		0.13–0.2
	1993–1997		0.8–0.95		0.15–0.3
	1997–2005	28.3	0.95–1.7	8.1	0.3–0.7
Krasnoyarsky region[20]	2001–2005	12.6	1.3	3.0	0.4
Novosibirsk	2003–2005	22.0		9.0	
Rostov-on-Don region[21]	2004–2005	14.6	1.1	4.3	0.2
Nizni Novgorod	2005	13.3		3.4	
Northern Portugal[24]	1979–1983		0.72		0.64
	1984–1988	13.6	1.58	9.9	0.98
Southern Portugal[25]	1991–1993		1.35		1.01–2.72
Spain, Galicia[23]	1976–1982				0.8
Italy, Bologna[22]	1972–1973	13.8	1.9		0.8
Norway[26]	1946–1955		0.7–1.4		
	1955–1960		1.1–2.7		
Norway[26]	1956–1963				0.1–0.4
	1964–1969				0.5–1.2
Japan[16]	1990			5.9	0.5

Age of the disease onset both in UC and CD corresponded to world trends. The maximum incidence peak in all regions was fixed at 20–29 and 30–39 years with a gradual decline in elderly groups (Figure 5).

IBD prevalence among urban and rural populations was investigated in three regions (Moscow region, Nizhni Novgorod region, and Rostov region) (Figures 6 and 7). The maximum difference between urban and rural populations was noted in the Rostov region, where UC prevalence was $19.5/10^5$ and $3.3/10^5$, correspondingly (urban/rural ratio = 6). In this region the difference in CD prevalence was twice lower (urban/rural ratio = 3.4). In the Nizhni Novgorod region an inverse regularity was noted: a large difference in CD prevalence between urban and rural populations (urban/rural ratio = 5.1) which was 2.5-fold higher than in UC (urban/rural ratio = 2). In the Moscow region both UC and CD prevalence among urban population slightly exceeded that among the rural population; the urban/rural ratio for both diseases was 1.1 (Figures 6 and 7). Despite these differences, the common trend in the regions examined conformed to that in other countries: the predominance of IBD among the urban population as compared to the rural one.

Comparing IBD prevalence in chief cities of the regions studied, it was shown that the prevalence did not differ significantly from each other. UC prevalence varied from $22/10^5$ to $31.1/10^5$, and CD prevalence from $7.5/10^5$ to $9.0/10^5$ inhabitants (Figure 8).

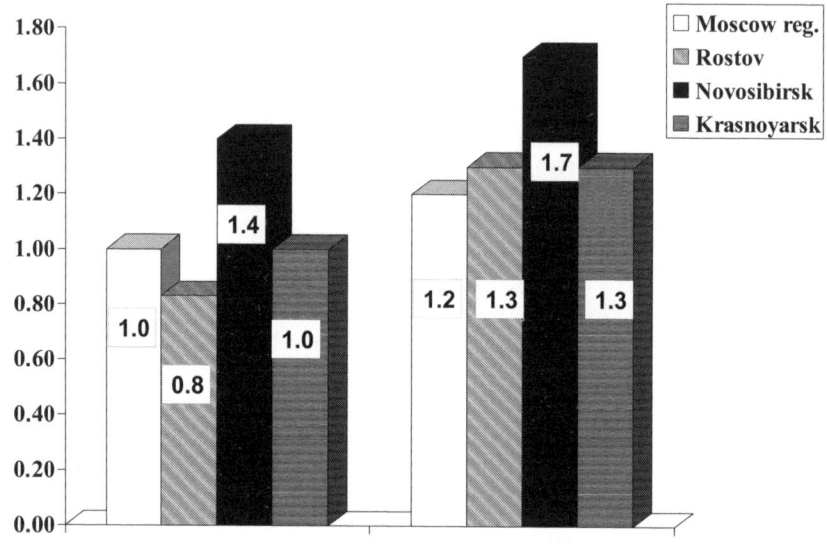

Figure 4 Female:male ratio in IBD in different regions of Russia

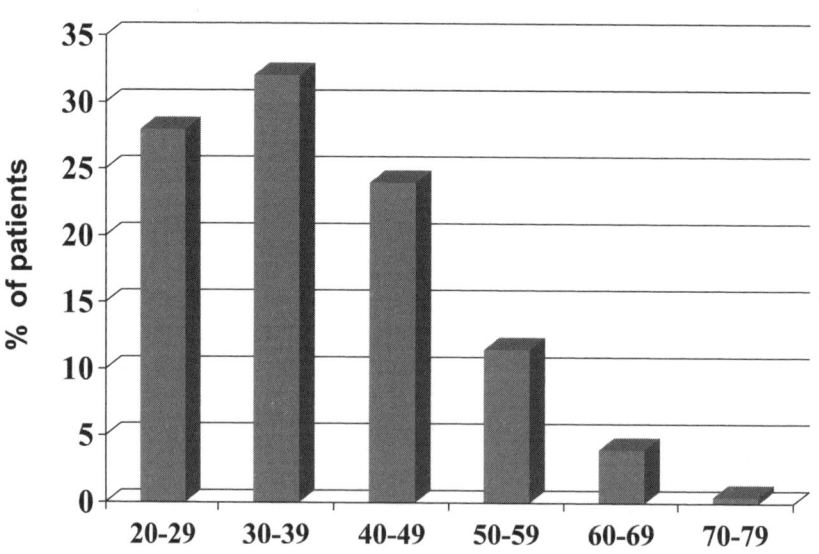

Figure 5 Distribution of UC and CD patients according to age of disease onset in all regions

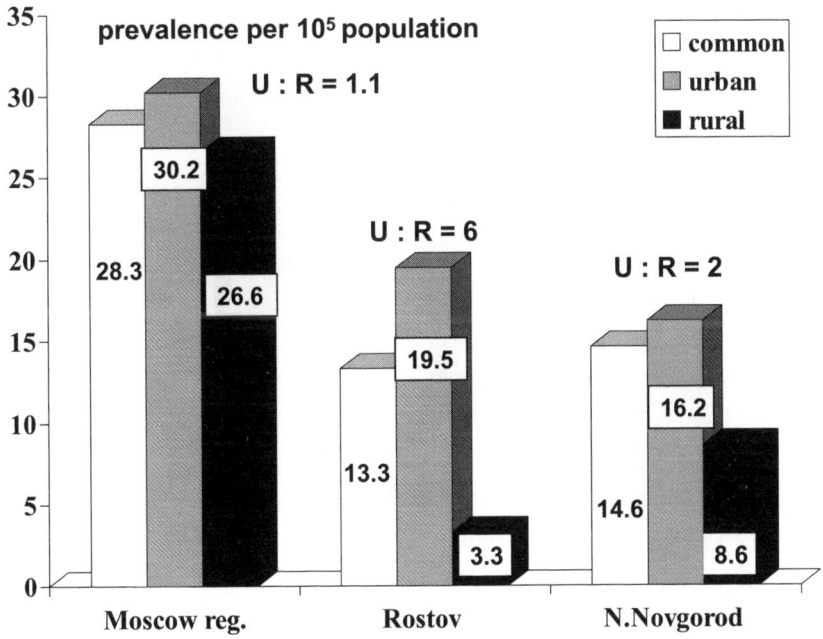

Figure 6 Prevalence of UC and urban:rural ratio in different regions

UC and CD incidence was studied in three regions. In the Moscow region epidemiological investigations were carried out from 1981 to 2005, the dynamics of incidence being studied over a period of 25 years. That investigation was both retrospective (1981–1993) and prospective (from 1994 to the present time). In the Krasnoyarsky region the incidence was studied retrospectively during 2001–2002 and prospectively during 2003–2005. In the Rostov region the study started only in 2004. The dynamics of UC and CD incidence in these regions during 5 years is shown in Figures 9 and 10. Incidence rates were low for both diseases. Minimum UC incidence in 2002 was found in the Krasnoyarsky region ($0.73/10^5$), in 2004 in the Rostov region ($0.74/10^5$), and maximum UC incidence in 2005 in the Moscow region ($1.7/10^5$). The lowest CD incidence was noted in 2004 in the Rostov region ($0.14/10^5$) and the highest in 2005 in the Moscow region ($0.7/10^5$). Figures 9 and 10 show a slow, gradual increase of IBD incidence. The most demonstrative are the data in the Moscow region for the 25-year period (Figure 11). UC incidence rate increased 2.8-fold, from $0.6/10^5$ in 1981–1984 to $1.7/10^5$ in 2005, and the CD incidence rate increased 5.4-fold (from 0.13 to $0.7/10^5$) for the same time period. CD incidence increased faster than UC incidences, and the UC/CD ratio decreased from 6 (1989–1996) to 2.4 (2005).

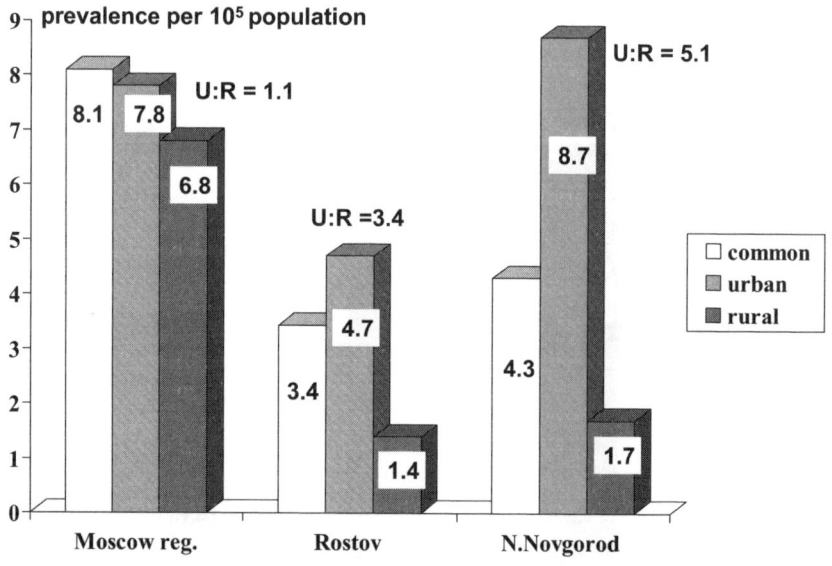

Figure 7 Prevalence of CD and urban:rural ratio in different regions

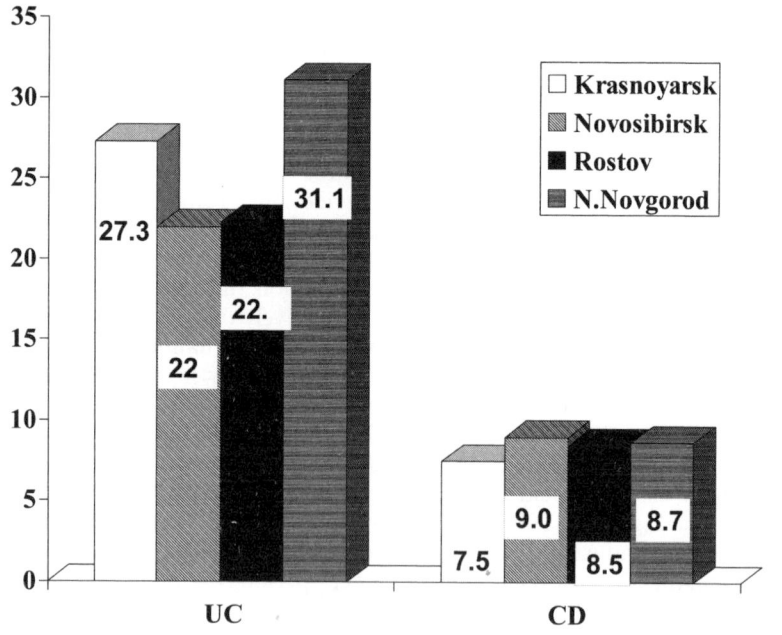

Figure 8 Prevalence of UC and CD in main cities of regions (per 10^5 population)

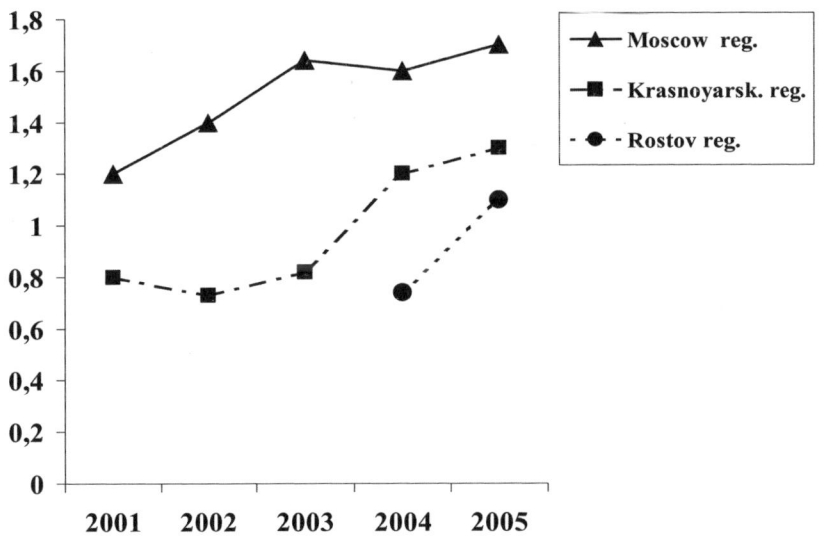

Figure 9 Incidence of UC in different regions of Russia in 2001–2005 (per 10^5 population)

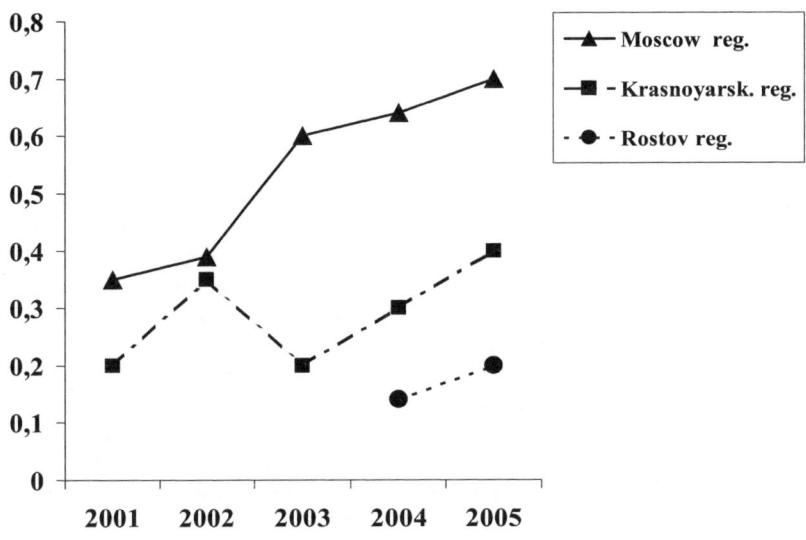

Figure 10 Incidence of CD in different regions of Russia in 2001–2005 (per 10^5 population)

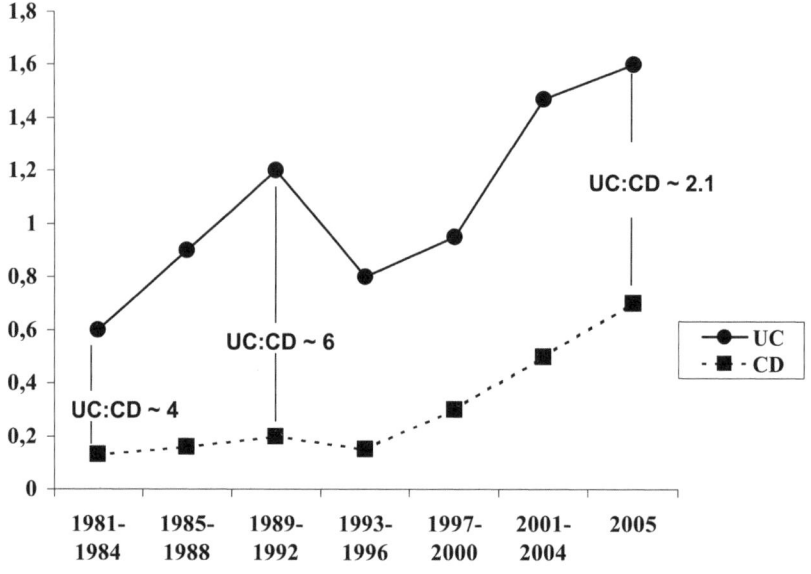

Figure 11 Dynamics of IBD incidence in Moscow region in 1981–2005 (per 10^5 population)

The frequency of complications in UC was equal in the three regions mentioned, and formed 20–22% (Figure 12). The most common UC complications were bleeding, toxic megacolon, colon perforation, and peripheral thromboses. A high frequency of colorectal cancer was noted – 3.5% (Figure 14). The frequency of complications in CD was significantly higher and differed among regions (Figure 13). The highest frequency of complications was found in Novosibirsk – 99.2%. Among complications the most frequent were stenoses, intestinal obstruction and fistulas (Figure 15).

The surgery rate in UC was 10.1–16.4% depending on the particular region (Figure 12), and that in CD was 31.1–48% (Figure 13). Mortality in both UC and CD varied from $0.1–0.4/10^5$ (Figures 12 and 13).

There was no difference in UC and CD prevalence and incidence depending on geographical location of the regions: neither north–south nor east–west. Both the Moscow and Nizhni Novgorod regions are located in the centre of the European part of Russia, latitude about 56° North, the Krasnoyarsky region and Novosibirsk in the east (eastern Siberia) – between the 55th and 56th parallels. Thus, four of the regions studied are at the same geographical latitude, but the prevalence in UC and CD in these regions is the same. It is of interest that Copenhagen is situated at the same latitude as Moscow, Nizhni Novgorod, Novosibirsk, and Krasnoyarsk, but IBD incidence in Copenhagen is one of the highest in the world. European countries with low UC and CD

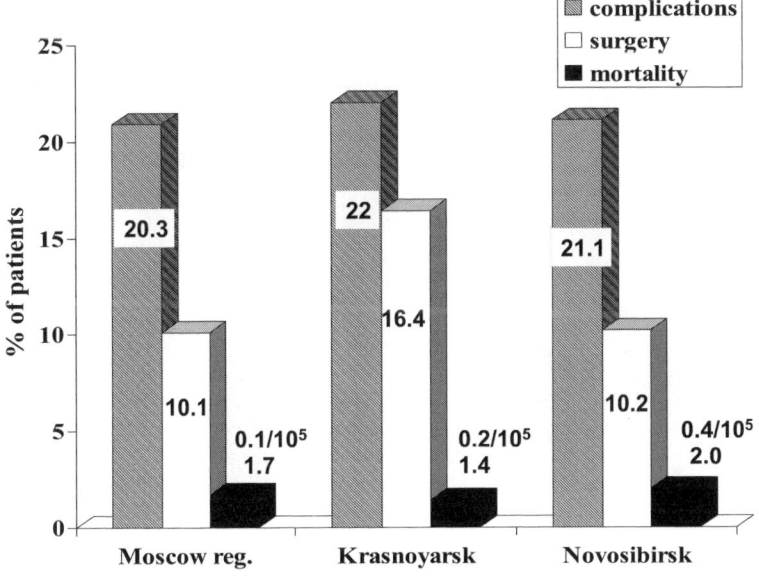

Figure 12 Complications, surgery and mortality* in UC in 2001–2005. *Mortality is indicated as a percentage of UC patients and per 10^5 population

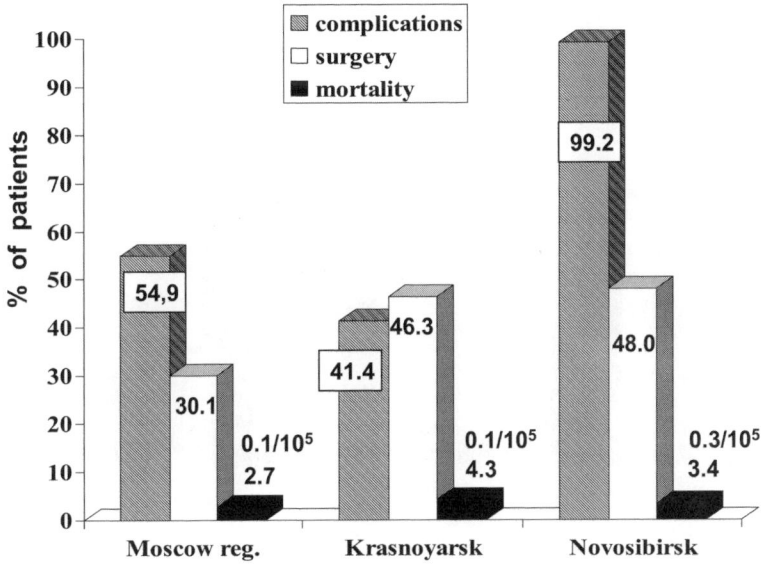

Figure 13 Complications, surgery and mortality* in CD in 2001–2005. *Mortality is indicated as a percentage of UC patients and per 10^5 population

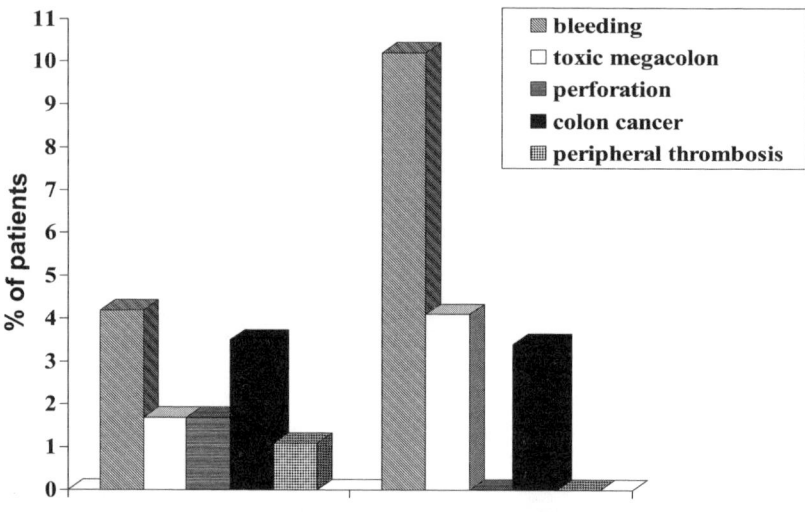

Figure 14   Frequency of complications in UC

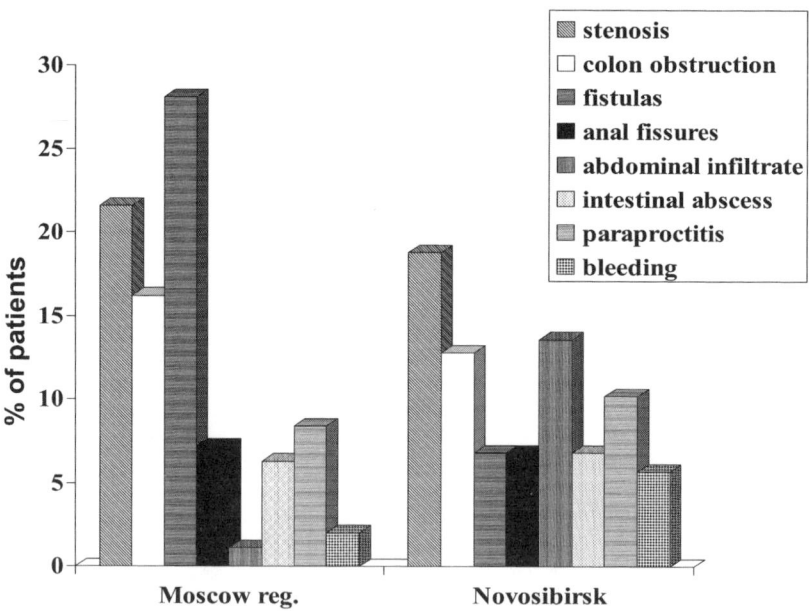

Figure 15   Frequency of complications in CD

incidence (Italy, Spain, and Portugal) are located southward of the most southern region examined in Russia – Rostov-on-Don. In spite of this fact the IBD incidence in these countries is higher than in the Rostov region.

CONCLUSION

- As shown above, the prevalence and incidences of UC and CD in all regions examined are approximately equal but 3–8-fold lower than those in Europe, the USA, and Canada.

- The prevalence and incidence of IBD in Russia corresponds more or less to early data from southern Europe (Spain, Portugal, Italy), Norway and from Japan.

- The prevalence of UC and CD is equal in different regions of Russia, except the Moscow region.

- The prevalence of IBD in urban inhabitants is 2–3-fold higher than in rural inhabitants in all regions excluding the Moscow region.

- In the Moscow region the prevalence of both diseases is 2-fold higher than in other regions, and the urban:rural prevalences do not differ from each other. This may reflect the influence of the Moscow megalopolis and urbanization of the population around Moscow.

- The female/male prevalence of UC does not differ significantly in all regions, but the female CD prevalence is significantly higher than the male one.

- UC and CD onset is around 20–40 years in all regions, as is the world trend.

- In the Moscow region the incidence of UC increased 3.5-fold and CD incidence 6.5-fold over a period of 25 years. The rise in incidence of CD was higher and the UC/CD ratio reduced from 6 to 2.

- The prevalence in the regions studied is very much the same despite differences in their geographical locations.

Acknowledgements

The author thanks the members of Russian IBD Study Group participants of this study:

Dr Inna Nikulina MD, PhD, senior researcher of the Moscow Regional Research Clinical Institute, for active participation and scientific assistance; Professor Anna Zlatkina, MD, Dr Med Sci, Moscow Regional Research Clinical Institute, the main gastroenterologist of the Moscow region, for initiation of this study and scientific support; Dr Irina Chechetkina, Krasnoyarsky State Medical Academy; Professor Nonna Nikolaeva MD, Dr Med Sci, the main gastroenterologist of Krasnoyarsky region, Krasnoyarsky State Medical Academy; Dr Vladislav Kosenko MD, Rostovsky State Medical

University; Professor Alexander Tkachev MD, Dr Med Sci, the main gastroenterologist of Rostovsky region, Rostovsky State Medical University; Professor Olga Alexeeva MD, Dr Med Sci, Director of the Volga Regional Gastroenterological Center; Professor Sergey Krishtopenko, MD, Dr Med Sci, Deputy director of the Volga Regional Gastroenterological Center; Dr Irina Svetlova, MD, PhD, associate professor, Novosibirsky State Medical University; Dr Ekaterina Valujskich, MD, Novosibirsky State Medical University; Professor Svetlana Kurilovitch, MD, Dr Med Sci, Novosibirsky State Medical University; Professor Marina Osipenko MD, Dr Med Sci, the main gastroenterologist of Novosibirsk, Novosibirsky State Medical University.

For support in the epidemiological study thanks to: Professor Gennady Vorobiev, Director of the Russian State Scientific Center of Coloproctology, President of the Russian Association of Coloproctology; Professor Gennady Onoprienko, Director of the Moscow Regional Research Clinical Institute; Professor Viacheslav Shumsky, Deputy Director of the Moscow Regional Research Clinical Institute; Professor Igor Khalif, Deputy Director of the Russian State Scientific Center of Coloproctology, Chair of the Russian IBD Study Group.

References

1. Irvine EJ, Farrokhyar F, Swarbrick ET. A critical review of epidemiological studies in inflammatory bowel disease. Scand J Gastroenterol. 2001;36:2–15.
2. Langholz E, Munkholm P, Nielsen OH et al. Incidence and prevalence of ulcerative colitis in Copenhagen county from 1962 to 1987. Scand J Gastroenterol. 1991;26:1247–56.
3. Marshall J, Hilsden R. Environment and epidemiology of inflammatory bowel disease. In: Satsangi J, Sutherland L, editors. Inflammatory Bowel Disease. Edinburgh: Churchill-Livingstone, 2003:17–28.
4. Loftus E. Crohn's disease in Olmsted County, Minnesota 1940–1993: incidence, prevalence, survival. Gastroenterology. 1998;114:1160–8.
5. Loftus E, Silverstein M, Sandborn W et al. Ulcerative colitis in Olmsted County, Minnesota, 1940–1993; incidence, prevalence, and survival. Gut. 2000;46:336–43.
6. Bernstein CN, Blanchard JF, Rawsthorne P, Wajda A. Epidemiology of Crohn's disease and ulcerative colitis in the central Canadian province: a population-based study. Am J Epidemiol. 1999;149:916–24.
7. Ekbom A, Helmick C, Zack M, Adami H-O. The epidemiology of inflammatory bowel disease: a large population-based study in Sweden. Gastroenterology. 1991;100:350–8.
8. Linberg E, Jarnerot G. The incidence of Crohn's disease is not decreasing in Sweden. Scand J Gastroenterol. 1991;26:495–500.
9. Tysk C, Jarnerot G. Ulcerative proctocolitis in Orebro, Sweden – a retrospective epidemiologic study, 1963–87. Scand J Gastroenterol. 1992;27:945–50.
10. Munkholm P, Langholz E, Nielsen JH et al. Incidence and prevalence of Crohn's disease in the county of Copenhagen, 1962–87: a sixfold increase in incidence. Scand J Gastroenterol. 1992;27:609–14.
11. Rubin G, Hungin A, Kelly P, Ling J. Epidemiological features of inflammatory bowel disease in North of England. Gastroenterology. 1999;110:A1004.
12. Taravela Veloso F. IBD in north Portugal. In: Monteiro E, Taravela F, editors. Inflammatory Bowel Disease. Dordrecht: Kluwer, 1994.
13. Ochoa V, Butron M, Cueto M, Pereira S. Epidemiology of IBD in Vigo health area, Spain In: Monteiro E, Taravela F, editors. Inflammatory Bowel Disease. Dordrecht: Kluwer, 1994.

14. Shivanada S, Lennard-Jones J, Logan R. Incidence of inflammatory bowel disease across Europe: is there a difference between north and south? Results of the European Collaborative Study of the Inflammatory Bowel Disease (EC-IBD). Gut. 1996;39:690–7.
15. Ekbom A. The changing face of Crohn's disease and ulcerative colitis. In: Targan S, Shanahan F, Karp L, editors. Inflammatory Bowel Diseases: From Bench to Bedside, 2nd edn. Dordrecht: Kluwer, 2003.
16. Yoshida Y, Murata Y. Inflammatory bowel disease in Japan: studies of epidemiology and etiopathogenesis. Med Clin N Am. 1990;74:67–89.
17. Blanchard JF, Bernstein CN, Wayda A, Rawsthorne P. Small-area variations and sociodemographic correlates for the incidence of Crohn's disease and ulcerative colitis. Am J Epidemiol. 2001;154:328–35.
18. Nikulina IV, Belousova EA, Zlatkina AR, Savov AM. Epidemiology of inflammatory bowel disease in Moscow region. In: Inflammatory Bowel Disease – Diagnostic and Therapeutic Strategies, Falk Symposium 154 (abstract 49).
19. Nikulina IV, Zlatkina AR, Belousova EA, Rumyancev VG. Assessment of clinico-epidemiology of inflammatory bowel disease in Moscow region. Russian J Gastroenterol Hepatol Coloproctol. 1997;2:67–71.
20. Nikolaeva NN, Chechetkina ID, Nikolaeva LV, Gigileva NL. The epidemiology of ulcerative colitis and Crohn's disease in Krasnoyarsky region. Russian J Gastroenterol Hepatol Coloproctol. 2004;5:496.
21. Kosenko VA, Tkachev AV, Dudareva LA. Epidemiology of ulcerative colitis in the Rostov area. In: Inflammatory Bowel Disease – Diagnostic and Therapeutic Strategies, Falk Symposium 154 (abstract 46).
22. Lanfranchi G, Michelini A, Bringola C. Uno studio epidemiologico sulle malattie inflamattorie intestinali nella provincia di Bolodna. G Clin Med. 1976;57:235–45.
23. Ruis V, Potel J. Crohn's disease in Galicia, Spain: 1968–1982. Front Gastrointestinal Res. 1986;11:94–101.
24. Taravela Veloso F, Carvalho J. Inflammatory bowel disease in north Portugal. In: Goebell H, Peskar BM, Malchow H, editors. Inflammatory Bowel Disease - -Basic Research and Clinical Implications. Lancaster:MTP Press, 1988:59.
25. Monteiro E, Freitas J, Soares C et al. Epidemiology of IBD in the south of Portugal: Almada, Seixal, Sesimbra. In Monteiro E, Taravela F, editors. Inflammatory Bowel Disease. Dordrecht: Kluwer, 1994.
26. Vatn M, Moum B, the IBSEN Study Group. IBD in Norway. In: Monteiro E, Taravela F, editors. Inflammatory Bowel Disease. Dordrecht: Kluwer, 1994.

Section II
Mechanisms of inflammatory bowel disease: 2nd session

Chair: GI VOROBIEV and RB SARTOR

8
State-of-the-Art Lecture:
Genetics and genomics: implications for clinical practice

A. S. PEÑA, M. L. LAINE, J. B. A. CRUSIUS, S. A. MORRÉ,
U. VAN DER VELDEN, F. LESSMANN, C. J. VAN DER PALEN,
A. J. VAN WINKELHOFF and B. G. LOOS

INTRODUCTION

Genetic predisposition contributes to the pathogenesis of most common diseases and several genes have been identified. Evidence for other susceptibility loci is also strong. Thus, the polygenic nature of inflammatory chronic diseases has been confirmed, but this does not follow Mendel's rules. The genes so far identified in Crohn's disease are involved in bacterial sensing such as CARD15[1-3]. Others are in the scaffolding of the intestinal epithelial cells, or in the transport of cations[1-3] or in the production of defensins[4]. These genes appear to be important for Caucasian patients only, and affect a subgroup of patients. This is difficult to understand and has delayed the implementation of genetic knowledge in clinical practice. Although substantial progress in the development of laboratory and analytical approaches to study non-Mendelian complex genetic disorders has been made, little is known of the interaction of several genes; first of genes which appear to function through complex networks and second the involvement of environmental factors and behavioural process that contribute to post-genomic regulatory events. These interactions are difficult to understand in spite of the accomplishments of the past few years.

The identification and characterization of the genetics and genomics of chronic inflammation are likely to contribute to understanding the basic aetiology of multifactorial diseases, such as inflammatory bowel diseases (IBD). This knowledge will improve risk assessment and influence therapeutics. Genetics identifies disease-related susceptibility genes while genomics identifies genes that belong to similar families based on their sequence homologies. The knowledge generated by genetics and genomics is now part of genomic science; this science is in the process of being integrated in

Table 1 Many common diseases are multifactorial and polygenic

– Multiple sclerosis	– Periodontitis
– Alzheimer's disease	– Rheumatoid arthritis
– Breast cancer	– Inflammatory bowel diseases
– Myocardial infarction	– Psoriasis
– Hypertension	– Primary sclerosing cholangitis
– Diabetes	
– Obesity	

the clinical setting. Through the use of genetics, clinical scientists will be able to profile variations between individuals' DNA to improve diagnostic skills, determine prognosis and predict responses to environmental and behavioural factors, as well as responses to particular drugs. This knowledge will contribute to a better understanding of common diseases which are multifactorial and polygenic (Table 1).

Transferring genomic science into a clinical setting is not easy. Technical and cultural challenges will have to be conquered to be able to use the new powerful genetic research tools. These tools are now available to classify the heterogeneity of disease and the individual responses to drugs. Also much of the generated genomic data of clinical relevance has been stored in a format that is inappropriate for use in routine diagnostic tests. The technology has not yet been established for rapid, inexpensive typing of most genomic biomarkers, with the exception of single-nucleotide polymorphisms (SNPs). For routine clinical practice, current methods need to be simplified to effectively use the available advanced technology networks.

The first chip-based diagnostic and chip-based risk assessment tools for prognosis are now available: the chip-based diagnostic tool for predicting cytochrome P450 enzymes responsible for the oxidative metabolism of many drugs is a useful indicator of therapy response. The chip-based risk assessment tool, e.g. the recently introduced IBDchip, permits assessment of prognosis in subgroups of patients suffering from Crohn's disease and ulcerative colitis[5]. These tools will be implemented if there is clear evidence for their clinical utility. This technology has to be supported by both physicians and health authorities. Specific training in this field will need to be provided to health-care professionals in order to effectively use these new tools. It is precisely at this interface that biomedical informatics is of ultimate relevance. As recently expressed by Martin-Sanchez et al., a characteristic of the 'post-genomic' era will be to correlate essential genotypic information with expressed phenotypic information[6].

Medical informatics as we have known the discipline in research and development of informatics-based methods has produced tools for medical and epidemiological research, patient care and health management. Bioinformatics has grown up with the human genome project. Bioinformatics handles genomics, proteomics and any other biological research data. These two disciplines have resulted in biomedical informatics (BMI), an emerging discipline that aims to make possible the necessary translation of multiple systems with different databases into a common database. BMI will play an important role in translating new insights in the pathophysiology of inflammatory processes and will help to develop new classification systems. It is also expected to provide information to design new treatment strategies[6–8].

To illustrate the state-of-the-art of the integration of genetics, genomics and BMI, in Amsterdam we are using as a model 'periodontitis', since this is also a common complex disease that requires the integration and analysis of multiple sources of data. Periodontitis offers a remarkable set of challenges to the new discipline BMI. The main challenge for BMI applied to complex diseases is the creation of a data warehouse (DW) for each disease to be studied. The INFOBIOMED consortium, a Network of Excellence of the European Union, has selected periodontitis as a pilot project (Figure 1). Periodontitis provides a good example of a chronic complex disease in which microbiological and genetic factors interact with environmental factors to determine disease susceptibility, severity of inflammation and evolution of the disease process.

PERIODONTITIS

Periodontitis is a chronic inflammatory disease of the supporting tissues of the teeth. These may show exposed root surfaces in swollen gums that easily bleed. The inflammatory process, a Th1 type of response, produces bone loss around the teeth which, after becoming loose, will eventually exfoliate. Patients with periodontitis experience problems with chewing due to tooth mobility and loss of teeth; they have bad breath and suffer from important subjective and objective aesthetic problems. Smoking is a risk factor strongly associated with periodontitis. In a study performed in Barcelona it was shown that smokers had 2.7 times, and former smokers 2.3 times, greater probabilities of having periodontitis than non-smokers. This was more evident after 10 years of smoking[9]. Diet and exercise are important in maintaining healthy gums[10–12] and stress enhances the risk of suffering from periodontitis (Figure 2)

The following oral bacterial species are recognized as periodontal pathogens: *Porphyromonas gingivalis*, *Prevotella intermedia*, *Tannerella forsythensis*, *Fusobacterium nucleatum*, *Actinobacillus actinomycetemcomitans* and the spirochaetal species *Treponema denticola*[13].

Genetic polymorphisms in a candidate gene approach have been explored as risk factors for periodontitis. There is limited evidence that some polymorphisms in the genes encoding interleukins (IL)-1, Fc gamma receptors (Fc gammaR), IL-10 and the vitamin D receptor, may be associated with periodontitis in certain ethnic groups, but the studies are underpowered[14].

These observations suggest that periodontitis may serve as a model for complex chronic inflammatory diseases, such as Crohn's disease and ulcerative colitis. A periodontitis data warehouse (PDW) has been structured with the INFOBIOMED network and allows an integrative research approach, in which the new field of BMI will contribute to new insights in chronic inflammatory and infectious diseases (Figure 3).

The development of DW tools that will become available for clinicians and researchers opens the path to new technical advances in data mining and visualization. The BMI approach will in the future assist IBD clinical scientists and clinicians in research.

	Participant name	Country
Fundació IMIM	Fundació IMIM *IMIM Foundation*	Spain
Institut Municipal d'Investigació Mèdica. IMIM	Institut Municipal d'Investigació Mèdica *Municipal Institute of Medical Research*	Spain
Instituto de Salud Carlos III	Instituto de Salud Carlos III *Carlos III Health Institute*	Spain
University of Leicester	University of Leicester	U.K.
University of Edinburgh	University of Edinburgh	U.K.
CUSTODIX	Custodix N.V.	Belgium
Universidad Politécnica de Madrid	Universidad Politécnica de Madrid *Polytechnic University of Madrid*	Spain
	Ἴδρυμα Τεχνολογίας και Ἐρευνας *Foundation for Research and Technology - Hellas*	Greece
ieeta	Universidade de Aveiro *University of Aveiro*	Portugal
	Center for Sundhedstelematik *Danish Centre for Health Telematics*	Denmark
INFORMA	Informa srl	Italy
HEINRICH HEINE UNIVERSITÄT DÜSSELDORF	Heinrich-Heine-Universität Düsseldorf *Heinrich-Heine-University Düsseldorf*	Germany
Erasmus MC	Erasmus Universiteit Medisch Centrum Rotterdam *Erasmus University Medical Center Rotterdam*	Netherlands
Hvidovre Hospital	Hvidovre Hospital, the Danish Hnpcc- Register, Hovedstadens Sygehusfællesskab	Denmark
ACTA	Academisch Centrum Tandheelkunde Amsterdam *Academic Centre for Dentistry Amsterdam*	Netherlands
AstraZeneca	AstraZeneca	Sweden

Figure 1   The EC-funded INFOBIOMED Study (Network of Excellence EC-IST 2001-35024)

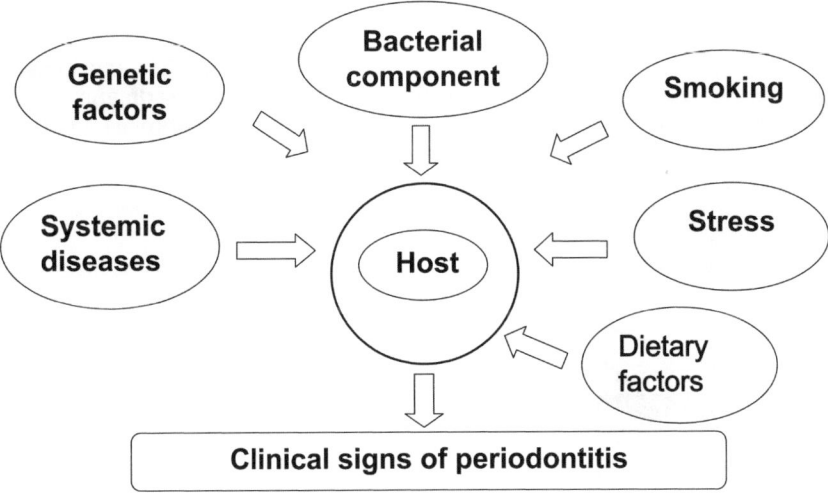

Figure 2   Periodontitis is a multifactorial disease

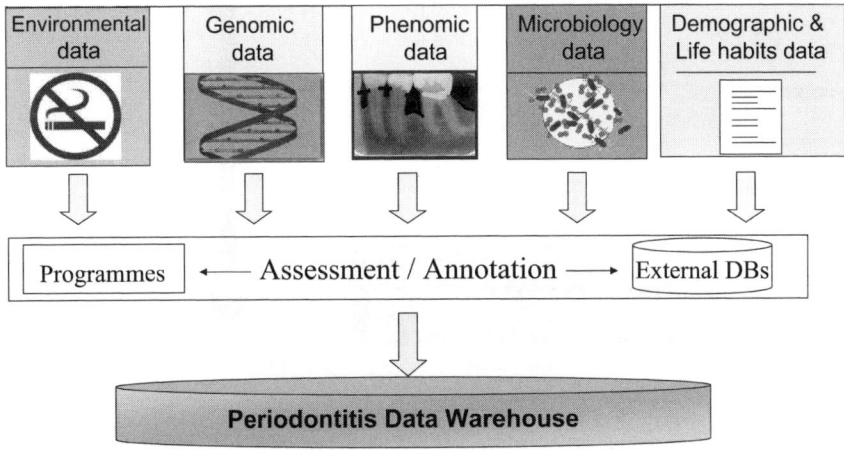

Figure 3   The main challenge for biomedical informatics applied to periodontitis is the creation of a data warehouse. DBs = databases

BIOMEDICAL INFORMATICS

BMI is the emerging discipline that aims to put bioinformatics and medical informatics together so that the discovery and creation of novel diagnostic and therapeutic methods is fostered[6]. In working with the model it appears that the challenges that BMI faces to be able to contribute to the advancement of the field can be summarized as follows (Figure 4):

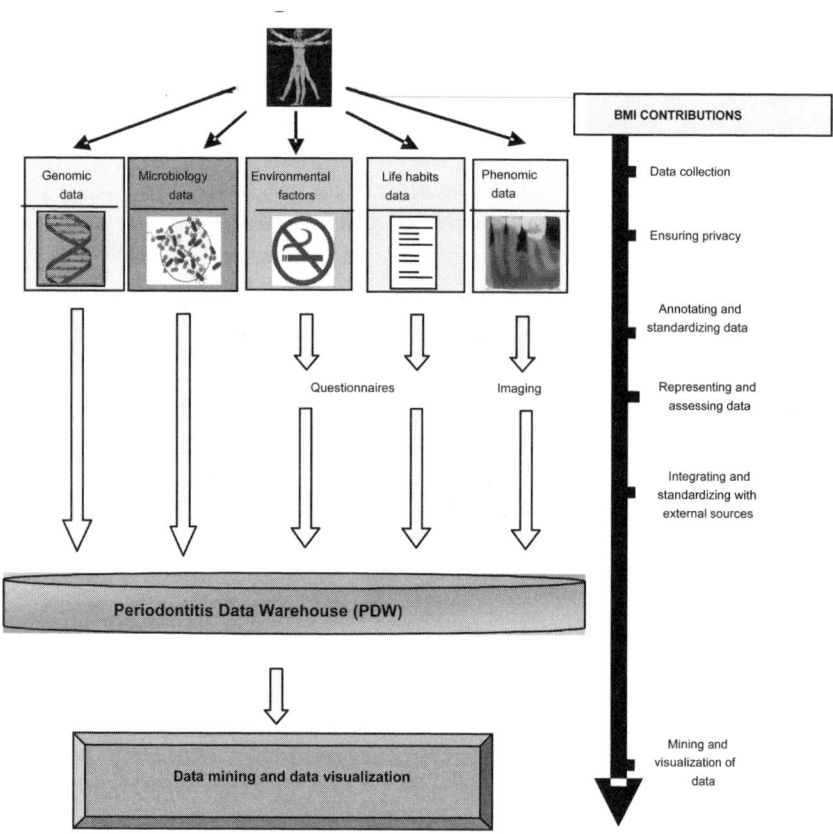

Figure 4 Development of data warehouse tools that will become available for clinicians and researchers opens the path to new technical advances in data mining and visualization

1. Data collection in daily clinical practice that responds to five distinct levels: genetic, environmental (smoking), infectious, disease phenotype, life habits.

2. Annotating and standardizing data of the different phenotypes determined by clinicians.

3. Annotating and standardizing data obtained by a dental image analysis (DIA) tool from dental X-rays. The radiographic data are kept in a particular protocol, 'DICOM', that can be accessed by any computer system in order to be able to analyse with multiple databases.

4. Ethical aspects such as ensuring privacy. The phenotype of the disease, genetic data, data on the infectious component and environmental factors generated by dentists and dental researchers, as well as researchers in the field of informatics, should be encoded to ensure anonymization. This process should be reversible to be able to give advice to the patient after the studies have led to useful therapeutic actions. In the interactive (reversible) pseudonymization model from Custodix[15], a transparent intermediary privacy protection engine is put between the users and the database web server (Figure 5).

5. Mining and visualization data analyse the different sets of data and then extract the meaning of the data. Data analysis and discovery learning algorithms produce a particular enumeration of models[16]. Data mining tools and knowledge discovery techniques are applied to the PDW.

The PDW has large quantities of heterogeneous data collected from diverse sources mentioned above, and this information is stored in specific categories so that it can be more easily retrieved, interpreted, and sorted by users (Figure 6).

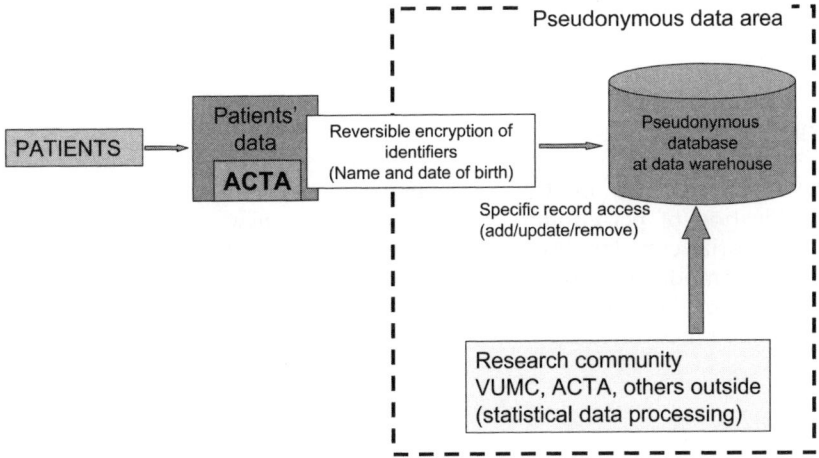

Figure 5 Privacy-enhanced data storage model of periodontitis ACTA (NL), Custodix (Belgium) and UPM (Spain)

Table 2 Main aims of data analysis, mining and visualization

– Clustering	– New classification of periodontitis
– Classification	– New clinical and genetic associations
– Association	– New scientific hypotheses on pathophysiology of periodontitis
	– New insights/pathways in other complex chronic inflammatory diseases

INSIGHT AND EXPECTED RESULTS

To identify interesting patterns and model profiles, to discriminate between patients with periondotitis with different prognoses, and to identify similarities across patient records and groups, similar records to clusters programmes are being developed by the Institute of Computer Science (ICS) and Hellas (Forth) in Greece under the leadership of V Moustakis and G Potomias.

The main message that we would like to pass on is that BMI has the tools to integrate the different branches of knowledge, but patience and dedication are necessary to achieve results, and expertise from different areas is required. The main aims of the data analysis, mining and visualization are shown in Table 2.

APPLICATION OF THE MODEL TO IBD

The management of chronic inflammatory diseases, such as IBD, is a major challenge for health systems in any country. The aetiology is multifactorial and polygenic. A classification based on molecular biology, genetic information, phenotype information and modern imaging systems is bound to produce new ways to identify subgroups of patients with different prognosis. Genetics genomics and BMI need to be integrated into current research in IBD.

CONCLUSIONS

The INFOBIOMED model is expected to deliver improvements in better classification of periodontitis, and to suggest a new understanding of a multifactorial complex disease. It is to be hoped that the experience gained with this model will form the basis to encourage clinical research in inflammatory bowel diseases. Table 3 summarizes the contribution of the approach to these diseases.

Figure 6 Example of the heterogeneity of the data that is integrated in a data warehouse

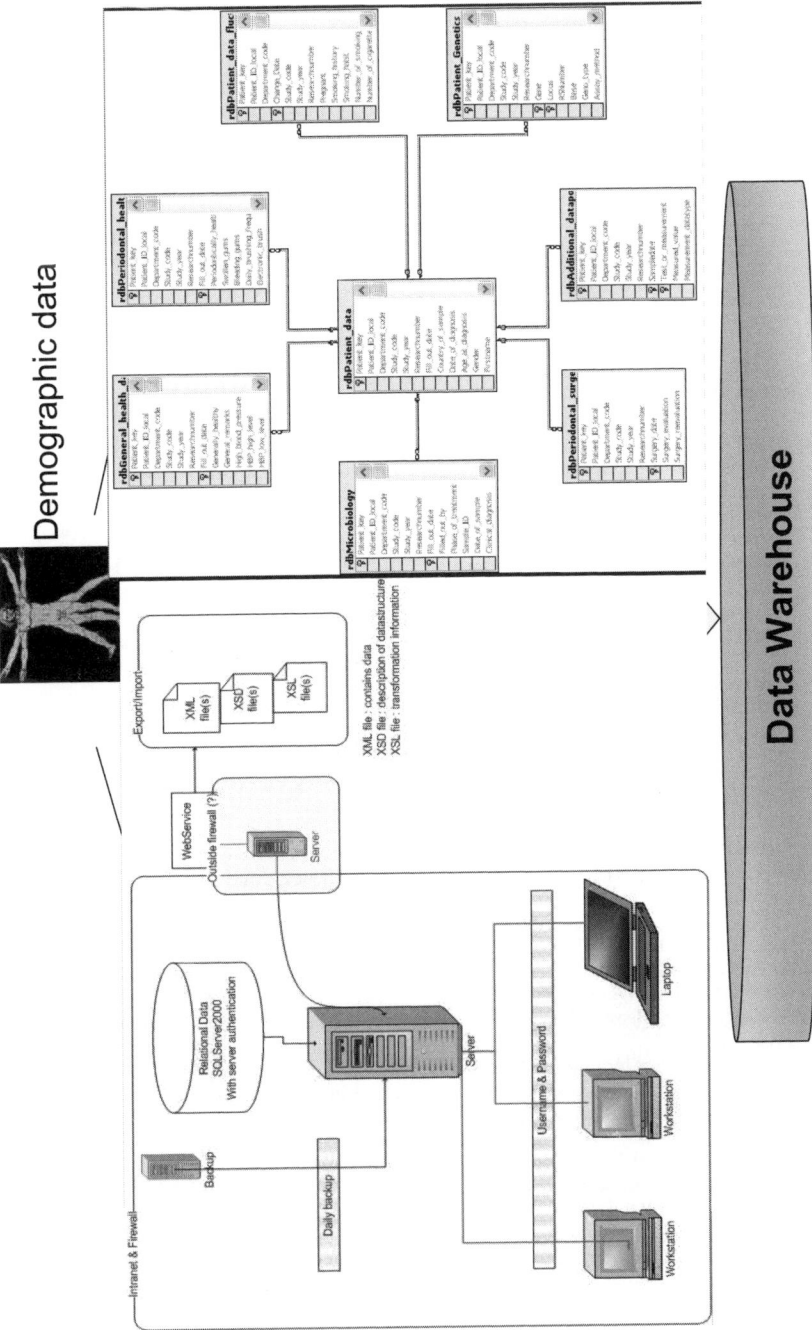

Table 3 Biomedical informatics will make possible the necessary translation of multiple systems with different databases into a common database

– Crohn's disease	– New comprehensive classification of
– Ulcerative colitis	inflammatory bowel disease
– Psoriasis	– New clinical–genetic associations
– Primary sclerosing cholangitis	– New scientific hypotheses on patho-physiology of Crohn's disease and ulcerative colitis
	– New insights/pathways in complex chronic inflammatory diseases

References

1. Hugot JP, Chamaillard M, Zouali H et al. Association of NOD2 leucine-rich repeat variants with susceptibility to Crohn's disease. Nature. 2001;411:599–603.
2. Ogura Y, Bonen DK, Inohara N et al. A frameshift mutation in NOD2 associated with susceptibility to Crohn's disease. Nature. 2001;411:603–6.
3. Hampe J, Cuthbert A, Croucher PJ et al. Association between insertion mutation in NOD2 gene and Crohn's disease in German and British populations. Lancet. 2001;357:1925–8.
4. Fellermann K, Wehkamp J, Herrlinger KR, Stange EF. Crohn's disease: a defensin deficiency syndrome? Eur J Gastroenterol Hepatol. 2003;15:627–34.
5. Sans M, Artieda M, Tejedor D et al. IBDCHIP: a new strategy to predict clinical course and development of complications in patients with inflammatory bowel disease (IBD). Gastroenterology. 2005;130 (Abstract).
6. Martin-Sanchez F, Iakovidis I, Norager S et al. Synergy between medical informatics and bioinformatics: facilitating genomic medicine for future health care. J Biomed Inform. 2004;37:30–42.
7. Sanz F, Diaz C, Martin-Sanchez F, Maojo V. Structuring European biomedical informatics to support individualized healthcare: current issues and future trends. Medinfo. 2004;11:803–7.
8. Eich HP, de la Calle G, Diaz C et al. Practical approaches to the development of biomedical informatics: the INFOBIOMED network of excellence. Stud Health Technol Inform. 2005;116:39–44.
9. Calsina G, Ramon JM, Echeverria JJ. Effects of smoking on periodontal tissues. J Clin Periodontol. 2002;29:771–6.
10. Al-Zahrani MS, Borawski EA, Bissada NF. Increased physical activity reduces prevalence of periodontitis. J Dent. 2005;33:703–10.
11. Al-Zahrani MS, Bissada NF, Borawski EA. Diet and periodontitis. J Int Acad Periodontol. 2005;7:21–6.
12. Al-Zahrani MS, Borawski EA, Bissada NF. Periodontitis and three health-enhancing behaviors: maintaining normal weight, engaging in recommended level of exercise, and consuming a high-quality diet. J Periodontol. 2005;76:1362–6.
13. van Winkelhoff AJ, Loos BG, van der Reijden WA, van der Velden U. *Porphyromonas gingivalis, Bacteroides forsythus* and other putative periodontal pathogens in subjects with and without periodontal destruction. J Clin Periodontol. 2002;29:1023–8.
14. Loos BG, John RP, Laine ML. Identification of genetic risk factors for periodontitis and possible mechanisms of action. J Clin Periodontol. 2005;32(Suppl. 6):159–79.
15. De Moor GJ, Claerhout B, De Meyer F. Privacy enhancing techniques – the key to secure communication and management of clinical and genomic data. Methods Inf Med. 2003;42:148–53.
16. Cios KJ, Moore GW. Uniqueness of medical data mining. Artif Intell Med. 2002;26:1–24.

9
Genetic factors in the inflammatory bowel disease

I. D. LORANSKAYA

Up to date the problem of the aetiology and pathogenesis of the inflammatory bowel diseases (IBD) remains one of the most important subjects of study. Results of epidemiological studies have shown that the genesis of IBD is strongly influenced by two groups of factors: hereditary predisposition and influence of the environment.

First reports on familial cases of the disease with this type of pathology[1] were made by JB Kirsner and JA Spencer in 1963. The role of genetic factors in IBD was proved by:

- Familial cases of Crohn's disease (CD) and ulcerative colitis (UC) are observed in 5–30% of patients (more often in 10–20% of cases)[2,3].

- The number of familial cases of the disease is higher in CD than in UC[4].

- First-degree relatives of UC patients have the highest risk of pathology development (10–20-fold) compared to healthy donors of the same age and sex[3,5,6].

- Cases of both CD and UC may be observed in one family, more often in cases when the disease started at an early age.

- A high frequency of IBD occurrence among Ashkenazi jews (2–4 times higher).

- Cases of IBD in twins occurs more often if they are monozygotic; the concordance of monozygotic twins is higher in CD[6]. However, the fact that concordance of monozygotic twins does not reach 100% testifies to the role of other factors in IBD pathogenesis.

- Association of IBD with a number of genetic syndromes (Turner's syndrome, glycogen storage disease type IB, Hermansky–Pudlak syndrome) and with hereditary predisposition diseases (primary sclerosing cholangitis, psoriasis, eczema, coeliac disease, ankylosing spondylitis).

During recent years there have been revolutionary studies in the genetics of IBD. The work was carried out in two main directions: the search for candidate genes and a patient's genome scanning[7]. The results of numerous studies make it possible to execute the analysis of genotype–IBD phenotype correlations.

The first area of investigation permitted determination of the IBD genetic markers. In 1996 Hugot et al.[8] found the locus of CD susceptibility on chromosome 16q – IBD1. In 1996 Satsangi et al.[9] found the locus of IBD susceptibility on chromosome 12q – IBD2. IBD3 – locus on chromosome 6p (HLA complex) determines the susceptibility to specific clinical phenotype in UC[10]. IBD4 – locus on chromosome 14q – association with CD. IBD5 – locus on chromosome 5q – association with IBD. IBD6 – locus on chromosome 19q – association with CD (?). The most impressive is the determination of the association of CD with the NOD2/CARD15 gene in chromosome 16 locus (IBD1).

In 2001 Hugot et al.[11] and Ogura et al.[12] proved the association of CD and the NOD2 gene on chromosome 16q in locus IBD1. NOD2 (nucleotide oligomerization domain) belongs to the NOD gene family and plays an important role in the origin of inflammation as a response to bacterial antigens. The NOD gene family is mainly expressed in monocytes, macrophages and B lymphocytes.

The NOD2 gene is responsible for activation of the nuclear NF-κB factor, which regulates expression of the majority of the anti-inflammatory cytokines and the response to the bacterial polysaccharide (an immune response to bacterial antigen).

CARD – caspase recruitment domain – the group of enzymes participating in the cell apoptosis process.

The association between NOD2/CARD15 gene mutations and CD supports the assumption that this disease is a pathological immune response to enteric microorganisms (or specific bacterial pathogens) with genetic determinacy. It is known that NOD2/CARD15 recognizes muramyl dipeptide – the obligatory component of the cell membrane of all bacteria living on Earth. However, there are many doubtful areas in the study of the gene CARD15 role in IBD:

- CARD15 mutations (Arg 702 Trp, Gly 908 Arg, Leu 1007 fsinsÑ) determine susceptibility to CD in specific racial and ethnic groups (no CARD15 mutations are revealed in Japanese or Afro-American populations or in Israeli Arabs).

- CARD15 mutations determine the development of CD phenotypes (ileitis, ileitis and right-sided colitis, strictures, penetrations); these are present in 20–27% of disease cases.

- It is important to prove the role of CARD15 mutations in cases of sporadic CD forms.

In Russia the study of the role of NOD2/CARD15 gene mutations for susceptibility to CD was undertaken for the first time. The trial included 51 CD patients and 54 healthy donors. DNA screening was carried out for mutations P268S, R702W and G908R by a PCR/RFLP method, and for ins3020C by a PCR/AFLP method. It was revealed that 29/51 (57%) patients had at least one mutation; of these 26% (13/51) had two mutations, 14% (7/51) had three; four patients (8%) had four mutations and one patient had five mutant alleles in the genotype. In the control group mutations were observed in 41% of cases; two mutations only in 13% of cases (7/54). Three and more mutations have not been observed.

The allele P268S frequency was 0.57 for patients and 0.44 for healthy people; for R702W it was 0.29 in patients and 0.02 in controls; for G908R it was 0.08 in patients and no mutations were found in controls; for ins3020C the figures were 0.49 and 0.08 correspondingly. Thus studies carried out in Russia have shown that R702W, G908R and ins3020C mutations in the NOD2/CARD15 gene are associated with a high risk of CD development. The role of P268S mutation has not been confirmed by our study.

The IBD3 locus includes genes of the main complex of human histocompatibility on chromosome 6p (HLA complex). The HLA complex plays an important role in human immune homeostasis, and carries out genetic control over immune reactions. Polymorphism of this system (more than 100 alleles) provides a high degree of individuality of a human being and of different ethnic populations. HLA-DNA genotyping in the PCR made it possible to study the genetic markers of IBD. It is shown that the DRB1*0103 gene is associated with UC and CD with colon lesion.

Genetic HLA markers determine the UC phenotype, the presence of extraintestinal manifestations and complications, as well as the necessity for a surgical procedure.

Study of antigens and genes of the HLA complex in IBD was carried out in Russia. (Table 1)[13–15].

The DRB1*0103 allele determines the severity of UC, the presence of extraintestinal manifestations and the necessity for surgical treatment[16].

We have studied the peculiarities of HLA II class allele distribution in UC and CD patients by HLA-DNA genotyping of DRB1, DQA1 and DQB1 loci allele polymorphism[17]. The control group comprised 147 healthy people. The genotyping embraces 13 alleles of locus DRB1, eight alleles of DQA1 locus and 10 alleles of DQB1 locus.

Table 1 HLA-markers for UC in Russia

	Positive associations	Negative associations
Ulcerative colitis		
Morozova[13]	B14, Cw4, DR3, DR5	Aw19, DR4
Pershko et al.[14]	DR3, B35	
Khidiyatov[15] (Bashkiriya))	DRB1*13	DRB1*04
Crohn's disease	A3, B14	Aw19

The analysis of distribution of DRB1 locus alleles showed that the HLA marker of predisposition to UC and CD is the DRB1*01 allele ($RR = 1.8$, $p = 0.0333$ for UC and $RR = 4.1$, $p = 0.0047$ for CD). In the UC group of patients, which was more numerous, the analysis of DRB1 allele association with the disease was carried out depending on the length of the pathological process (lesion) in the colon, the age of patients at the onset of the disease and its clinical form (Table 2).

It was determined that the unbiased resistance marker in left-sided UC is the DRB1*04 allele ($RR = 0.12$, $1/RR = 8.3$, $p = 0.0306$). Resistance to this form of the disease is eightfold higher with this allele than without it.

The predisposition marker of distal forms of UC is allele DRB1*08 ($RR = 3.5$, $p = 0.0167$).

Study of the peculiarities of allele distribution of the DRB1 locus in UC patients depending on the age of onset of the disease revealed that the positive association with young age (up to 30) has the DRB1*01 allele ($RR = 2.4$, $p = 0.0400$). For patients with onset of the disease after the age of 30–50 years the genetic marker of predisposition will be DRB1*08 ($RR = 3.1$, $p = 0.0383$), and the resistance marker is DRB1*04 ($RR = 0.13$, $1/RR = 7.7$, $p = 0.0096$), which has a high negative linkage.

A marked positive association with a specific age of onset of the disease was observed in the distribution analysis of the allele frequencies of the DRB1 locus in the homozygotic state. Thus the DRB1*11 homozygotic allele is the marker of disease onset for 30–50-year-old patients ($RR = 6.0$, $p = 0.0236$). At the same time the homozygosity on the DRB1*15 allele is a manifested association with disease onset in those 51–70 years of age ($RR = 36.5$, $p = 0.0100$). The risk of developing the disease at this age in the presence of homozygosity on the DRB1*15 allele is 36.5-fold higher than in its absence.

Results of HLA-DNA typing in patients with different clinical forms of UC revealed that in the chronic continuous form of the disease the predisposition marker is DRB1*01 allele ($RR = 2.5$, $p = 0.0483$), and the resistance marker is DRB1*11 ($RR = 0.17$, $1/RR = 5.9$, $p = 0.0307$). The chronic recurring form of the disease has its own manifested resistance marker DRB1*04 ($RR = 0.1$, $1/RR = 9.7$, $p = 0.0031$), indicating a high degree of resistance to this form of UC.

As a result of the data acquired it was observed that the DRB1*01 allele is the predisposition marker of the onset of disease at young ages, and of the chronic continuous form of UC; DRB1*08 allele is positive for distal forms of the pathology and its onset in patients of 30–50 years of age. At the same time DRB1*04 is the left-sided colitis resistance marker and the marker of the onset of the disease in those 30–50 years of age and its chronic recurring form. The allele DRB1*11 is the resistance marker for the chronic continuous form of UC.

It was also observed that the DRB1*11 allele in the homozygotic state is the predisposition marker for disease onset at the age of 30–50, and homozygosity on allele DRB1*15 confers the high risk of UC onset at the age of 51–70.

Study of allele distribution of the loci DQA1 and DQB1 in UC and CD patients has not revealed any connection with the diseases. Therefore we have again confirmed the genetic heterogeneity of UC.

Perinuclear antineutrophil cytoplasmic antibodies (pANCA) are considered to be the subclinical markers of genetic predisposition in IBD. pANCA are

Table 2 Association analysis of locus DRB1 alleles in UC with different clinical forms of the disease

		HLA genes DRB1	Patients (n = 116)	Controls (n = 294)	RR	1/RR	p-Value
Localization:							
Left-sided intestinal lesion	n = 28	DRB1*04	0.0	12.2	0.12	8.3	0.0309
Distal forms	n = 58	DRB1*08	12.1	3.7	3.5	–	0.0167
Onset of disease:							
Up to 30 years old	n = 40	DRB1*01	17.5	8.2	2.4	–	0.0400
30–50 years old	n = 56	DRB1*04	1.8	12.2	0.13	7.7	0.0096
30–50 years old	n = 56	DRB1*08	10.7	3.7	3.1	–	0.0383
30–50 years old	n = 28*	(DRB1*11)	14.3	2.7	6.0	–	0.0236
51–70 years old	n = 10*	(DRB1*15)	20.0	0.7	36.5	–	0.0106
Type of disease:							
Chronic continuous	n = 38	DRB1*01	18.4	8.2	2.5	–	0.0483
Chronic continuous	n = 38	DRB1*11	2.6	13.9	0.17	5.9	0.0307
Chronic recurring	n = 68	DRB1*04	1.5	12.2	0.11	9.1	0.0031

n, number of patients seen.

N, number of tested HLA haplotypes.

RR, relative risk.

p, reliability of association.

found in more than 70% of patients with UC and their healthy relatives. In CD the pANCA are positive only in 10–15% of patients with clinical phenotype similar to UC.

The enteric barrier defect is genetically determined for CD and is observed in patients' first-degree relatives (the CD genetic marker)[18,19].

For the first time the enteric barrier function in IBD (70 patients: 55 UC and 15 CD) was studied with the help of the immune enzymatic method of determination of ovalbumin in the blood under the egg (food) load[17]. The enteric barrier function was defective in 92% of cases of CD and 67% of UC patients. In the UC group the level of ovalbumin in the blood was manifestedly higher in severe forms of the disease in those with food intolerance and intestinal bacterial overgrowth (Figures 1–4).

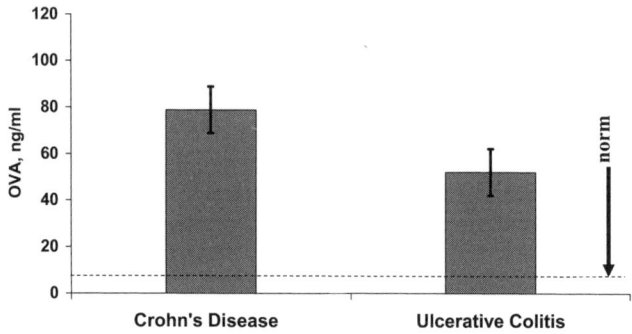

Figure 1 Permeability of the intestinal barrier for OVA in CD and UC

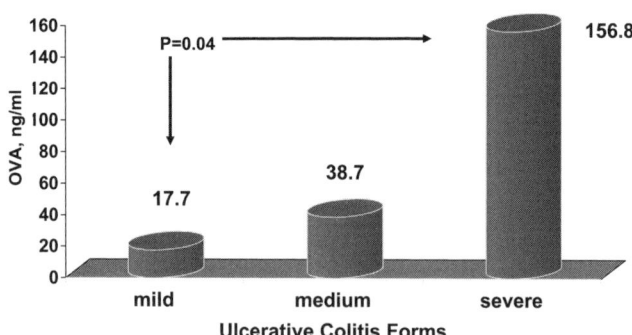

Figure 2 OVA permeability in UC of different levels of severity

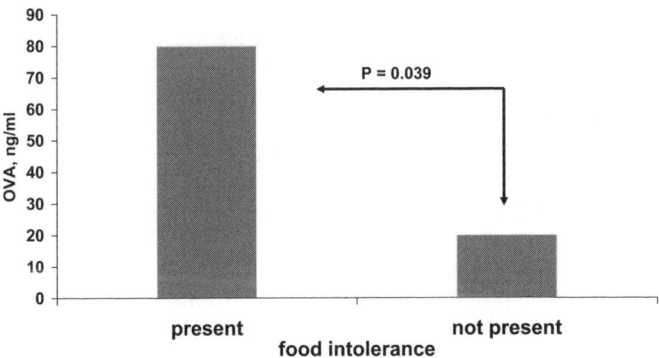

Figure 3 Permeability of the intestinal barrier for OVA in UC (as per food intolerance)

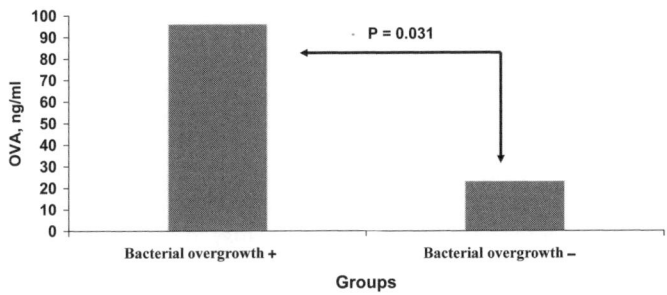

Figure 4 OVA permeability in UC

At present active studies of other gene candidates of predisposition to IBD are ongoing[7,16,20–25].

Chromosome 2: gene family IL-1 (IL-1α, IL-1β, IL-1ra)

Chromosome 3:
Region HLA class II – MICA and MICB genes (gene family encoding the expression of stress glycoproteins in epithelium)
Region HLA class III – TNF-α gene – predisposition to CD and severe UC forms: GNA12 protein gene, MLH-1 gene.

Chromosome 5: OCTN (cation transporter genes) – determines the epithelial barrier function.

Chromosome 7: MUC-3 – encodes mucosa secretion; MDR-1 (multidrug resistance gene) – membrane-transporting protein.

Chromosome 10: DLG5 (*Drosophila* discs large homologue 5).

Chromosome 19: ICAM-1 gene (intercellular adhesion molecule) – determines neutrophil migration into the inflammatory area.

Ulcerative colitis is a disease characterized by a high risk of the development of colon cancer. Changes in cell genetics – chromosome aberrations, chromatic balance, chromosomal instability – precede dysplasia and neoplasia.

A high expression of REG 1α protein (regeneration gene) is observed in the colon mucosa of UC patients which evidently plays an important role in the development of colorectal cancer[26]. DNA damage in the form of microsatellite instability (MSI) is accompanied by higher levels of DNA reparation enzyme activity – AAG and APE1 – in the area of inflammation, which also increases the risk of development of neoplasia.

Studies of the proliferative activity of epithelial mucosa of the colon were carried out with the help of computer microspectrophotometry of colon tissue samplings taken from different sectors of the colon of 50 patients suffering from the disease for more than 10 years[17]. Microspectrophotometry of epithelial nuclei obtained mean values of integral brightness of the cell nuclei of the investigated clones which were related to diploid standard (2c), acquired on the basis of measuring lymphocyte nuclei of the same histological cut. The DNA content indices in cell nuclei were expressed in ploidy units (c). Proliferative activity (PA) was treated as the increase of the DNA content in nuclei over 2c.

It was revealed that in the group of UC patients the highest intensity of proliferation was observed in the caecum (DNA $4.6 \pm 0.9c$, PA = 2.6 ± 0.5); little less in the transverse colon (DNA $3.5 \pm 0.75c$, PA = 1.5 ± 0.4) and sigmoid colon (DNA $3.3 \pm 0.3c$, PA = 1.3 ± 0.15).

Thus we have identified a tendency to an increase in proliferative activity in the colon mucosa epithelium from the sigmoid to the caecum section in UC. The DNA content in the caecum epithelium is close to the DNA index of severe dysplasia of the large intestine (5.2c) and in colonocytes of sigmoid bowel and transverse colon it correlates with this index for benign tumours and for transition conditions with dysplasia features present in an organ (3.6c).

The acquired data support the necessity for a dynamic follow-up of UC patients with the aim of early verification of neoplastic processes. Therefore, substantial progress made in the study of IBD genetic markers makes it possible to envisage, in the near future, success in the study of pathogenesis, in forecasting the course and determining effective methods of treating this pathology.

References

1. Kirsner JB, Spencer JA. Family occurrences of ulcerative colitis, regional enteritis, and ileocolitis. Ann Intern Med. 1963;59:133–44.
2. McConell RB, Vadheim CM. Inflammatory bowel disease. In: King RA, Rotter JI, Motulsky et al., editors. The Genetic Basis of Common Diseases. New York: Oxford University Press, 1995:326–48.
3. Peeters M, Vermeire S, Rutgeerts P. Genetics and IBD: what to tell our patients today? Falk Symposium, 1998;106:11.
4. Binder V, Orholm M. Familial occurrence and inheritance studies in inflammatory bowel disease. Neth J Med. 1996;48:53–6.
5. Polito JM, Chieds B, Mellits ED et al. Crohn's disease: Influence of age at diagnosis on site and clinical type of disease. Gastroenterology. 1996;3:580–6.
6. Satsangi J, Jewell DP. The genetics of inflammatory bowel disease. Gut. 1997;40:572–4.
7. Russell RK, Wilson DS, Satsangi J. Unravelling the complex genetics of inflammatory bowel disease. Arch Dis Child. 2004;89:598–603.

8. Hugot JP, Laurent-Puig P, Gower-Roussean C et al. Mapping of a susceptibility locus for Crohn's disease on chromosome 16. Nature. 1996;379:821–2.
9. Satsangi J, Parkes M, Louis E et al. Two stage genome-wide search in inflammatory bowel disease provides evidence for susceptibility loci on chromosomes 3, 7 and 12. Nat Genet. 1996;14:199–202.
10. Satsangi J, Welsh KI, Bunce M et al. Contribution of genes of the major histocompatibility complex to susceptibility and disease phenotype in inflammatory bowel disease. Lancet. 1996;347:1212–17.
11. Hugot JP, Chamaillard M, Zouali H et al. Association of NOD2 leucine-rich repeat variants with susceptibility to Crohn's disease. Nature. 2001;411:599–603.
12. Ogura Y, Bonen DK, Inohara N et al. A frameshift mutation in NOD2 associated with susceptibility to Crohn's disease. Nature. 2001;411:603–6.
13. Morozova NA. Clinical and genetic correlations in IBD. Candidate disseration. Moscow, 1997, p.24.
14. Pershko AM, Tkachenko EI, Grinevich VB. Clinical and genetic associations of HLA-antigens and UC clinical forms. Mater. 4 Russian Gastroenterology Week. Moscow, 1998, No. 292.
15. Khidiyatov II. Optimization of diagnostics and treatment patients with UC. Avtoref. dokt. diss. Ufa, 1999, p.33.
16. Watts DA, Satsangi J. The genetic jigsaw of inflammatory bowel disease. Gut. 2002;50 (Suppl. III):31–6.
17. Loranskaya ID. Non-specific colitis and IBS: pathogenesis, diagnostic and prognosis. Diss. dokt. M., 2001, p.185.
18. Hollander D, Vadheim CM, Brettholz E et al. Increased intestinal permeability in patients with Crohn's disease and their relatives. Falk Symposium, 1993;72:8.
19. Peeters M, Geypens B, Claus D et al. Clustering of increased small intestinal permeability in families with Crohn's disease. Gastroenterology. 1997;113:802–7.
20. Cho JH. Advances in the genetics of inflammatory bowel disease. Curr Gastroenterol Rep. 2004;6:467–73.
21. Duerr RH. Genetics of inflammatory bowel disease. IBD. 1996;2:48–60.
22. Duerr RH. The genetics of inflammatory bowel disease. Gastroenterol Clin N Am. 2002;31:63–76.
23. Mathew CG, Lewis CM. Genetics of inflammatory bowel disease: progress and prospects. Hum Mol Genet. 2004;13:161–8.
24. Satsangi J. Genetic heterogeneity within inflammatory bowel disease. Falk Symposium, 1998;106:10.
25. Trinh TT. The promise and perils of interpreting genetic associations in Crohn's disease. Gut. 2005;54:1354–7.
26. Sekikawa A, Fukui H, Fujii S. Possible role of REG I^2 protein in ulcerative colitis and colitic cancer. Gut. 2005;54:1437–44.

10
Genotype-based classification of inflammatory bowel disease phenotype

D. P. JEWELL

INTRODUCTION

For many years there has been much discussion regarding the precise disease entity of ulcerative colitis (UC) and Crohn's disease (CD). Are they two distinct diseases? Are they a spectrum of the same pathological process? Is proctitis the same disease as extensive UC? How many diseases are encompassed by a clinical picture of 'CD'? These are just a few questions that have been raised, and no clear answers have emerged until recently when genetic studies have offered the promise of being able to define disease by genetic analysis. Furthermore, the natural history and behaviour of inflammatory bowel disease (IBD) is also partly determined by genetic factors, which has given rise to the possibility of being able to predict the course of disease based on genetic analysis.

Family studies in the early 1990s provided strong presumptive evidence that a genetic component was involved in the aetiopathogenesis of both UC and CD, with a greater involvement in CD. The problem was how to find a gene when one did not know what to look for in diseases that were clearly not inherited along Mendelian principles. The introduction of microsatellite technology which allowed diseases to be linked to certain regions of a chromosome provided the necessary methodology and the first genome-wide searches in IBD were published in 1996. These confirmed that there were indeed susceptibility genes underlying the two diseases and that both diseases were polygenic. How many genes are involved is still unclear, but there are at least nine regions across the human genome which have been linked to UC, CD or both. In 2001, one gene was identified on chromosome 16 for CD which is known as CARD15 or NOD2. How mutations in this gene influence disease pathogenesis is unclear, and there is evidence for loss of function, gain of function, impaired intracellular killing of bacteria and reduced defensin secretion by Paneth cells. Since the CARD15 protein recognizes a muramyl dipeptide moiety of peptidoglycan found in the walls of both Gram-positive and Gram-negative bacteria, it has the potential for having a major role in innate immunity, and it is possible that mutations within the gene could lead to a variety of functional outcomes.

The genetic studies to date have tended to provide evidence for genetic mutations affecting phenotype rather than overall susceptibility to IBD. The exception is the TNFSF gene, in which mutations have been associated with CD in both Western and Oriental populations[1]. This chapter will provide a short review of the genotype–phenotype studies that have been performed.

DISEASE DISTRIBUTION

Following the discovery that mutations in the NOD2 gene were associated with CD, a large cohort of patients were studied in order to explore the genotype–phenotype relationships in more detail. The study clearly showed that the mutations were found in those patients with ileal CD and to a lesser degree in those with ileocolonic disease. For patients with isolated colonic disease, the NOD2 mutations were no commoner than in the control population. This finding has been widely replicated and a meta-analysis confirmed the association with odds ratios of 2.20 (95% CI 1.84–2.62), 2.99 (2.38–3.74) and 4.09 (3.23–5.18) for the three common SNPs (SNPs 8, 12, 13) in non-Jewish Caucasians. The frequency of these NOD2 risk alleles is slightly higher in Jewish patients but is extremely low in Asian populations. The OR in carriers of at least two risk alleles was 17.1 (10.7–27.2). It is unclear why possession of one or more of these CARD15/NOD2 mutations puts patients at risk of developing ileal CD. However, the recent finding that the CARD15/NOD2 protein can be found in Paneth cells, predominantly found in the distal ileum, and that patients possessing one or more of these mutations fail to secrete alpha-defensins 5 and 6 from these cells, offers insight into possible mechanisms.

Colonic CD appears to be influenced by genes within the HLA region on the short arm of chromosome 6. Thus, HLA-DRB1*0103 which is only present in about 2% of the Caucasian control population is found in up to 32% of patients with isolated CD. The odds ratios range from 5.1 to 18.5. The very tight linkage disequilibrium across the HLA region makes it difficult to be sure whether association with a particular allele is genuine or whether it is is just in linkage disequilibrium with a more relevant gene. However, the association with Crohn's colitis is seen with both the DRB1*0103–DQB1*0301 and the DRB1*0103–DQB1*0501 haplotypes, suggesting that the DRB1*0103 allele is indeed involved in disease pathogenesis.

HLA alleles are also associated with ileal CD. The strongest and most replicated association is with DRB1*07 in patients who do not possess CARD15 mutations. In large studies from the UK, Canada and Spain, the odds ratios were 1.5, 1.9 and 2.6, respectively. Although these odds ratios are quite low they are similar to those observed in CD patients carrying a single CARD15 mutation. The association has not been observed in Japan, but the allele frequency in the control population is less than 1%, which would therefore require a very large cohort of patients in order to detect an association with a similar odds ratio to that found in Caucasians.

For UC, the association with HLA-DRB1*0103 has been widely replicated. This allele is present in about 8–10% of patients compared with 2% in the normal population, but the allele frequency rises to 15% or so in patients with extensive disease. As with Crohn's colitis, it seems highly likely that DRB1*0103 is involved in determining the extent of disease, but it is not clear by what mechanism, although it presumably involves antigen processing and hence the adaptive immune response.

DISEASE BEHAVIOUR

Both diseases are clinically very heterogeneous, especially CD, and why different patients often have very different types of disease is not clear. There are suggestions that at least some of this heterogeneity can be explained by different genetic factors. Stricturing CD has been associated with the CARD15 mutations in several studies and confirmed in the meta-analysis. However, caution is needed before accepting this finding completely because stricturing CD is mostly seen in the ileum, and the question becomes whether CARD15 mutations are associated with stricturing disease independently of the association with ileal disease. Some studies have tried to overcome this problem by using multiple logistic regression analyses, but the numbers of patients going into these analyses have been small. The other problem is that clinical observation indicates that, although many patients with stricturing disease will continue to develop further strictures during the course of their disease, the phenotype is not completely stable and such patients can change to fistulizing disease and vice-versa. With regard to perianal disease, patients with CD who are homozygous for the 250 kb haplotype on chromosome 5 are more likely to develop perianal fistulas than those with the wild-type haplotype.

The severity of the inflammation may also be under genetic influence, especially for colonic disease. Thus, the HLA class 2 allele, DRB1*0103, is present significantly more often in patients with either Crohn's colitis or UC who have severe disease and come to colectomy. However, the proportion of patients carrying this allele is not sufficiently great to be clinically useful in terms of being able to predict which patient might require colectomy – 12–15% will possess DRB1*0103 compared to about 8% with milder disease and 2% of healthy individuals.

Patients with ulcerative proctitis have long been known to be a mixed group. When followed over time, 55–65% will always have distal disease whereas the others will show progression of disease to affect greater parts of the colon after 10 years or more of having the disease. The reasons why some patients do not extend their disease are unknown. However, Ahmad et al.[6] have studied a large cohort of these patients who have remained stable for at least 10 years, and have shown an association with a haplotype of polmorphisms in the promoter region of TNF-α compared to patients with more extensive disease. There is no obvious biological explanation for this and, indeed, it is likely that the haplotype is on an extended haplotype within the class 3 region which presumably contains the relevant gene. The tight linkage disequilibrium across this gene dense region on chromosome 6p makes precise gene detection extremely difficult.

EXTRAINTESTINAL MANIFESTATIONS

The recognition that genetic make-up might determine whether an individual is likely to develop extraintestinal manifestations has provided intriguing insights into the pathogenesis of these clinical features. If the genetic associations turn out to be true, and they remain to be replicated in larger independent cohorts, then it is clear that patients not carrying the relevant 'at-risk' alleles are unlikely to develop these extraintestinal manifestations however severe their disease is. Thus, activity indices that include extraintestinal manifestations as part of the index become redundant and invalid – that includes the Crohn's Disease Activity Index, the Harvey–Bradshaw Index, and many of the UC activity indices.

Table 1 summarizes the data that have been published so far. The rare class 2 HLA allele, DRB1*0103, appears to predict many of these extraintestinal manifestations. However, once again, the mechanisms are not known, and it is not clear whether this is the relevant allele or whether it is in tight linkage disequilibrium with a more relevant allele. For ankylosing spondylitis the expected association with HLA B27 holds, but is not nearly as strong as seen in idiopathic ankylosing spondylitis where 95% of patients will carry this allele.

Table 1 Genetic associations of the extraintestinal manifestations (EIM) of IBD

EIM related to IBD activity[2,3]	
Arthropathy type 1	HLA DRB1*0103 (38%)
Arthropathy type 2	HLA B44 MICA-9 (95%)
Erythena nodosum	TNF-α – 1031C (67%)
Uveitis	HLA DRB1*0103, B27
Recurrent mouth ulcers	HLA DRB1*01013, B27
EIM unrelated to IBD activity[4,5]	
Ankylosing spondylitis	HLA B27 (65%)
Primary sclerosing cholangitis	Various class II and MIC-A alleles

CONCLUSIONS

Over the past 10 years it has become clear that not only is there a strong genetic influence underlying the susceptibility to CD and UC, especially for CD, but that there is also marked genetic heterogeneity. Careful genotype–phenotype analysis has provided insight into explaining the well-known clinical heterogeneity. However, at the present time it is not possible to be sure of the exact identity of the genes in question, apart from CARD15, and so a molecular classification is still a hope for the future. Nevertheless, is it possible that genetic analysis at diagnosis might predict the course of disease in terms of severity, natural history, extraintestinal manifestations and response to treatment? The evidence discussed briefly in this chapter suggests that this may be possible for some aspects of the diseases. The development of a DNA microarray chip to test this in large cohorts is now in progress and, supported by a substantial grant from the European Community, it will be possible to test the accuracy of genetic predictions. Obviously there will be ethical issues to address if a poor prognosis is predicted. However, since environmental factors including the gut flora are at least equal to genetic factors in determining the natural history of disease, any prediction from genetic information alone is unlikely to be clinically useful.

References

1. Yamazaki K, McGovern D, Ragoussis J et al. Single nucleotide polymorphisms in TNF SF15 confer susceptibility to Crohn's disease. Hum Mol Genet. 2005;14:3499–506.
2. Orchard TR, Thiyagaraja S, Welsh KI, Wordsworth BP, Hill Gaston JS, Jewell DP. Clinical phenotype is related to HLA genotype in the peripheral arthropathies of inflammatory bowel disease. Gastroenterology. 2000;118:274–8.
3. Orchard TR, Chua CN, Ahmad T, Cheng H, Welsh KI, Jewell DP. Uveitis and erythema nodosum in inflammatory bowel disease: clinical features and the role of HLA genes. Gastroenterology. 2002;123:714–18.
4. Smale S, Natt RS, Orchard TR, Russell AS, Bjarnason I. Inflammatory bowel disease and spondylarthropathy. Arthritis Rheum. 2001;44:2728–36..
5. Donaldson PT. Genetics of liver disease: immunogenetics and disease pathogenesis. Gut. 2004;53:599–608.
6. Ahmad T, Armuzzi A, Neville M et al. The contribution of human leucocyte antigen complex genes to disease phenotype in ulcerative colitis. Tissue Antigens. 2003;62:527–35.

11
Role of the intestinal barrier in inflammatory bowel disease

S. ZEISSIG, F. HELLER and J.-D. SCHULZKE

INTRODUCTION

In general, inflammatory processes in the intestine including chronic inflammatory bowel disease (IBD) are accompanied by altered barrier function. This has two main consequences. First, small solutes and water can flow into the lumen and cause *leak flux diarrhoea*. The second consequence regards larger molecules such as antigens, which under normal conditions cross the epithelial barrier only in small amounts, which allows for immune tolerance induction. However, if the intestinal barrier is impaired, uptake of increased amounts of antigens may aggravate or even initiate inflammation. Besides altered tight junctions, other structural changes in the epithelium such as epithelial cell apoptosis, erosion/ulcer type lesions and transcytosis can also play a role and should be considered. In some regions along the gastrointestinal tract M cells, the follicle-associated epithelium (FAE) above Peyer's patches and transepithelial extrusions of antigen-presenting cells (APC) can contribute to the transport of antigens through the epithelial barrier. This chapter gives an overview of: (a) changes observed in barrier properties in IBD, (b) regulation of intestinal barrier function during inflammation and (c) antibody therapy targeting epithelial dysfunction in IBD.

EPITHELIAL BARRIER FUNCTION IN IBD

Crohn's disease

Crohn's disease (CD) is an autoimmune disease with inflammation of the small and/or large intestinal mucosa leading to significant diarrhoea. Possible mechanisms for this epithelial dysfunction comprise reduced absorption and a defect in epithelial barrier function. Therefore, epithelial barrier function, as well as tight junction structure and epithelial apoptosis, were studied in forceps biopsies obtained during endoscopy from the inflamed sigmoid colon of CD patients. Specimens were chosen which exhibited mild to moderate disease activity with an endoscopic appearance of hyperaemia, oedema and granularity, and a histological score with an intact epithelium without erosions or ulcer-type lesions. Alternating current impedance spectroscopy was applied to determine the epithelial resistance as a proportion of total transmural resistance. This is important, since the subepithelial resistance is *in vivo* not part of the barrier. Hence the majority of subepithelial tissue is located below the blood capillaries. Discrimination between epithelial and subepithelial resistance is crucial, since both parameters change in opposing directions in CD. In a statistical analysis epithelial resistance turned out to be decreased by 41%, which in conventional Ussing experiments would have been masked by the increase of subepithelial resistance due to inflammatory cell infiltration and submucosal oedema. Thus, taken together the inflamed colonic mucosa in CD is characterized by a significant loss of barrier function.

A possible explanation for this change in barrier properties would be altered tight junction (TJ) structure within the epithelium. Before going into the details of TJ structure in CD, it should be mentioned that it has been shown for several epithelia that large differences in resistance are associated with only small differences in the number of horizontally oriented TJ strands following a logarithmic correlation[1]. This held true also for CD, where the pronounced decrease in epithelial resistance was paralleled by a rather small reduction in epithelial cell tight junction complexity (Table 1). Furthermore, strand discontinuities were more frequent in CD than in controls (Table 1). In this manner, strand discontinuities are important in enabling macromolecules, including food antigens and bacterial lipopolysaccharides, to pass the epithelial barrier.

Table 1 Barrier function, tight junctions and apoptosis in Crohn's disease

	Epithelial resistance	TJ strand count	Strand discontinuities	Apoptotic rate
Control	39 ± 4 Ω.cm2 (10)	7.2 ± 0.2 (6)	0.2 ± 0.1 (6)	1.0 ± 0.1 % (10)
Crohn's disease	23 ± 3 Ω.cm2 (10)**	4.7 ± 0.2 (6)***	2.9 ± 0.6 (6)***	2.8 ± 0.3 % (8)***

In sigmoid colon of controls and patients with Crohn's disease, epithelial resistance was measured by alternating current impedance spectroscopy. Furthermore, epithelial TJ were characterized by measuring the number of horizontally oriented strands in the main compact meshwork of the TJ (strand count) and the frequency of strand discontinuities (per micrometre strand length) by freeze-fracture electron microscopy. Finally, apoptotic rate was determined within the epithelium using TUNEL staining. All values are means $\pm$ SEM, number of patients is given in parentheses.

**p < 0.01 versus control, ***p < 0.001 versus control.

To obtain an insight into the molecular structure of the changes in TJ strands in CD, we analysed TJ proteins by Western blotting and densitometry in plasma membrane fractions prepared from endoscopic biopsies. This showed that occludin, claudin-5 and claudin-8 were down-regulated in CD, while claudin-1 and claudin-4 were almost unchanged. In contrast, claudin-2 was not down-regulated but even up-regulated; however, in contrast to the other claudins, this represents a pore-forming TJ protein. In addition, claudin-5 and claudin-8 were distributed off the TJ in confocal laser-scanning microscopy (data not shown).

Contribution of epithelial apoptosis and epithelial lesions to barrier disturbance in CD

In addition to changes in epithelial TJ, there was evidence for up-regulation of epithelial apoptosis not only in ulcerative colitis (UC)[2] but also in CD (Table 1). However, epithelial lesions such as erosions were not observed (data not shown), which is in sharp contrast to our previous investigation in UC[3] and may explain why the extent of barrier disturbance is more pronounced in UC than in CD, while TJ morphometry and apoptotic rate in the epithelium are similar.

Transcytotic macromolecule transfer through the epithelium may contribute to antigen uptake in CD

There is increasing evidence in the past few years that antigens can be taken up to a significant amount through the transcellular route by endocytotic uptake and transcytosis. This mechanism seems to be intensified in CD, as indicated by electron microscopy studies using ovalbumin and horseradish peroxidase[4,5]. The mechanisms which regulate this transport during inflammation, however, are still unknown, but could also include proinflammatory cytokines (cf. below). The relative contribution of these different barrier defects to the overall barrier impairment in Crohn's disease, however, needs further experimental exploration.

Ulcerative colitis

There are significant changes in epithelial TJ structure and function not only in CD but also in UC, which have recently been described in detail by our group[6,7]. In addition, apoptotic rate was also found to be up-regulated in UC and contributed to the barrier defect[7]. As the result of these apoptotic events and an IL-13-dependent arrest in epithelial restitution ability (see below), epithelial lesions such as microerosions are frequent in UC even in early inflammatory stages[3].

PROINFLAMMATORY CYTOKINES CAN REGULATE INTESTINAL BARRIER FUNCTION

Tight junctions are down-regulated by proinflammatory cytokines

Intestinal inflammation including IBD is usually associated with elevated cytokine release in the mucosa. In has been shown in several cell line models, animal models and cytokine knockout models that proinflammatory cytokines, especially tumour necrosis factor alpha (TNF-α), interferon gamma (IFN-γ) and interleukin-13 (IL-13), can impair the epithelial barrier of the intestine. TNF-α expression is up-regulated in intestinal diseases, including IBD. Serosal addition of TNF-α (100 ng/ml) decreased R^t in the colonic epithelial cell line HT-29/B6 (Table 2). This effect was dose-dependent, was not reversible as long as TNF-α was present in the bathing medium, and it could be mimicked by serosal addition of (activating) antibodies against the p55 TNF-α receptor[8].In this way no cytotoxic effects were observed in lactate dehydrogenase release assays and immunofluorescence localization studies with anti-ZO-1 antibodies revealing no evidence for disruption of the monolayer after TNF-α treatment. In freeze-fracture electron microscopy, TJ complexity was decreased by TNF-α, as indicated by a decrease in the number of strands from 4.7 to 3.4. A combination of TNF-α with IFN-γ even acted synergistically on the epithelial barrier (Table 2).

A comparable effect on the TJ was also observed with IL-13, an important Th$_2$-effector cytokine which has been shown to contribute to the inflammatory response in UC. It can decrease epithelial resistance after 24 h in HT-29/B6 cell monolayers and acts synergistically with TNF-α on barrier function (Table 2). This is due to both a change in TJ strand composition with an increase in claudin-2 and induction of epithelial apoptosis. Furthermore, IL-13 can cause arrest of epithelial restitution (data not shown).

Table 2 Proinflammatory cytokine effects on epithelial barrier function

Cytokine	Concentration	Duration (h)	Resistance in % of initial value
Control (no cytokine)		24	98 ± 5
IFN-γ	1 U/ml	24	98 ± 1 NS
IFN-γ	10 U/ml	24	86 ± 5 NS
IFN-γ	100 U/ml	24	83 ± 7 NS
IFN-γ	1000 U/ml	24	79 ± 5**
TNF-α	5 ng/ml	24	69 ± 9**
TNF-α	100 ng/ml	24	18 ± 1**
TNF-α + IFN-γ	5 ng/ml + 10 U/ml	24	23 ± 4***
IL-13	10 ng/ml	24	76 ± 2***
IL-13 + TNF-α	10 ng/ml + 5 ng/ml	24	47 ± 1***

In HT-29/B6 cell monolayer, the influence of proinflammatory cytokines on electrical resistance was determined. NS, not significantly different from control.

**$p < 0.01$, ***$p < 0.001$.

EFFECT OF THERAPEUTIC AGENTS ON INTESTINAL BARRIER FUNCTION

The increasing amount of information on epithelial barrier features at cellular and molecular levels, as well as on their disturbance and regulation during inflammation, has raised the expectation that repair of barrier function becomes possible in IBD as the result of therapeutic intervention. This is indeed the case with anti-inflammatory therapy strategies which can heal the inflamed mucosa. In contrast, several distinct agents shown to improve barrier function in cell or animal models, including glutamine[9,10], butyrate[11], probiotics[12,13] and TGF-β have shown only limited importance when applied to IBD patients[14].

Anti-inflammatory therapy strategies can improve epithelial barrier function

That anti-inflammatory therapy can improve epithelial barrier function is in principle true for every therapeutic agent of this group of therapeutics, and can be assumed to directly correlate with the anti-inflammatory efficacy. Data to support this have usually been obtained using *in-vivo* permeability tests with drinking solutions containing various permeability markers including lactulose/rhamnose-ratio, PEG-400 or ^{51}Cr-EDTA. On the one hand this is indicated by a correlation of CD activity and intestinal permeability[15,16]. On the other hand this is supported by data from patients with active CD either before and after steroid therapy or before and after application of elemental diets[17,18].

Along this line of evidence there is now also direct evidence for anti-TNF-α antibodies to improve epithelial barrier function in CD[19]. While TJ structure was little affected 2 weeks after a single infusion of Remicade® (infliximab), apoptotic rate recovered almost completely in most of the patients. As the result of this change in apoptotic rate, epithelial resistance as measured by impedance spectroscopy was also almost normal again in endoscopic biopsies from these CD patients.

References

1. Claude P. Morphological factors influencing transepithelial permeability: a model for the resistance of the zonula occludens. J Membrane Biol. 1978;39:219–32.
2. Sträter J, Wellisch I, Riedl S et al. CD95 (APO-1/Fas)-mediated apoptosis in colon epithelial cells: a possible role in ulcerative colitis. Gastroenterology. 1997;113:160–7.
3. Gitter AH, Wullstein F, Fromm M, Schulzke JD. Epithelial barrier defects in ulcerative colitis: characterization and quantification by electrophysiological imaging. Gastroenterology. 2001;121:1320–8.
4. Schürmann G, Brüwer M, Klotz A, Schmidt KW, Senninger N, Zimmer KP. Transepithelial transport processes at the intestinal mucosa in inflammatory bowel disease. Int J Colorect Dis. 1999;14:41–6.
5. Söderholm JD, Streutker C, Yang PC et al. Increased epithelial uptake of protein antigens in the ileum of Crohn's disease mediated by tumour necrosis factor alpha. Gut. 2004;53: 1817–24.

6. Schmitz H, Barmeyer C, Fromm M et al. A decrease in tight junction complexity contributes to the severely impaired epithelial barrier function in ulcerative colitis. Gastroenterology. 1999;116:301–9.

7. Heller F, Florian P, Bojarski C et al. Interleukin-13 is the key effector Th2 cytokine in ulcerative colitis that affects epithelial tight junctions, apoptosis, and cell restitution. Gastroenterology. 2005;129:550–64.

8. Schmitz H, Fromm M, Bentzel CJ et al. Tumor necrosis factor-alpha (TNF-α) regulates the epithelial barrier in the human intestinal cell line HT-29/B6. J Cell Sci. 1999;112:137–46.

9. Gennari R, Alexander JW. Arginine, glutamine, and dehydroepiandrosterone reverse the immunosuppressive effect of prednisone during gut-derived sepsis. Crit Care Med. 1997;25:1207–14.

10. Li J, Langkamp-Henken B, Suzuki K, Stahlgren LH. Glutamine prevents parenteral nutrition-induced increases in intestinal permeability. J Parent Ent Nutr. 1994;18:303–7.

11. Butzner JD, Parmar R, Bell CJ, Dalal V. Butyrate enema therapy stimulates mucosal repair in experimental colitis in the rat. Gut. 1996;38:568–73.

12. Czebrucka D, Dahan S, Mograbi B, Rossi B, Rampal P. *Saccharomyces boulardii* preserves the barrier function and modulates the signal transduction pathway induced in enteropathogenic *E. coli*-infected T84 cells. Infect Immun. 2000;68:5998–6004.

13. Madsen K, Cornish A, Soper P et al. Probiotic bacteria enhance murine and human intestinal epithelial barrier function. Gastroenterology. 2001;121:580–91.

14. Akobeng AK, Miller V, Stanton J, Elbadri AM, Thomas AG. Double-blind randomized controlled trial of glutamine-enriched polymeric diet in the treatment of active Crohn's disease. J Pediatr Gastroenterol Nutr. 2000;30:78–84.

15. Adenis A, Colombel JF, Lecouffe P et al. Increased pulmonary and intestinal permeability in Crohn's disease. Gut. 1992;33:678–82.

16. Andre F, Andre C, Emery Y, Forichon J, Descos L, Minaire Y. Assessment of the lactulose-mannitol test in Crohn's disease. Gut. 1988;29:511–15.

17. Sanderson IR, Boulton P, Menzies I, Walker-Smith JA. Improvement of abnormal lactulose/rhamnose permeability in active Crohn's disease of the small bowel by an elemental diet. Gut. 1987;28:1073–6.

18. Zoli G, Care M, Parazza M et al. A randomized controlled study comparing elemental diet and steroid treatment in Crohn's disease. Aliment Pharmacol Ther. 1997;11:735–40.

19. Zeissig S, Bojarski C, Bürgel N et al. Downregulation of epithelial apoptosis and barrier repair in active Crohn's disease by TNFalpha antibody treatment. Gut. 2004;53:1295–302.

Section III
Management of inflammatory bowel disease: 1st session

Chair: AI PARFENOV and WJ SANDBORN

12
Histological evaluation of the activity of ulcerative colitis in its initial stage of development

V. Y. GOLOFEEVSKY

INTRODUCTION

At present it is obvious that histological study of the mucus of the large intestine is a priority for estimation of the many specific particularities of development variations of ulcerative colitis (UC). The purposes of histological analysis are: determination of activities of the disease, estimation main morphological change, realization of the differential diagnosis, well-timed correct treatment, estimation of efficiency of treatment and time of the onset of histological remissions. So histological estimation of the mucus of the colon is particularly necessary at the time of primary determination of the diagnosis of UC, and particularly important in an acute attack of the disease. We propose that correct interpretation of histological data under primary diagnostics of UC can greatly influence the choice of drugs (5-ASA, systemic or topical glucocorticoids, immunosuppressants), their doses and regimes of treatment.

MAIN 'CLASSIC' MORPHOLOGICAL CHANGES OF UC

From literature data[1-3] it is known that the main pathohistological manifestations of UC are: damage to the arterioles, venules and capillaries (Figures 2 and 3; normal mucosa, Figure 1); inflammation, neutrophil infiltration (Figure 4); damage to crypt and crypt abscesses (Figure 5); hypersecretion of mucus (Figure 6); atrophy and fibrosis (Figure 7).

However, these changes are not always specific to each patient and do not always confirm our experience.

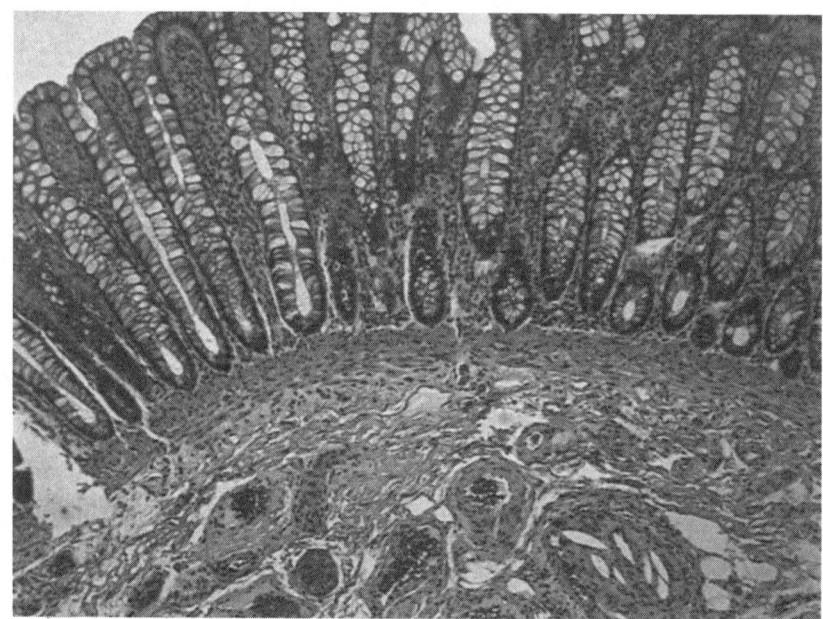

Figure 1 Normal mucosa of colon

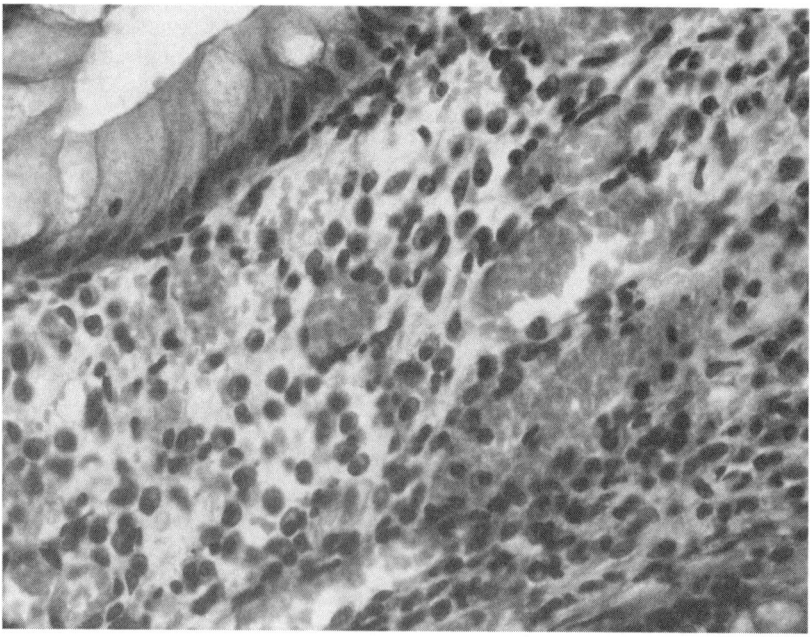

Figure 2 Damage to the capillaries

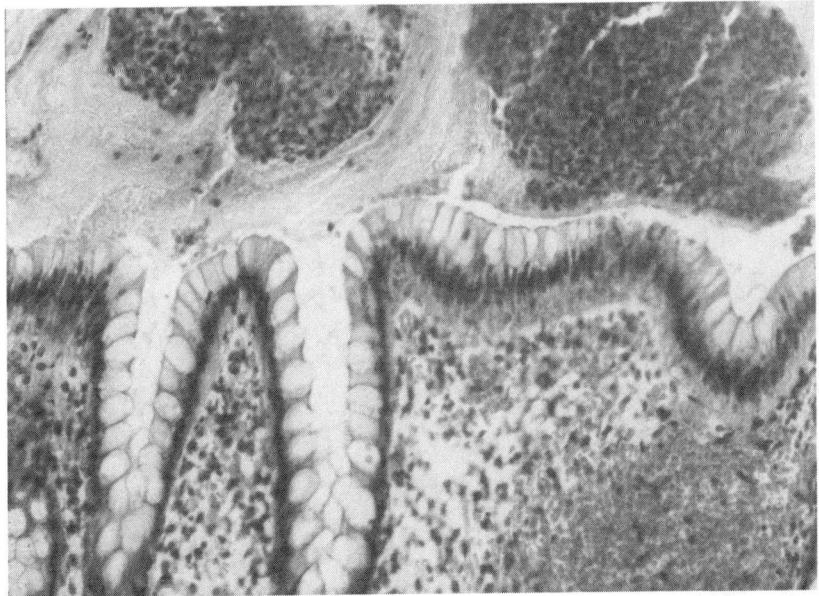

Figure 3 Erythrocytopedesis and haemorrhage

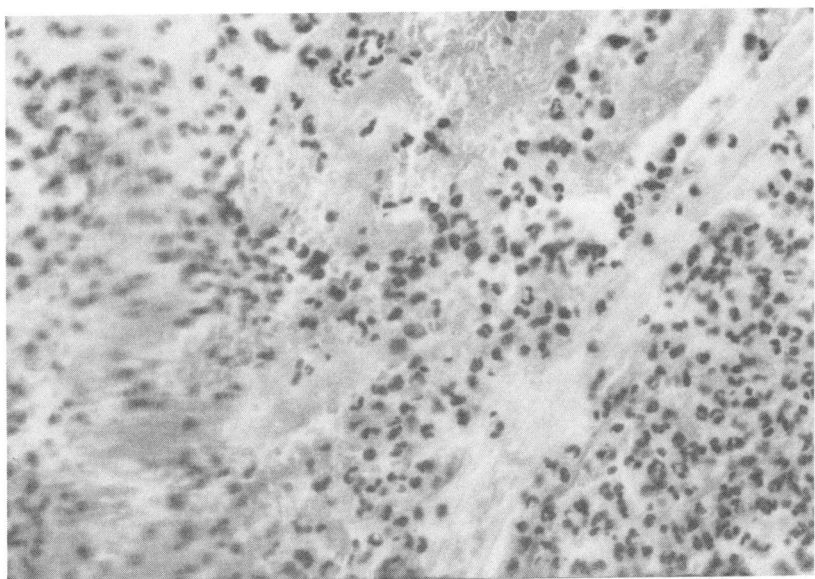

Figure 4 Neutrophil infiltration

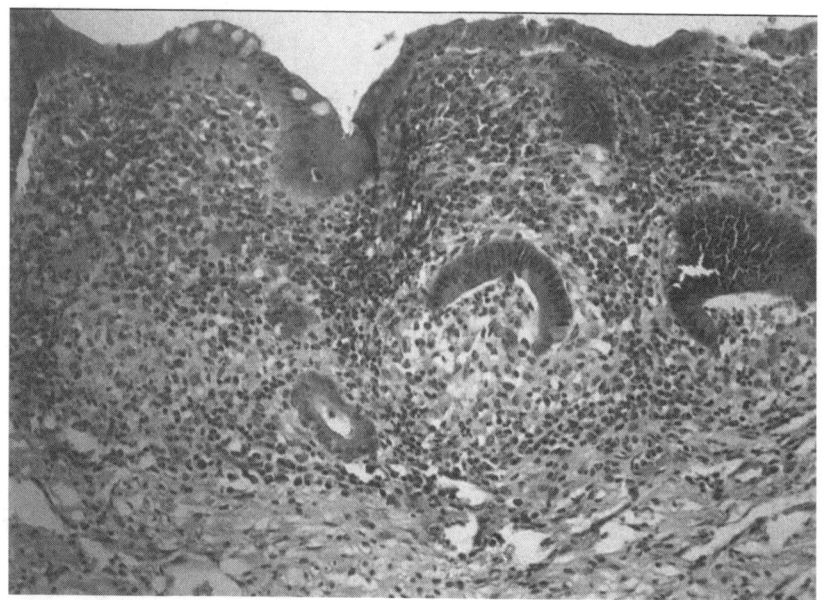

Figure 5 Atrophy and crypt abscesses

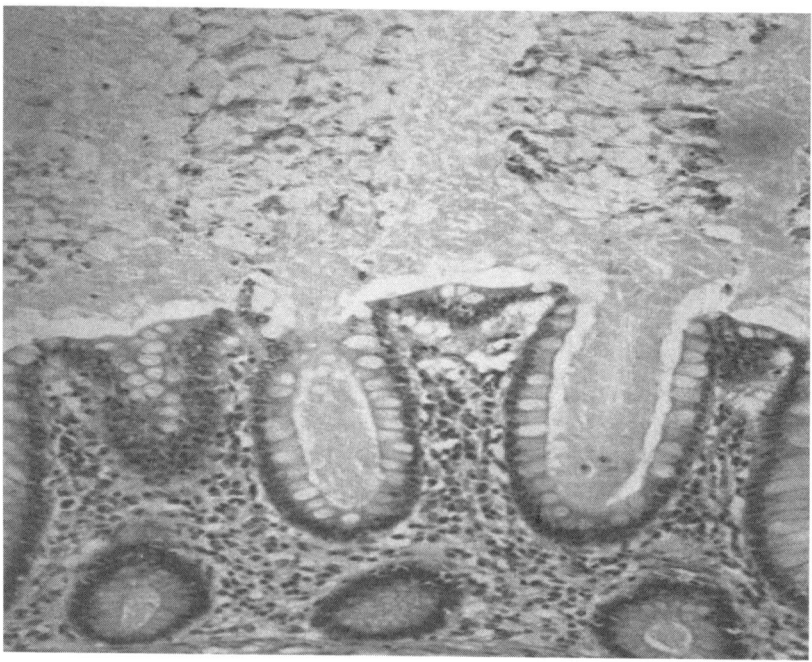

Figure 6 Hypersecretion of mucus

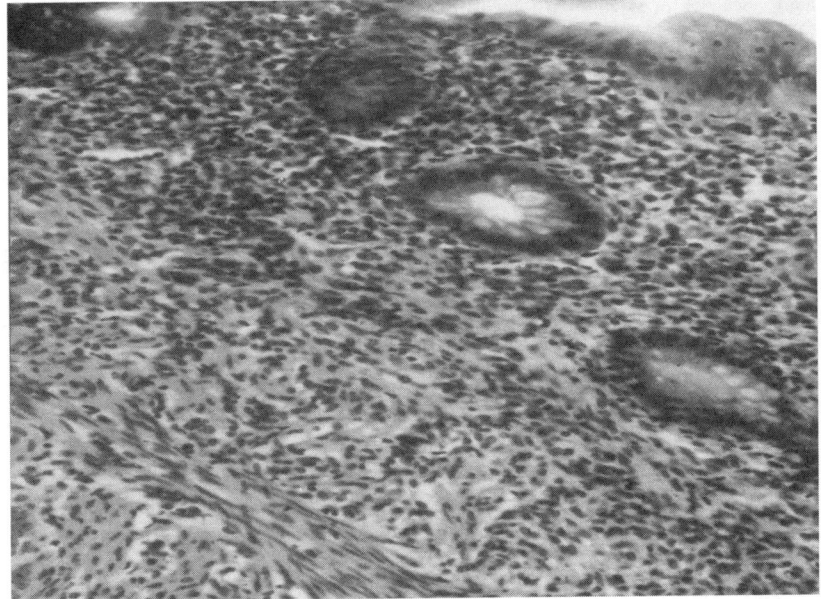

Figure 7 Atrophy and fibrosis

Patients in our study

During 1996–2005 we observed 112 women of 18–47 years old, who have presented with a primary attack of left-side UC. The health state in the majority of patients (87%) was in mild- and middle danger (diarrhoea attacks were noted up to 10–15 times over 24 h; the average blood loss was equal to 50–100 ml over 24 h, and duration of anamnesis was up 2 months). During rectosigmoidoscopy three or four biopsies were taken.

During the study we developed a scale of the extent of histological activities of UC (Table 1).

RESULTS AND DISCUSSION

After histological analysis, four groups were selected: In the first group of 22 cases (19.6%) the presence of crypt epithelium dystrophy in the mucosa was revealed, as well as damage to the microcirculation (capillary dilation, sludge, haemorrhage, oedema), and the presence in the infiltrate of a large number of eosinocytes (Figure 8). Anamnesis was particularly short in the patients of this group (from several days to 1 month).

In the second group of 44 cases (39.0%) purulent-destructive changes were discovered (predominantly infiltration with neutrophil leucocytes with secretion of cation proteins in the layer of mucosa above the epithelium, crypt abscesses).

Table 1 Scale of the extent of histological activities of ulcerative colitis

Signs	Degree	Points	k
Dystrophy colonocytes	None	0	
	Moderate	1	7
	Expressed	2	
Atrophy	None	0	
	Moderate	1	4
	Expressed	2	
Neutrophile infiltration	None	0	
	Moderate	1	7
	Expressed	2	
Eosinophile infiltration	None	0	
	Moderate	1	5
	Expressed	2	
Lymphocyte and plasmocyte infiltration	Moderate	0	
	Expressed	1	5
Crypt abscesses	None	0	
	Moderate	1	8
	Expressed	2	
Microcirculation	Moderate expansion capillary	1	
	Expressed expansion, sludge	2	6

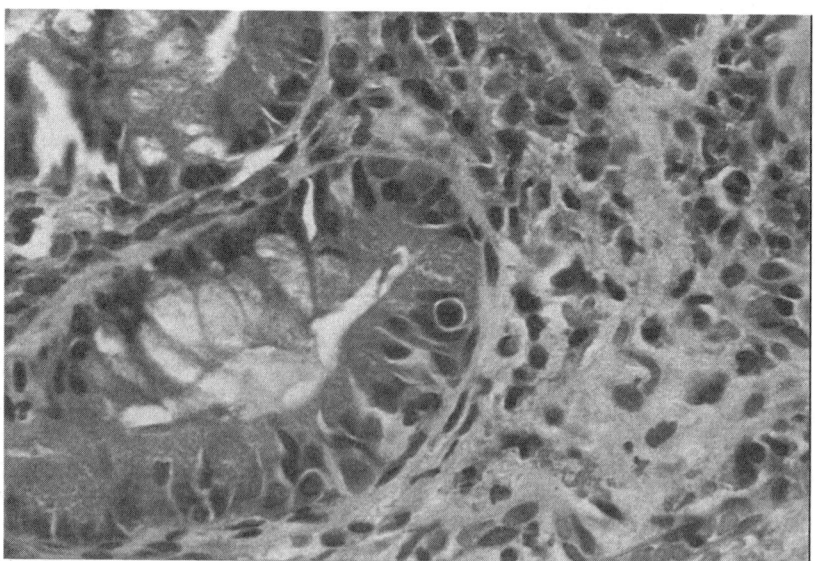

Figure 8 Eosinophil infiltration

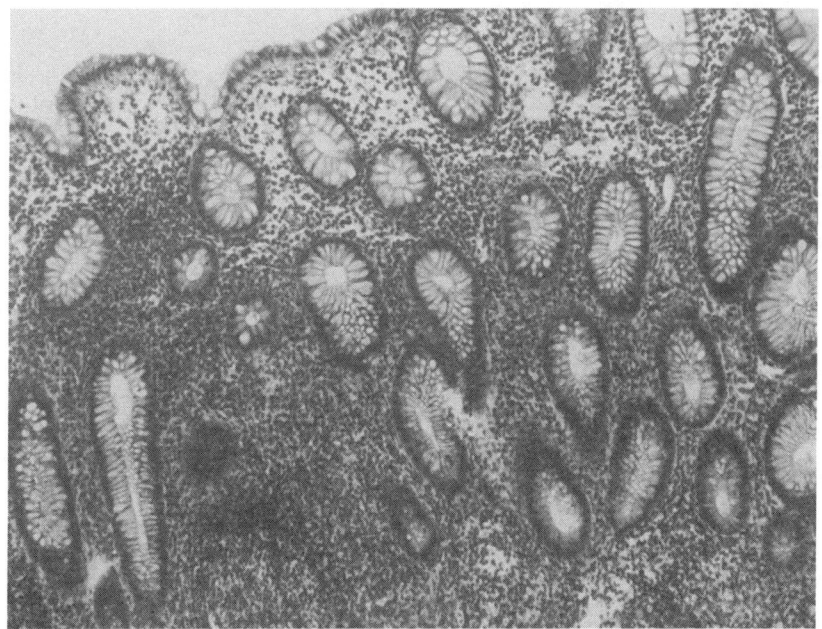

Figure 9 Lymphocytic infiltration, lymphoid follicles

In the third group of 9 cases (7.9%) with minimal clinical manifestation the presence of predominantly lymphoplasmacyte infiltration, lymphoid follicles (Figure 9), or fibrosis and atrophy was noted. Crohn's disease was excluded in this group of patients.

The fourth group of 37 cases (33.2%) was notable for mixed morphological changes.

Consequently, it is possible to select, as a minimum, three histological variants (or stages) of primary UC: capillaries–toxitic stages; destruction stages; atrophic–fibrotic stages.

It is possible that separation of these variants can promote the choice of the methods, modes and doses of treatment which, combined together, indicates a need for a study in a larger cohort.

The other approach to choice of treatment and determination of the real periods of the approach to remissions can be calculation of the index of histological activities of UC. The method is simple. The method including count value (k) each symptom and estimation signs in points. We have defined the following ranges of histological activity: serious relapse, 61–81 points; moderate relapse, 42–60 points; incomplete remission, 23–41 points; remission, 0–22 points.

We have defined that histological remission approaches for 4–5 weeks to later clinical remission and for 2–3 weeks later endoscopic remission.

DIFFERENTIAL DIAGNOSIS

It is therefore obvious that correct histological estimation promotes making a differential diagnosis of UC with Crohn's disease, lymphocytic colitis, collagenous colitis, and indeterminate colitis, as well as discovering different degrees of dysplasia.

CONCLUSION

The results of this study indicate that patients with UC in its initial stage of development can show various combinations of pathological changes in colon mucosa. Overall, the main tactics when considering choice of treatment of UC must be built on estimation of histological activities of the pathological process with provision for its localizations and extent. The main criterion of remission must be histological remission. Histological study can serve in an objective way not only for determination of remission, but also in helping in the choice of doses supporting medicine.

References

1. Aruin L, Kapuller L, Isakov V. Morphological Diagnostics of the Diseases of the Stomach and Bowels. Moscow; 1998.
2. Belousova E. Ulcerative Colitis and Crohn's Disease. Moscow; 2002.
3. Roth M, Bernhardt V. Inflammatory Bowel Diseases. Freiburg; 2006.

13
Crohn's disease of the small intestine: versions of the clinical picture and problems of differential diagnosis

L. B. LAZEBNIK and A. I. PARFENOV

INTRODUCTION

Crohn's disease (CD) of the small intestine (regional granulomatosis enteritis) is one of the internal organ diseases that is difficult to diagnose. The absence of clear symptoms, the presence of extraintestinal manifestations and the difficult visual observation of most of the small intestine lead to diagnostic difficulties in CD. This disease was described about 75 years ago by BB Crohn, L Ginsberg and GD Oppenheimer, but to date its unusual clinical picture is still being investigated.

This chapter gives a retrospective analysis of small intestinal CD diagnosis, as well as an analysis of clinical, X-ray, and endoscopic signs of this disease. The aim of this retrospective analysis is to improve early diagnosis of the disease.

One hundred and twenty patients with CD of the small intestine (66 men and 54 women, 23–77 years old; 53% being 20–30 years old) formed only 1.2% of the other intestinal diseases observed in the small intestine pathology department of our Institute during the past 15 years (1991–2005)[1]. This fact proved the rarity of CD. The fact that the disease was diagnosed in 82.5% of patients only in 2–7 years after the first clinical symptoms testified to the difficulty of diagnosis.

Some versions of CD were defined during investigation of the first clinical symptoms of the disease and its clinical course.

VERSIONS OF THE CLINICAL PICTURE

Localization and the acuteness of the pathological process, intensity and extent of inflammation, complications and extraintestinal manifestations mainly affect the clinical picture of small intestinal CD; 74 patients (61.7%) had inflammation in the terminal part of the ileum.

Inflammation had spread to the caecum in 32 patients with terminal ileitis, to the ascending colon in eight patients and to the duodenum in three patients. Three patients (2.5%) had granulomatous duodenitis. So 97.5% of patients with CD of the small intestine had inflammation of the distal part of the ileum, and 33.3% of patients had inflammation of the colon (especially caecum) at the same time.

ACUTE VERSION OF CD

The acute version of CD was found in 36 patients (30%). These patients were hospitalized with abdominal pain attack (mainly in the right iliac region) in the surgical department. Thirty patients were operated with urgent indications. Resection of changed intestine was performed in patients with inflammation of the terminal ileum, which sometimes spread to the caecum, and in those with peritonitis, due to perforation or necrosis of the changed intestine part. Resection of the terminal ileum part was performed in 17 patients, resection of the terminal ileum part and segment of jejunum was performed in nine patients, resection of ileum and right hemicolectomy was performed in four patients. No operation was performed in six patients, who had had a less acute initiation of the disease. The chronic course of CD was observed in these patients later.

CHRONIC RELAPSING CD

The primany chronic version

The fever, acceleration of erythrocyte sedimentation and leukocytosis, that testify to some inflammation, were the first clinical signs in 38 patients (31.7%).

Inflammation of the intestinal wall was mainly restricted by submucous intestinal base for a long time according to retrospective analysis. Chronic diarrhoea, sometimes with blood and abdominal pain attacks, which are typical of the intestinal contraction, were observed in patients after a few months or years. These symptoms are signs of a transmural lesion of the intestinal wall.

Anaemia, oedema, due to hypoproteinaemia, chronic diarrhoea and body weight decrease are signs of an intestinal lesion of considerable size, and the development of enteropathy with protein loss.

Stenosing version

Uncertain abdominal pain and extraintestinal manifestations (unclear fever, joint pain, erythema nodosum, etc.) were the symptoms of CD for a long time in 46 patients (38.3%). Diagnosis was unclear for many years. CD had evidently begun in childhood in three patients, since these patients showed physical deficiencies as well as sexual retardation. Sometimes it was possible to palpate infiltrate in the abdominal cavity. Later, the symptoms of intestinal obstruction increased: there were pain attacks, especially in the right iliac region, with vomiting, abdominal distention, loud rumbling, and retention of stool and flatus. It was possible to observe peristalsis with high 'toruses'. Most of the patients with CD had diarrhoea, but the mechanisms of its pathogenesis were different.

Patients with an ileal lesion have a changed intestinal absorption of bile acids, and they mostly have cholegenic diarrhoea (cholerrhoea). Strictures of small intestine, intestinal stasis and bacterial dissemination promote the hypersecretion of water and electrolytes in the intestinal lumen.

EXTRAINTESTINAL MANIFESTATIONS

Extraintestinal and systemic signs were revealed in 27 patients (22.5%). Well-known[2] osteal and articular syndromes (arthritis, spondylitis, sacroileitis), dermal and mucosal syndromes (erythema nodosum, stomatitis) and ophthalmic syndromes (iridocyclitis, keratoconjunctivitis) were found especially often. We have observed these uncommon extraintestinal manifestations also.

Patient T (45 years old) was examined in our Institute with severe myopathy of unclear aetiology. The results of his small intestinal investigations with videocapsule are presented in Figures 1–3. Videoendoscopic examination of this patient was performed in the Institute of Surgery of RAMS named after

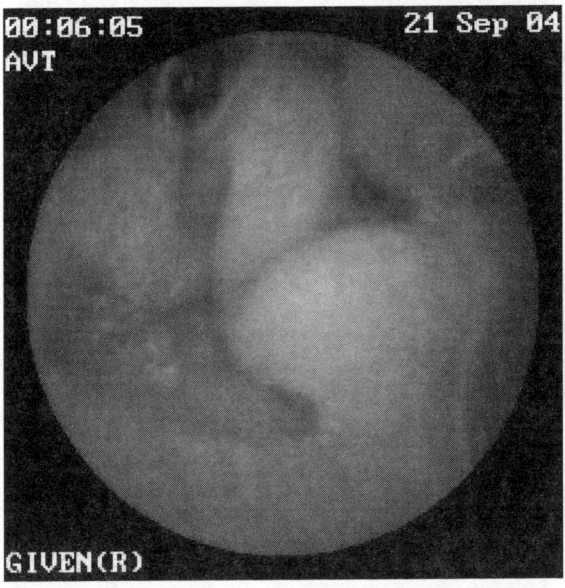

Figure 1   Videocapsule: erosions of the small intestine of patient T with Crohn's disease

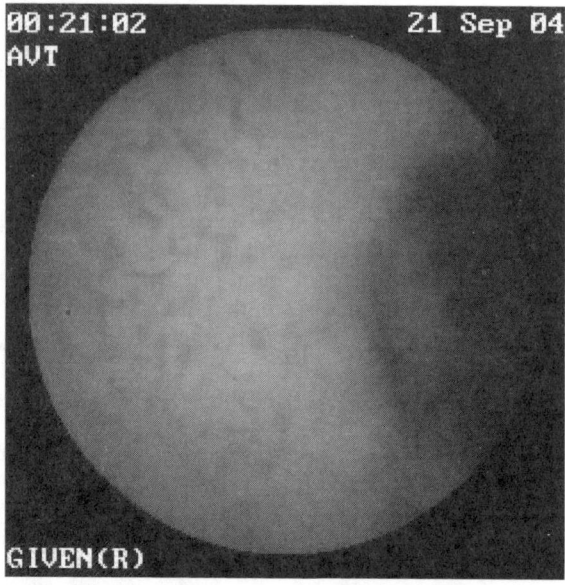

Figure 2 Videocapsule: erosions of the small intestine of patient T with Crohn's disease

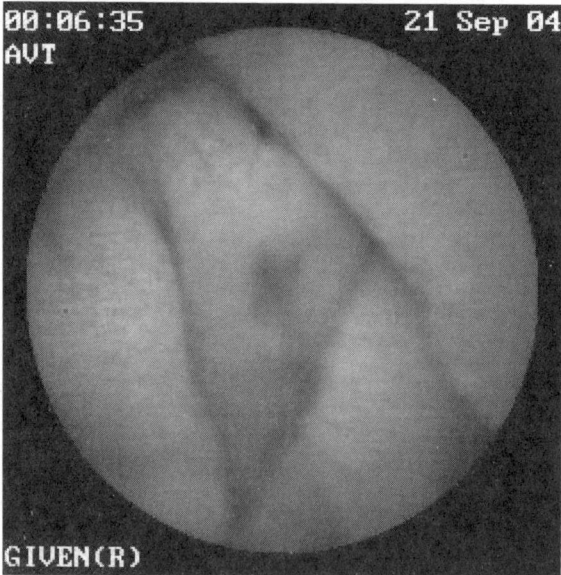

Figure 3 Videocapsule: erosions of the small intestine of patient T with Crohn's disease

AV Vishnevskyi. This examination revealed multiple erosions of the jejunum. The granulomatous inflammation in the middle part of the jejunum, that is typical of CD, was revealed with intestinoscopy. Treatment with metipred and pentas was effective. Pain in muscles had disappeared, and morphological remission was obtained. Another of our patients is a woman P, 50 years old. She had pains in her bones for 10 years. Osteoporosis was revealed with densimetry. Multiple stones in the gallbladder and kidneys were found in the year 2003. Pains in the eyeball appeared in January 2004.

Subacute fibrinous iridocyclitis of the right eye was diagnosed; this was treated with good effect in the ophthalmic hospital. The patient was hospitalized in the Institute of Gastroenterology for non-urgent cholecystectomy. A moderate painful infiltrate in the right iliac region size 3 × 10 cm, with solid-elastic consistency, was found. Ultrasonographic examination revealed irregular thickening of the terminal part ileum walls. The surrounding tissues were infiltrated and oedematic (Figures 4 and 5). X-ray examination of the ileocaecal region demonstrated the terminal part of the jejunum as a narrow (up 0.5 sm) irregular twist zone. Relief was disorderly, but evacuation through this zone was not disturbed (Figure 6).

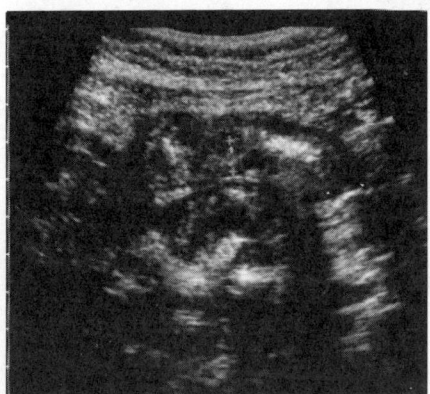

Figure 4   Ultrasonographic picture of iliac region of patient P. The walls of the terminal part of the ileum on the length 8 cm are irregular, thickening from 5 to 8 mm with hypoechoic structure

Ilioscopy

The intestinal mucus membrane was severely hyperaemic, oedematic, with a patch that resembled pus with pseudopolypous formations which form specific irregular relief (Figure 7).

The painful infiltrate with solid-elastic consistency and size 3–4 cm that was connected with skin and slightly raised above the region of the left cheek had formed during the patient's examination. A single superficial rounded ulcer (aphthae) with size 0.3 cm, that had a severe thin red border and a slight yellow

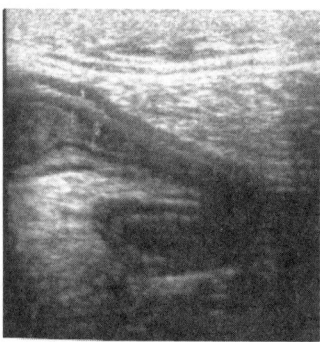

Figure 5 Ultrasonographic picture of the right iliac region of patient P. Surrounding tissues are infiltrated and oedematic

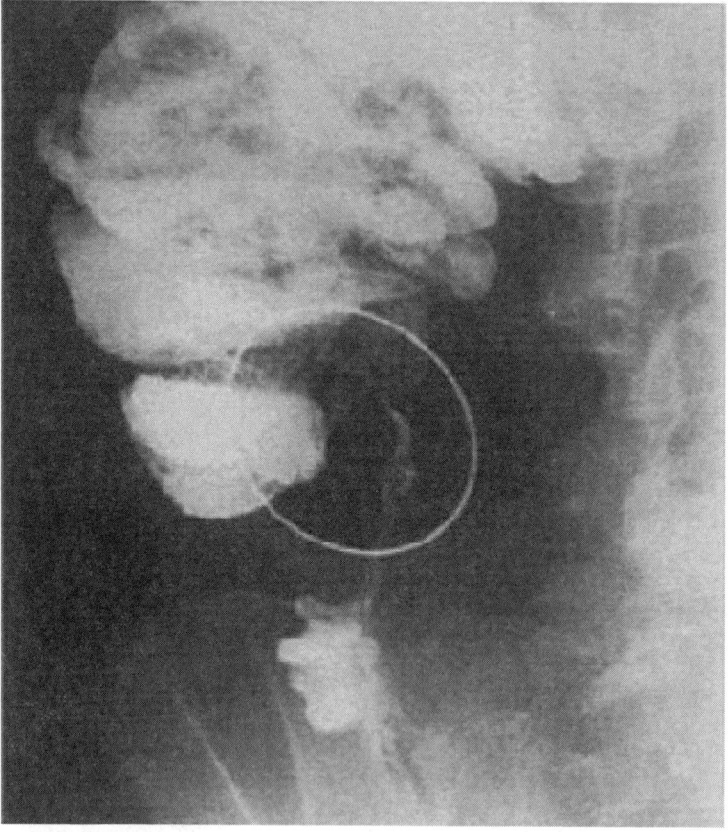

Figure 6 Roentgenogram of patient P with retrograde barium filling-up of large intestine and ileum. Severe contraction of ileum in terminal part. Crohn's disease of ileum

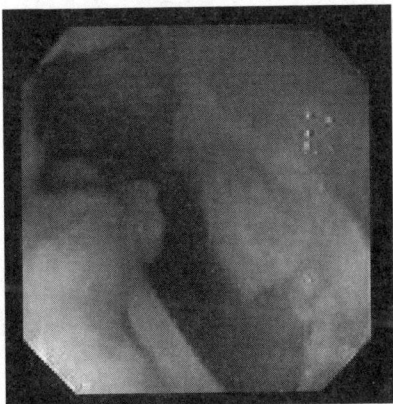

Figure 7 Ileoscopy of patient P. The mucus membrane of the small intestine is severely hyperaemic and oedematic, with a patch that resembles pus with pseudopolypous formations which form specific irregular relief

Table 1 The rare extraintestinal manifestations of Crohn's disease

Localization	Typical signs
Skin	Vesiculo-pustular, erythematous, ulcerative-destructive granulomatous lesion[3] Syndrome Svite (acute dermatosis, pyoderma)[4,5] Sarcoidal cicatrices[5]; vasculitis Sheilein–Genokha[6]
Mucus membranes	Granulomatous kxeilit, vulvit[7]; stomatitis[8] Metastases of Crohn's disease[9,10]
Muscles	Myopathy[11]
Vessels	Chronic aortitis[12]; Takayasu disease[13]
Lungs	Granulomatous tracheobronchitis[13]; sarcoidosis[14]
Liver	Granulomatous hepatitis; cholestatic hepatitis[15]
Biliary tract	Primary sclerosing cholangitis[16]
Kidneys	Nephrotic syndrome, amyloidosis[17]
Nervous system	Peripheral neuropathy; epileptic attacks; depression[18] Vasculitis of the central nervous system[19]

patch on its base, was revealed on the mucus membrane of the mouth cavity in the infiltrate's projection.

The patient was treated with metipred 48 mg/day, dexsamethasone by vein through a dropper 60 mg/day, Salofalk 1.5 g/day and abdominal pains ceased, the infiltrate of the left cheek had disappeared in 3–4 days, and the infiltrate in the right iliac region had disappeared in 10 days.

So CD in this patient was manifested with iridocyclitis, osteoporosis, cholelithiasis and urolithiasis, as well as with metastatic lesions of skin and subcutaneous fatty tissue.

The rate of CD activity may be determined using a special index: index Best[21], index Van Geesa[22], and index of severity and activity (SAF)[23] have been suggested at different times. The index of activity by Best is graded at 0 in healthy persons, less than 150 in persons with slight activity, and more than 150 in patients with severe activity.

DIAGNOSIS

The right diagnosis in patients with acute version CD was usually revealed using laparoscopy or laparotomy, that were performed because of the supposed diagnosis of acute appendicitis. The compact hyperaemic part of the intestine, enlarged lymphatic nodes of radix mesenterii and complications (perforation, abscess, stenosis) were found during the operation. In these cases it is necessary to perform differential diagnosis with iersiniosis, that may manifest with acute terminal ileitis. It is necessary to perform special serological examinations.

Sarcoidosis-like granulomas with Pirogov–Langhans cells in the submucosal base, severe infiltration of the intestinal wall with lymphoid cells (Figure 8) and ulcers up to the serous membrane (Figure 9) were revealed in the operative material of the intestinal wall in 40% of patients.

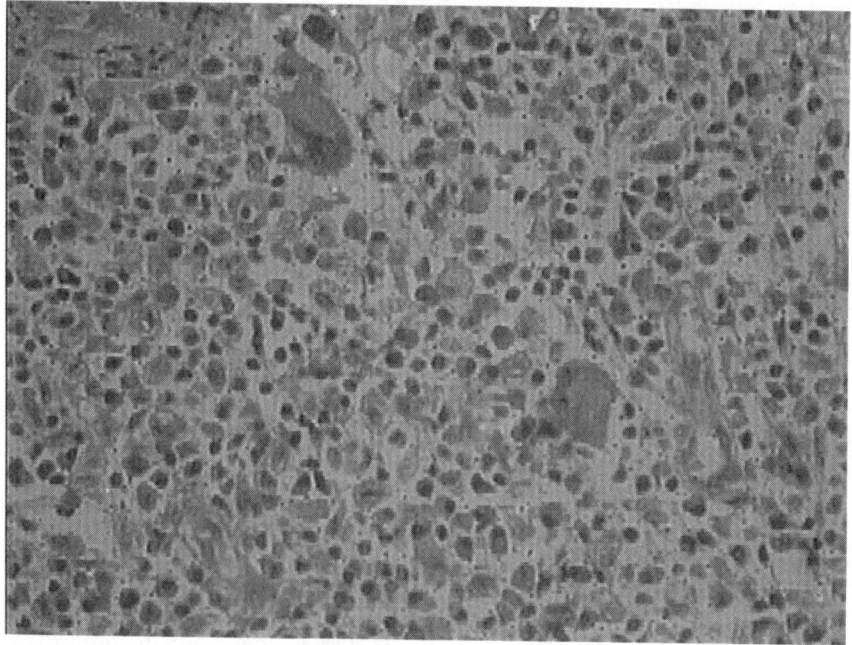

Figure 8 Microphoto: Crohn's disease. Granulomas. Staining with haematoxylin and eosin; original magnification × 500. Operative material

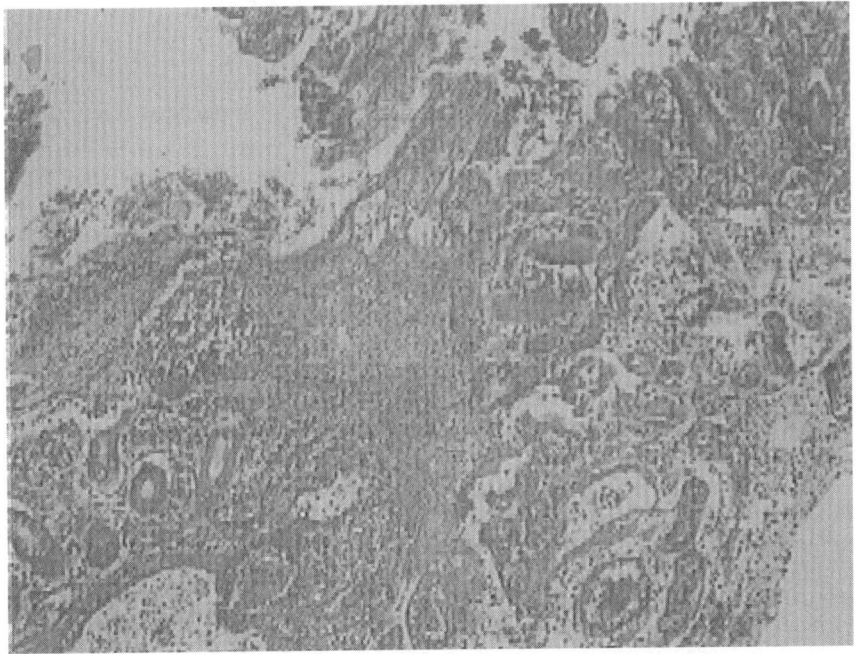

Figure 9 Microphoto: Crohn's disease. Fissured ulcer. Staining with haematoxylin and eosin; original magnification × 120. Operative material

Diagnosis in patients with the stenosing version and the primary chronic version of CD is very difficult, and disease is usually diagnosed 3–5 years after the appearance of the first clinical symptoms. The loss of body weight may be very significant up to cachexia. Poor absorption and increased protein catabolism due to inflammation are the reasons for the trophicity disturbance.

Sometimes it is possible to see the asymmetry of the abdomen due to the protruding belly in the right lower region. The mild infiltrate due to oedematic and compacted intestinal wall or interintestinal abscess is revealed with palpation.

Iron deficiency or B_{12}-deficiency anaemia, disturbance of bleeding time, and decrease of prothrombin may be revealed during analysis of blood. A steady lowering of protein may be observed in patients with lesions of the small intestine due to severe protein exudation in the intestinal lumen.

X-ray examination of stomach and small intestine may be performed only in the absence of partial small intestinal obstruction. The line of narrowing intestinal parts, that are divided by normal segments, is the usual picture of granulomatous enteritis. Diagnosis is very difficult in early stages. However, it it is possible to find superficial aphthae or linear ulcers in the distal part of the ileum using the method of double-contrast with barium enema or during the usual movement of barium sulphate.

According to the classification of Herlinger and Medlinte[20], based on X-ray and morphological changes, there are three stages of CD. The first stage is the early changes. Typical signs are thickening and straightening of folds due to submucous oedema and the presence of multiple small superficial ulcers up to 0.1–0.2 cm, surrounded by infiltrative torus. The intestinal wall is elastic. The second stage is the intermediate changes. The presence of nodular relief, ulcerations, rigidity of mesenterial margin and the presence of pseudodiverticula on the other margin are typical signs of this stage. The intestinal wall is significantly thickened; the intestinal lumen is normal. There are nodular defects of equal size with diameter <1 cm due to submucous oedema with atrophy and cicatrization of the mucus membrane. The third stage is the stage of significant changes. The ulcerative and nodular relief of mucus (symptom 'cobbled road'), the presence of deep fissural ulcerations with spasm and lumen narrowing, that resembles cord, are typical signs of this stage. The distance between intestinal loops is increased; intestinal walls are thickened and rigid.

The signs of the first stage of CD were revealed in 7.5% of patients. One of these patients had absence of visual ulcerations that had made the X-ray diagnosis difficult, but after 1 year an X-ray picture of this patient had demonstrated significant changes; one more segment was revealed in one of the proximal intestinal loops with the signs of early changes.

The second stage of CD was revealed in 22.5% of patients; 70% of patients had demonstrated an X-ray picture of the third stage. The signs of jejunal obstruction (fixed intestinal loops with gas) were revealed on X-ray of the abdominal cavity in the right lower quadrant in these patients. The intestinal lumen was significantly narrowed in all these patients. Alternation of the intestinal parts with different stages of lesions and the normal intestinal segments was revealed in all patients in the third stage of CD.

At the present time ultrasonographic examination is used for diagnosis of CD. The typical thickening of the intestinal wall and the increase of lymphatic nodes in the small intestinal mesentery are revealed using this method. The endoscopic method with histological examination of the small intestinal mucus membrane is limited, since only 10–50 cm of ileum may be examined with retrograde ileoscopy in most patients. Intestinoscopy with a special fibroscope is used to examine the upper part of the small intestine.

There is usually severe oedema of the intestinal mucus membrane, which thickens, with ulcerations, rough folds and multiple haemorrhages. The deformation and narrowness of the stomach, typical changes of mucus membrane relief due to submucous nodes, and the presence of pseudodiverticula etc. are observed in patients with granulomatous process in the stomach or duodenum. The granulomas, that resemble sarcoids, were very rarely revealed with histological examination of bioptats (only in single cases). Macroscopic changes in the intestinal walls have major significance for the diagnosis of CD.

DIFFERENTIAL DIAGNOSIS

The diagnosis of CD is especially suspected in the young patients with diarrhoea, fever, loss of body mass, permanent pains in the right iliac region and especially with infiltrate in the same region. Differential diagnosis with acute appendicitis, iersiniosal ileitis, necrotic enteritis due to *Clostridium perfringens* and eosinophilic gastroenteritis must be performed in patients with the acute version of CD.

The anamnesis with exacerbations is more prolonged in patients with CD versus patients with appendicitis. Videolaparoscopy of the organs of the abdominal cavity significantly simplifies this differential diagnosis.

The first clinical symptoms of iersiniosal ileitis are very similar to the symptoms of CD. Definite serological and bacteriological reactions are used in these cases[24]. Repeated X-ray and endoscopic examinations are performed in doubtful cases. The intestinal changes are reversible in patients with iersiniosal ileitis versus patients with CD.

Differential diagnosis with follicular ileitis, non-sclerosing ileitis, chronic non-granulomatous ulcerous ileitis (jejunoileitis) and eosinophilic gastroenteritis is very difficult.

Nodular lymphoid hyperplasia, which forms irregular relief of mucus membrane in the region of Peyer's patches and in the terminal part of the ileum, is a typical sign of follicular ileitis. Acute follicular ileitis develops in children with measles and other infectious diseases. The clinical picture resembles acute appendicitis with pains in the right iliac region, vomiting, fever and leukocytosis. Hyperaemia and oedema of the terminal part of the ileum on the length 10–20 cm, induration and increase of mesenterial lymphatic nodes are revealed with laparotomy. This special treatment is not necessary in patients with acute follicular ileitis versus patients with CD, and it disappears without any medicine in a few days. Subacute follicular ileitis develops in a few weeks; the typical signs are diarrhoea, nausea, vomiting and fever up 38°C. Infiltrate is sometimes revealed in the right iliac region. The round pseudopolypous formations (nodous lymphoid hyperplasia) are revealed with X-ray and endoscopic examination in the distal iliac region. Tuberculosis, iersiniosis, viral or other infections are the reasons for subacute follicular ileitis.

Mild pains in the right iliac region and severe nodular lymphoid hyperplasia are typical signs of chronic follicular ileitis (Figure 10). The changes of relief are the same as in patients with Crohn's disease; the main difference is the absence of sclerosal changes of the intestinal wall. Chronic follicular ileitis is usually named non-sclerosal ileitis[25]; its aetiology is usually unknown; sometimes it may be iersiniosal ileitis.

Chronic ulcerous non-granulomatous ileitis (jejunoileitis)

This is a rare disease of unknown aetiology. Chronic diarrhoea, enteropathy with protein loss, cachexia, and pain in abdomen that resembles colic are the typical signs of the condition. Fever, anaemia, leukocytosis, hypoproteinaemia and secondary hypogammaglobulinaemia are very often revealed also. Total or subtotal atrophy of mucus membrane with ulcers and mainly

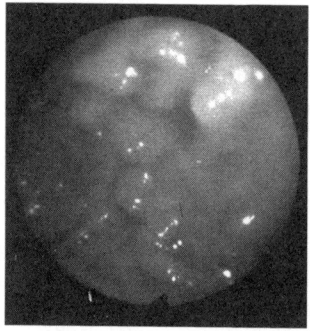

Figure 10 Ileoscopy. Terminal ileitis with nodal lymphoid hyperplasia

lymphoplasmocyte infiltration of the propria lamina small intestine mucus membrane are revealed using histological examination of bioptats. The number of crypts is decreased.

Granulomatous proliferation or parasitogenic inclusions are absent; a gluten-free diet is not effective. The corticosteroids promote remission. The prognosis of non-granulomatous ileitis is indefinite but spontaneous remission sometimes occurs.

Eosinophilous gastroenteritis

Eosinophilous gastroenteritis, with segmentary intestinal lesions, severe oedema and thickening of intestinal wall, resembles CD.

Macroscopic changes in the mucus membrane ('cobbled road') fissures, ulcers and erosions that are not typical of eosinophilous enteritis, but are typical in patients with CD, are the differential criteria to diagnosis in such patients.

Epitheliocellular granulomas and the absence of mucus membrane infiltration with eosinophils are typical signs with microscopic examination in patients with CD, and CD is necessary to differentiate with granulomatous inflammation of small intestine of known aetiology. The aetiology may be tuberculosis, vascular lesions, mycosis, sarcoidosis, lymphogranulomatosis or parasitogenic invasions.

CONCLUSIONS

The advantage of gastroenterology is the accessibility of visual and histological examination of gastroenterological organs, including the small intestine. The intestine may be observed inside and outside using modern endoscopic methods. It is possible to observe the intestinal walls and surrounding tissues with ultrasonography and computer tomography.

So it seems that the problems of intestinal diagnosis are solved; but the diagnosis of terminal ileitis, and especially of jejunoileitis, is very complex. The first reason for this is the clinical training of physicians. Usually a doctor diagnoses the diseases that he or she knows. So the doctor must first know the clinical signs of CD, and must search with roentgenologists, endoscopists and other specialists, for this disease in patients who have typical clinical signs.

References

1. Adler G. Crohn's disease and ulcerative colitis [translation from German]. M:Geotar. Med. 2001.
2. Krikunov VP, Goloviznin MV. Seronegative spondyloarthritis in patients with nonspecific ulcerative colitis and Crohn's disease. In: Rheumatic Diseases. Medicine. 1997:331–5.
3. Matheson BK, Gilbertson EO, Eichenfield LF. Vesiculopustular eruption of Crohn's disease. Pediatrics. 1996;13:127–30.
4. Gonzalvez Perales JL, Tamarit Orti R, Ballester Fayos J et al. A case of Sweet's syndrome associated with Crohn's disease. Gastroenterol Hepatol. 1997;20:134–7.
5. Travis S, Innes N, Davies MG et al. Sweet's syndrome: an unusual cutaneous feature of Crohn's disease or ulcerative colitis. Eur J Gastroenterol Hepatol. 1997;9:715–20.
6. Schlehaider UK, Suckow M, Rosenthal P et al. Cutaneous reactions in Crohn disease. Vasculitis in various skin segments. Hautarzt. 1997;48:328–31.
7. Rogers RS 3rd, Bekic M. Diseases of the lips. Semin Cutan Med Surg. 1997;16:328–36
8. Dunlap CL, Friesen CA, Shultz R. Chronic stomatitis: an early sign of Crohn's disease. J Am Dent Assoc. 1997;128:347–8.
9. Chiba M, Iizuka M, Horie Y et al. Metastatic Crohn's disease involving the penis. J Gastroenterol. 1997;32:817–21.
10. Sangueza OP, Davis LS, Gourdin FW. Metastatic Crohn's disease. South Med J. 1997;90:897–900.
11. Heuss D, Hauser I, Riess R. Atypical inflammatory myopathy associated with Crohn's disease. Clin Neuropathol. 1996;15:150–4.
12. Wackerlin A, Zund G, Maggiorini M et al. Aortic valve insufficiency in Crohn's disease. Schweiz Med Wochenschr. 1997;127:935–9.
13. Houman MH, Doghri A, Boubaker J et al. Takayasu disease in Crohn's disease: an exceptional association. Ann Gastroenterol Hepatol (Paris). 1996;31:337–40.
14. Fellermann K, Stahl M, Dahlhoff K et al. Crohn's disease and sarcoidosis: systemic granulomatosis? Eur J Gastroenterol Hepatol. 1997;9:121–4.
15. Hilzenrat N, Lamoureux E, Sherker A et al. Cholestasis in Crohn's disease: a diagnostic challenge. Can J Gastroenterol. 1997;11:35–7.
16. Rasmussen HH, Fallingborg JF, Mortensen PB et al. Hepatobiliary dysfunction and primary sclerosing cholangitis in patients with Crohn's disease. Scand J Gastroenterol. 1997;32:604–10.
17. Kullmann F, Kullmann M, Leser HG et al. Nephrotic syndrome as the initial symptom of Crohn disease. Z Gastroenterol. 1996;34:757–62
18. Elsehety A, Bertorini TE. Neurologic and neuropsychiatric complications of Crohn's disease. South Med J. 1997;90:606–10.
19. Brohee P, Violon P, Mavroudakis N et al. Central nervous system lesions associated with Crohn's disease. J Neuroimaging. 1997;7:195–8.
20. Herlinger H, Medlinte D. Clinical Radiology of the Small Intestine. Philadelphia: Saunders. 1989:295–335.
21. Best WR, Becktel JM, Singleton JW et al. Development of a Crohn's disease activity index. National Cooperative Crohn's disease study. Gastroenterology. 1976;70:439–44.
22. van Hees PAM, van Elteren PH, van Lier HJJ et al. An index of inflammmatory activity in patients with Crohn's disease. Gut. 1980;21:279–86.
23. Goebell H. Different activity indices in Crohn's disease and their possible role. In: H. Goebell et al., editors. Inflammatory Bowel Diseases: Basic Research and Clinical Implications. Lancaster: MTP Press, 1988:253–8.
24. Parfenov AI. Diseases of Ileocecal Region. Moscow:Anakharsis. 2005:103–38.
25. Von Ernst Hafter. Praktische Gastroenterologie. 5. Neuberarbetete Auflage. Stuttgart: Georg Thième Verlag, 1973:288–90.

14
Distal colitis as a special pattern of ulcerative colitis

I. L. KHALIF and N. S. MALAKHOVA

As is well known, ulcerative colitis (UC) always starts with a lesion of the rectum[1–5]. The development of the disease is such that some patients have a total lesion of the large intestine, and in some patients the inflammation can have a limited character for a long period of time. In patients with initially localized UC (proctitis and proctosigmoiditis) the inflammation during the patient's life can be localized only to distal sections, while in others the inflammation can extend to proximal sections of the large intestine.

Recently we have formed the opinion that UC is a heterogenic disease that includes different clinical subgroups, distal forms being one of them.

Distal UC, irrespective of its small area of lesion of the large intestine, has all the negative properties characteristic of UC: limited or complete loss of the capacity for work, chronic continuous character with resistance to basic anti-inflammatory preparations in 25–50% of cases, the necessity of surgical treatment in 14–16% of cases due to inefficiency of conservative therapy, and development of complications threatening the life of a patient[1,6,7].

For the period 1980–2003 a total of 832 patients of age groups from 15–73 years were observed at the Centre, with the initial diagnosis 'distal UC form'. The average age of patients was 44 ± 5 years. In the majority of patients – 600 (72.1%) – UC developed when they were 20–49 years old. There were 369 (44.4%) men and 463 (55.6%) women. By the time of the first consultation in the Centre 219 (26.3%) patients had proctitis and 613 (73.6%) had proctosigmoiditis. The length of the illness was from 3 months to 27 years. More than half of patients – 426 (51.2%) – had a duration of disease from 6 months to 10 years (thus the average duration of the disease was 5.25 ± 1.25 years). An acute form of UC was observed in 96 patients (11.5%), a chronic recurring form in 493 (59.3%) patients, and a chronic continuous form in 243 (29.2%) patients. In proctitis cases the chronic uninterrupted clinical course prevailed – 123 (56.2%) cases. A chronic recurring clinical course was observed in 73 (33.3%) cases, and an acute clinical course in 23 (10.5%) cases. On the contrary in proctosigmoiditis the chronic recurring clinical course prevailed – 420 patients (68.5%). A chronic continuous course was found in 120 (19.6%) cases and an acute course was observed in 73 (11.9%) cases. As far as the severity of exacerbations was concerned the mild form prevailed – 498 patients (59.9%), moderate in 302 patients (36.3%), and severe exacerbation in 32 patients (3.8%).

Perianal lesions were observed in some patients. For the whole duration of observation they were detected in 75 (9.01%) out of 832 cases. Anal fissures were observed in 14 patients (18.66%), a pararectal fistula after the paraproctitis autopsy in 46 patients (61.33%), and the combination of anal fissure and fistula occurred in 15 patients (20%).

Transformation of the disease into the extensive form occurred in 118 (14.18%) patients with the initial diagnosis of distal UC form (Table 1).

Table 1 Transformation frequency of distal form of UC into the extensive form

Types of distal form of UC	Number of patients (n = 118)	Percentage
Left-sided proctitis	5	4.23
Total proctitis	8	6.77
Left-sided proctosigmoiditis	45	38.12
Total sigmoiditis	60	50.84

It is worth mentioning that on the whole transformation occurred in proctosigmoiditis in 105 patients, which constituted 89%. Transformation into the extensive lesion of the large intestine occurred in 13 patients (11%) with the initial diagnosis 'UC in the form of proctitis'. Thus essential differences have been revealed in the frequency of transformation of UC depending on its form – proctitis or sigmoiditis ($p < 0.05$).

By the transformation date the age of patients varied from 15 to 70 years of age – 43.5 ± 5 on average (Table 2). The largest group of patients was from 20 to 49 years old (34.5 ± 3.5 years). This group constituted 83 patients (70.3%).

Table 2 Distribution of patients between age groups by the time of distal UC transformation into extensive forms

Age at the time of UC transformation (years)	Number of patients (n = 118)	Percentage
15–19	2	1.69
20–29	22	18.65
30–39	34	28.81
40–49	27	22.89
50–59	18	15.25
60–69	8	6.77
70 and older	7	5.93

Table 3 Duration of UC prior to its development into extensive forms

Duration of UC by the time of transformation	Number of patients (n = 118)	Percentge
3–6 months	2	1.69
6 months–1 year	18	15.25
1–5 years	49	41.52
6–10 years	24	20.33
11–15 years	12	10.16
16–20 years	10	8.47
> 20 years	3	2.54

The duration of the disease by the time of transformation was from 3 months to 20 years, the average was 10.15 ± 2 years (Table 3).

Most frequently the transformation occurred during the period from 1 to 5 years anamnesis (3 ± 0.5 years on average). This group included 49 patients (41.5%): 11 of them (22.4%) were 20–29 years old (24.5 ± 0.5 years of age on average); 20 patients (40.81%) were 30–39 years old (34.5 ± 0.5 years of age on average); 15 patients (30.61%) were 40–49 years old (44.5 ± 0.5 years of age on average); one patient (2%) was 17, and two patients (4%) were 60–69 years old (64.5 ± 0.5 years of age on average).

The severity of exacerbation of UC in patients with subsequent transformation into the extensive forms during the first visit to the Centre is shown in Table 4.

Table 4 Severity of exacerbation of UC in patients with subsequent transformation into extensive forms at the time of the first visit to the Centre

Severity of exacerbation of UC	Number of patients (n = 118)	Percentage
Mild	28	23.7
Moderate	86	72.8
Severe	4	3.5

We observed a tendency towards severity of exacerbation with UC trasformation into extensive forms (Table 5). Thus the attack of the disease during or after which transformation into the extensive form of UC was registered had moderate or severe forms.

In accordance with previous reports perianal lesions are not characteristic of UC, but their frequency rate amounts to 3–5%[8,9]. The frequency rate of perianal lesions in the distal form of UC with its subsequent trasformation into the extensive forms has not been studied. The data acquired in our study on the higher frequency rate of perianal lesions (9.01%) in the general structure of the distal UC form as compared to 3–5%, are new and noteworthy. In the assessed 118 patients with transformation into extensive forms of UC, 61 had

Table 5 Severity of exacerbation of UC on the time of transformation

Severity of exacerbation on the time of transformation	Number of patients (n = 118)	Percentage
Moderate	69	58.47
Severe	49	41.53

perianal lesions (51.7%). The data acquired on the high rate of perianal lesions in patients with transformation into the extensive forms of UC demonstrate the aggressive pathomorphism of the distal UC form in the presence of perianal lesions.

We have carried out a comparative analysis of the clinical manifestation in three groups of patients. In the first group 714 patients had the distal UC form during the whole trial period. In the second group were 74 patients with transformation into extensive UC, but without subsequent surgical procedure. In the third group there were 44 patients with transformation into extensive UC with subsequent surgical treatment.

Earlier reports[6] state that UC starts to manifest itself with blood in the normal faeces and then stool becomes more and more frequent. Such an initial stage of the disease correlates with its subsequent resistant severe clinical course. On the contrary, when the disease begins with diarrhoea, with the subsequent appearance of blood in faeces, such a course is more often observed in mild forms which show a good response to basic anti-inflammatory therapy. In view of this we decided to specify initial symptoms of the disease: 'presence of blood in faeces' and 'diarrhoea' and study their occurrence in distal UC (Table 6). On the basis of the analysis of occurrence of these two symptoms in the trial groups it was revealed that the initial presence of blood in the normal faeces and then the more frequent stool was observed in 518 patients, which constituted 62.2%. The occurrence of this symptom did not vary significantly in trial groups of patients; therefore it was not associated with the subsequent severity of the course of the disease.

Table 6 Comparative analysis of the clinical manifestation features of the disease in distal UC patients

Manifestation features	First group (n = 714)	Percentage	Second group (n = 74)	Percentage	Third group (n = 44)	Percentage
Starting with blood in the faeces	448	62.7	41	55.4	29	65.9
Starting with diarrhoea	266	37.3	33	44.6	15	34.1

We carried out a comparative analysis of the initial severity of the disease in the aforementioned three groups of patients at their first visit to the Centre of Coloproctology. Analysis of the data obtained demonstrated that the first group of patients is characterized by the mild form at the initial stage – 470 patients (65.8%) as compared to the second and third groups, where mild forms of UC at the first visit to the Centre totalled 28 patients (23.7%). Correspondingly in the second and third groups the number of cases having the moderate course of the disease was higher (about 3 times as high) and was observed in 86 patients (72.8%). In the first group the manifestation of the disease of moderate severity was observed in 216 patients (30.2%), and the severe initial stage of the disease was about the same in all three groups (2.7–4.6%).

The disease after transformation into extensive forms showed a moderate severe and severe character together with a chronic continuous course of illness. Of 118 patients 44 (37.3%) demanded surgery due to inefficiency of treatment and development of enteric complications of the disease (Table 7).

Table 7   Indications for surgery after transformation into extensive UC

Indications for surgery	Number of patients (n = 44)	Percentage
Melaena	14	31.8
Hormone dependence	15	34.2
Hormone resistance	15	34.2

In the group of patients with the initial diagnosis as UC in the form of proctosigmoiditis (832 patients) surgical treatment was necessary only for 44 patients (6.2%) after transformation into the extensive form. For patients with the initial diagnosis – UC in the form of proctitis – there was no need for surgical treatment either before or after its transformation into extensive forms.

None of 832 patients developed malignization.

The essence of the disease is pathomorphological changes in the colon mucosa; that is why the next stage of the UC distal form study was analysis of the endoscopic and morphological chatacteristics of the colon mucosa.

Microscopic changes of the intestinal wall in UC patients with extensive lesions are comprehensively described in the literature[2,10–13]. Analysis of the morphological basis of the disease stays acute for early detection of dysplasia and colon cancer and prediction of the course of the disease. Taking into consideration the possibility of transformation of distal UC, the absence of unbiased criteria that permit us to determine the risk group of patients of such a course of the disease prior to the inpatient stage of treatment, we have undertaken research aimed at estimating the necessity of histological biopsy tests of samples from all sections of the colon, and not only the section(s) affected by a lesion (rectum or rectum and sigmoid intestine) in each separate case of distal UC.

To estimate the necessity of step-by-step biopsy for each patient with the distal form of UC we have studied 76 distal UC patients (proctitis and proctosigmoiditis), comprising 36 women and 40 men. They have undergone total colonoscopy with biopsy of all sections of the large intestine. Samples were taken from the caecum, ascending, transverse, and descending colon; sigmoid intestine and rectum; and also from the section 5 cm proximal to the visually detected border of inflammation in the intestine.

As the result of comparison of endoscopic and morphological methods of checkup four types of change were determined in the large intestine:

- An isolated lesion of the rectum, or both the rectum and the sigmoid intestine, with proved morphological absence of the lesion of proximal sections of the colon – 27 patients (35.5%).

- An isolated lesion of the rectum, or both the rectum and the sigmoid intestine, with morphological features of inflammation of all sections of the large intestine – 26 patients (34.2%).

- A segmentary lesion of the intestine (distal sections of the large intestine and the lesion focus in the caecum) and morphological features of inflammation in all sections of the large intestine – 18 patients (24.0%).

- An isolated lesion of the rectum, or the rectum and the sigmoid intestine, and morphological features of inflammation in the caecum – five patients (6.3%).

Therefore only 27 patients (35.5%) with a distal UC lesion have morphological proof of the absence of the lesion in the upper sections of the large intestine.

In more than half of cases in the trial, i.e. 44 patients (58.2%), morphological tests of biopsy material taken from all sections of the large intestine revealed slight or moderately developed inflammation in all sections of the large intestine. During the follow-up period of 2 years, three patients (6.8%) with the presence of morphological changes in the visually intact proximal sections of the colon have developed clinically manifested inflammation (transformation). This permits us to consider morphological changes in visually intact sections of the large intestine as an unbiased group criterion of UC transformation into its extensive forms.

It is worth paying attention to the group of patients with a 'segmentary' lesion of the large intestine (in distal sections and in the caecum). Such a lesion is one of the features of Crohn's disease; however, it is not a substantial criterion for diagnosis. Clinical, endoscopic and morphological features of such patients mainly correspond to the UC diagnosis. We believe that patients with such lesions should be considered as having a low-grade differentiation colitis, or one of the possible indicative features of the subsequent transformation of the distal form of UC.

In case of morphological detection of inflammation characteristic of UC in all sections of the large intestine, and not only in those with visually detected changes, patients have to receive both local and systemic basic therapy and regular check-ups. It is important to consider such patients as a risk group of possible transformation into the extensive forms of UC.

The presence of the focus of inflammation in the mucus of the caecum revealed by pathomorphological examination of patients with visible distal lesion and the absence of visible features of inflammation in the caecum demands further diagnosis to differentiate between Crohn's disease and low-grade differentiation colitis.

Patients with a visible or pathomorphological 'segmentary' lesion of the large intestine need to undergo systemic and local basic therapy.

References

1. Adler G. Crohn's disease and ulcerative colitis. Geotar Med. 2001:220.
2. Aruin LI, Kapuller LL, Isakov VA. Morphologic diagnostics of gastric and intestinal diseases. Triada. 1998:496.
3. Belousova EA. Ulcerative colitis and Crohn's disease. Tver': Izdatel'stvo Triada. 2002:128.
4. Hanauer SB. Inflammatory bowel disease. N Engl J Med. 1996;334:841–8.
5. Kirsner JB. Inflammatory Bowel Disease, 6th edn. 2004:754.
6. Belousova EA. Drug-resistant inflammatory bowel disease: clinical characteristics and prognostic possibilities. Thesis for PhD Moscow, 1982:38.
7. Targan SR, Shanahan F. Inflammatory Bowel Diseases: From Bench to Bedside. 1994:795.
8. Khalif IL. Clinical and immunological investigation into ulcerative colitis. Thesis for PhD Moscow, 1982:26.
9. Shivananda S, Hordijk ML, Ten Kate FJW et al. Differential diagnosis of inflammatory bowel disease. A comparision of various diagnostic classifications. Scand J Gastroenterol. 1989;24(Suppl. 170):167–73.
10. Tcherbakov IG. The pathological morphology of the mucous membrane in the gastric intestinal tract acute bacteriologic and viral intestinal infections and chronic colitis. Thesis for PhD Moscow, 1996:38.
11. Farmer RG, Easley KA, Rankin GB. Clinical patterns, natural history, and progression of ulcerative colitis. A long-term follow-up of 1116 patients. Dig Dis Sci. 1993;38:1137–46.
12. Geboes K. Histopathology of Crohn's disease and ulcerative colitis. In: Satsangi J, Sutherland LR (eds). Inflammatory Bowel Diseases. London: Churchill Livingstone. 2003: 255–76.
13. Seldenrijk CA, Morson BC, Meuwissen SGM, Schipper NW, Lindeman J, Meijer CJL. Histopathological evaluation of colonic mucosal biopsy specimens in chronic inflammatory bowel disease: diagnostic implications. Gut. 1991;32:1514–20.

15
Implications of dysplasia in the prevention of ulcerative colitis-associated colon cancer

J. D. LEWIS

INTRODUCTION

Colorectal cancer is a potentially life-threatening complication of inflammatory bowel disease (IBD). Patients with long-standing disease involving large portions of the colon have the highest risk of developing colorectal cancer. There are two basic strategies to prevent colon cancer in patients with IBD – prophylactic total colectomy or serial surveillance colonoscopies with colectomy reserved for those patients with dysplasia detected on random or targeted biopsies. Most patients opt for surveillance in favour of prophylactic colectomy. This chapter will discuss several controversies surrounding the use of surveillance colonoscopy to prevent colorectal cancer-related morbidity and mortality.

THE PATHWAY TO COLON CANCER IN PATIENTS WITH ULCERATIVE COLITIS

The biology of non-IBD-related sporadic colon cancer has been well studied. Through a series of acquired genetic mutations, normal colonic mucosa progresses to an adenomatous polyp and ultimately to invasive cancer[1]. Removal of the dysplastic adenomatous polyp essentially eliminates the risk of those dysplastic cells progressing to cancer. Strong evidence supports the theory that removal of all identifiable polyps in patients without IBD results in a substantial reduction in the risk of subsequent colon cancer[2].

For patients with IBD the biological pathway to colon cancer is different. Rather than progressing through a precancerous stage as a discrete polyp, IBD-related colon cancer is believed to develop in the setting of a more diffuse process. The chronic inflammation in the colon is often referred to as a field defect such that precancerous changes may occur diffusely throughout the diseased bowel. While many of the acquired genetic mutations in IBD-related colon cancers are similar to those observed in sporadic colon cancer, the sequence of these mutations is often quite different[3,4]. Nonetheless, these mutations result in characteristic histological changes which can be categorized as low-grade dysplasia, high-grade dysplasia or invasive cancer.

The core concept behind surveillance colonoscopy with random biopsy is that flat dysplasia can be viewed as a precursor lesion to invasive colon cancer. The biological model proposes that, through a series of acquired genetic mutations, normal colonic tissue progresses to low-grade dysplasia, then high-grade dysplasia, and subsequently invasive cancer. Under this model, if we are able to identify patients with precancerous dysplasia, surgery could be performed before invasive cancer develops, while those patients without precancerous dysplasia could retain their colon. As such, essentially all guidelines recommend colectomy for high-grade dysplasia. However, because the data on the risk of subsequent colon cancer among patients with only low-grade dysplasia, particularly unifocal low-grade dysplasia, are less clear, guidelines are less specific about the appropriate management of low-grade dysplasia[5]. Some have argued that patients with low-grade dysplasia can be followed with frequent surveillance colonoscopies[6,7].

CAN A PROGRAMME OF SURVEILLANCE COLONOSCOPY PREVENT MORBIDITY AND MORTALITY FROM COLON CANCER?

The strongest evidence of efficacy comes from randomized controlled trials. Unfortunately, not all clinical questions are suitable to being answered in a clinical trial. To date a randomized trial of surveillance colonoscopies in patients with long-standing extensive ulcerative colitis has not been completed and is unlikely to ever happen. Such a study would require a very large sample size and a long duration of follow-up. Furthermore, because surveillance colonoscopy has become a standard component of many physicians' clinical practice, randomizing some patients to no-screening might raise ethical questions. Thus, it appears that decisions on the effectiveness of cancer surveillance with serial colonoscopies will need to be made from observational data.

Several observational studies have addressed outcomes of surveillance colonoscopy programmes in patients with ulcerative colitis. In a case–control study Eaden and colleagues suggested that colonoscopy surveillance may be effective at reducing colon cancer incidence[8]. In their study of 102 patients with ulcerative colitis (UC) and colon cancer and 102 UC patients without colon cancer, patients with colon cancer were far more likely than controls to have undergone one or two colonoscopies during follow-up. These differences persisted after adjusting for a measure of the frequency of flares of disease and a similar difference was not seen with barium enema. This latter finding suggests that the detection of dysplasia at colonoscopy may have led to more early colectomies, before colon cancer had time to develop. It is notable that they did not observe a dose response with regard to number of colonoscopies, as the magnitude of the protective effect was smaller for more than two colonoscopies during follow-up. In addition, the authors were not focusing exclusively on surveillance colonoscopies with random and targeted biopsies. Nonetheless, these data suggest that use of colonoscopy may be effective at reducing colorectal cancer incidence.

For several reasons colon cancer mortality is as important to study at colon cancer incidence. First, colectomy is the definitive method of reducing colon cancer incidence. In addition, treatment of early-stage colon cancer is the same as for dysplasia (i.e. colectomy) and the expected cancer-free survival excellent. Thus, the goal of screening programmes may be viewed as prevention of advanced-stage colon cancer. To that end, Choi and colleagues examined the stage of cancers diagnosed among patients who were and were not participating in a surveillance programme[9]. In their study of 41 patients with UC-related colon cancer, 37% vs 14% of cancers were Dukes stage A if the patient was or was not in a surveillance programme, respectively ($p = 0.04$). While such studies are often criticized for potential lead-time bias, the strong correlation between colon cancer stage and cancer-related mortality argues that a stage shift to earlier cancer with surveillance is a clinically important finding.

Karlen and colleagues tried to directly answer the question of whether surveillance colonoscopy could reduce the risk of cancer-related mortality in a case–control study[10]. Patients who died of colon cancer were far less likely to have undergone one or more surveillance colonoscopies (odds ratio = 0.29), although this was not statistically significant. However, the presence of a dose response provided further evidence of the protective effect.

Taken as a whole, these studies suggest that the use of surveillance colonoscopy can prevent colon cancer-related morbidity and mortality, but that the intervention is far from perfect. Despite the use of surveillance colonoscopy, most IBD-related cancers are diagnosed at Dukes stage B or higher[10].

HOW TO RESPOND TO THE FINDING OF COLONIC DYSPLASIA

Given that the goal of surveillance colonoscopy is to identify lesions that predict the development of colon cancer in the near future, understanding the risk of concurrent or subsequent colon cancer in patients with dysplasia is critical. Over a decade ago Bernstein and colleagues summarized the available literature on this question[11]. Their data estimated that 43% of patients with a dysplasia-associated lesion or mass (DALM), 32–42% of patients with high-grade dysplasia, and 8–19% of patients with low-grade dysplasia have or will develop colon cancer in the near future. For patients with the finding of indeterminate for colon cancer and without dysplasia, the risk of subsequent colon cancer was 9% and 2%, respectively. These data clearly support the recommendation for immediate colectomy in patients with high-grade dysplasia or DALM lesions, but raise a question about the need for colectomy in patients with low-grade dysplasia.

In response to this controversy, several additional studies have focused on outcomes among patients with low-grade dysplasia. Despite a number of additional studies being completed, a definitive answer to this question has remained elusive. One study[12] reported high rates of progression to colon cancer, two reported modest rates of progression to colon cancer (6% and 10%)[7,13], while one study reported no cancers among 60 patients with low-grade dysplasia followed for an average of 10 years[6].

There are several potential explanations for these discrepant results. All of the studies have been relatively small, thus limiting the precision of the cancer incidence estimates. Furthermore, and perhaps equally as important, the clinical challenge of defining low-grade dysplasia is real. It is well documented that inter-rater agreement on the finding of low-grade dysplasia can be low[7,14]; thus, what one study refers to as low-grade dysplasia may have been categorized as either high-grade dysplasia, indefinite for dysplasia, or no dysplasia in other studies.

What then should the clinician do when faced with a finding of low-grade dysplasia? The conservative answer is to recommend colectomy, recognizing that some patients will be unwilling to accept this recommendation. These patients should understand that a strategy of waiting for a more advanced finding on surveillance colonoscopy or symptoms may lead to diagnosis of cancer at a more advanced stage[12]. Furthermore, some patients have progressed from low-grade dysplasia to invasive cancer without an intervening diagnosis of high-grade dysplasia despite continued surveillance colonoscopies.

ADENOMATOUS POLYP-LIKE LESIONS – A UNIQUE FORM OF DYSPLASIA IN IBD PATIENTS

In recent years it has been recognized that not all raised dysplastic lesions are equal. The classic DALM lesion is associated with a very high prevalence of synchronous colon cancer and is a clear indication for total colectomy. However, some raised dysplastic lesions are sporadic adenomatous polyps that might have developed even in the absence of IBD. These lesions are separate from the neoplastic process associated with chronic IBD.

Removal of adenomatous polyps in patients without IBD can reduce the subsequent risk of colon cancer[2]. Most data suggest that these adenoma-like mass lesions, sometimes referred to as ALM, do not portend an elevated risk of synchronous or subsequent colon cancer among patients with IBD as well, as long as the ALM is removed in its entirety. Several cohort studies of patients with ALM have documented very low rates of subsequent colon cancer following removal of the ALM. After initial reports by several groups[15,16], concern was raised that these studies had relatively short follow-up periods. However, long-term follow-up in one of these cohorts has provided additional evidence of the safety of removing ALM[17]. After an average of 7 years of follow-up the cumulative risk of colon cancer was only 4%, which is consistent with what one might expect in the absence of any dysplasia. Although this study included only 24 patients with ALM, the low incidence of colon cancer is reassurance that removal of ALM is safe.

The challenge for the clinician is to distinguish ALM from DALM. When a lesion develops outside of the area affected by the IBD, such as in the caecum in a patient with left-sided ulcerative colitis, the lesion can be confidently labelled as an ALM. For lesions developing within a diseased area of the colon this distinction is more challenging. Although various molecular and histological features have been suggested, there is no gold standard for this distinction[4]. The seminal studies describing the safety of continued surveillance after removing ALM made the distinction of ALM versus DALM on the basis of clinical judgement. Central to this judgement is the absence of flat dysplasia near the base of the polyp or elsewhere in the colon. However, the visual appearance of the polyp, the patient's age, and the opinion of the pathologist should also be considered when deciding whether a lesion is a DALM or ALM.

CONCLUSION

Colon cancer remains an important and potentially lethal complication of IBD. Although randomized controlled trial data are lacking, the body of evidence supports the effectiveness of colon cancer surveillance with serial colonoscopy and random colon biopsies to reduce colon cancer-related morbidity and mortality. Central to this strategy is referral of high-risk patients for total colectomy, specifically those with dysplasia. Whether low-grade dysplasia should always result in a recommendation for colectomy is less clear. The available data generally support the theory that patients with low-grade dysplasia have a risk of subsequent colon cancer greater than that observed among patients without dysplasia, although less than that observed in patients with high-grade dysplasia or DALM. Furthermore, some data suggest that delayed colectomy in these patients increases the risk for advanced-stage cancer. As such, if the primary goal is to reduce colon cancer-related morbidity and mortality, it is prudent to recommend colectomy for patients with any grade of dysplasia. In contrast to flat dysplasia and DALM, the available data suggest that it is safe to entirely remove ALM and continue with periodic colonoscopic surveillance.

References

1. Fearon ER, Vogelstein B. A genetic model for colorectal tumorigenesis. Cell. 1990;61:759–67.
2. Winawer S, Zauber A, Ho N et al. Prevention of colorectal cancer by polypectomy. N Engl J Med. 1993;329:1977–81.
3. Lewis JD, Deren JJ, Lichtenstein GR. Cancer risk in patients with inflammatory bowel disease. Gastroenterol Clin N Am. 1999;28:459–77.
4. Odze RD. Adenomas and adenoma-like DALM in chronic ulcerative colitis: a clinical, pathological, and molecular review. Am J Gastroenterol. 1999;94:1746–50.
5. Lewis JD. The many faces of low-grade dysplasia [comment]. Gastroenterology. 2003;125:1531–3.
6. Befrits R, Ljung T, Jaramillo E, Rubio C. Low-grade dysplasia in extensive, long-standing inflammatory bowel disease: a follow-up study. Dis Colon Rectum. 2002;45:615–20.
7. Lim CH, Dixon MF, Vail A, Forman D, Lynch DA, Axon AT. Ten year follow up of ulcerative colitis patients with and without low grade dysplasia. Gut. 2003;52:1127–32.
8. Eaden J, Abrams K, Ekbom A, Jackson E, Mayberry J. Colorectal cancer prevention in ulcerative colitis: a case–control study. Aliment Pharmacol Ther. 2000;14:145–53.

9. Choi PM, Nugent FW, Schoetz DJ Jr, Silverman ML, Haggitt RC. Colonoscopic surveillance reduces mortality from colorectal cancer in ulcerative colitis [see comments]. Gastroenterology. 1993;105:418–24.

10. Karlen P, Kornfeld D, Brostrom O, Lofberg R, Persson PG, Ekbom A. Is colonoscopic surveillance reducing colorectal cancer mortality in ulcerative colitis? A population based case–control study [comment]. Gut. 1998;42:711–14.

11. Bernstein CN, Shanahan F, Weinstein WM. Are we telling patients the truth about surveillance colonoscopy in ulcerative colitis? [see comments]. Lancet. 1994;343:71–4.

12. Ullman T, Croog V, Harpaz N, Sachar D, Itzkowitz S. Progression of flat low-grade dysplasia to advanced neoplasia in patients with ulcerative colitis [see comment]. Gastroenterology. 2003;125:1311–19.

13. Ullman TA, Loftus EV Jr, Kakar S, Burgart LJ, Sandborn WJ, Tremaine WJ. The fate of low grade dysplasia in ulcerative colitis. Am J Gastroenterol. 2002;97:922–7.

14. Odze RD, Goldblum J, Noffsinger A, Alsaigh N, Rybicki LA, Fogt F. Interobserver variability in the diagnosis of ulcerative colitis-associated dysplasia by telepathology. Modern Pathol. 2002;15:379–86.

15. Rubin PH, Friedman S, Harpaz N et al. Colonoscopic polypectomy in chronic colitis: conservative management after endoscopic resection of dysplastic polyps [see comment]. Gastroenterology. 1999;117:1295–300.

16. Engelsgjerd M, Farraye FA, Odze RD. Polypectomy may be adequate treatment for adenoma-like dysplastic lesions in chronic ulcerative colitis [see comments]. Gastroenterology. 1999;117:1288–94; discussion 1488–91.

17. Odze RD, Farraye FA, Hecht JL, Hornick JL. Long-term follow-up after polypectomy treatment for adenoma-like dysplastic lesions in ulcerative colitis [see comment]. Clin Gastroenterol Hepatol. 2004;2:534–41.

16
Chemopreventive effect of aminosalicylates

H. HERFARTH

INTRODUCTION

Colorectal cancer represents a serious risk for patients suffering from left-sided colitis or pancolitis[1–3]. Risk factors include primary sclerosing cholangitis, young age of onset, and a family history of colorectal cancer. Probable risk factors are a high intestinal inflammatory activity, backwash ileitis and folate deficiency. Several clinical strategies aim at the prevention of colorectal cancer in ulcerative colitis: (UC):

1. Surveillance colonoscopy is recommended 8 years and 15 years after the onset of the disease in patients with pancolitis and left-sided colitis, respectively.

2. Prophylactic proctocolectomy if dysplasia is detected.

3. Chemoprevention employing 5-aminosalicylic acid (5-ASA) or, in the presence of primary sclerosing cholangitis, ursodeoxycholic acid.

Additionally other factors such as smoking, prolonged steroid use, and regular intake of aspirin and other non-steroidal anti-inflammatory drugs (NSAID) may also influence the risk for the development of colorectal cancer in UC[4] (Table 1). Besides the above-mentioned risk and protective factors for the development of colorectal cancer in patients with UC, one should also keep in mind that extensive Crohn's colitis also represents a risk factor for colorectal cancer in patients suffering from Crohn's disease, which, however, is much less well defined[5,6].

CHEMOPREVENTION IN COLORECTAL CANCER

Chemoprevention is defined as the use of specific pharmacological or nutrient agents to prevent, reverse, or inhibit the process of carcinogenesis. Interest in chemoprevention for colorectal cancer evolved from large epidemiological

Table 1 Protective factors associated with colorectal cancer in ulcerative colitis

Variables	Odds ratio	95% CI
Smoking	0.5	0.2–0.9
Surveillance colonoscopy		
1–2	0.4	0.2–0.7
>2	0.3	0.1–0.8
5-ASA use		
1–5 years	0.4	0.2–0.9
6–10 years	0.6	0.3–1.4
>10 years	0.6	0.3–1.3
Steroid use >1 year	0.4	0.2–0.8
Aspirin	0.3	0.1–0.8
NSAID	0.1	0.03–0.5

Variables associated with colorectal cancer were registered in 188 patients with ulcerative colitis-related cancer and matched controls in a retrospective case–control study[4].

Table 2 Aspirin prevents adenoma recurrence in patients with previous resection of colorectal cancer

	Aspirin 325 mg/day n = 259	Placebo n = 258
>1 Adenoma (%)	17*	27
Number of adenomas (mean ± SD)	0.3 ± 0.9**	0.5 ± 1.0
RR (95% CI)	0.65 (0.46–0.91)	

A total of 517 randomized patients had at least one colonoscopic examination a median of 12.8 months after randomization[8].

*$p < 0.004$; **$p < 0.003$ vs placebo; RR = relative risk.

studies demonstrating significantly lower rates of colorectal cancer in individuals consuming regular aspirin or other NSAID[7]. Prospectively, placebo-controlled, double-blind clinical trials demonstrated a protective effect of regular therapy using aspirin in groups of patients with an increased risk for colorectal cancer[8–10] (Table 2). The main mechanism by which aspirin and NSAID exert their chemopreventive effects is by inhibiting the enzyme cyclooxygenase (COX), which is involved in the metabolism of arachidonic acid and the production of prostaglandins[11]. COX consists of two isoforms: the constitutively expressed COX-1 isoform, which plays a role in cellular homeostasis and occurs throughout the whole gastrointestinal tract, and the COX-2 isoform, which is normally present in low levels in the synovium, the central nervous system, the kidneys and the ovaries, but is little expressed in the gastrointestinal tract. COX-2 activity is only up-regulated after induction by various cytokines or growth factors. Studies analysing human tissue sections of colorectal cancer, as well as induced colorectal cancers, in animal models demonstrate both an increase in the activity of COX-2 and in the concentration of prostaglandin E2 in such tumours. The protective mechanism of a COX-2 inhibition by NSAID against the development of a colorectal cancer has been demonstrated in several experimental animal models[12]. Oshima et al., for example, impressively demonstrated that, in an animal model of familial adenomatous polyposis (ApcΔ716 knockout mouse), the development of colonic adenomas was almost completely suppressed if a COX-2 mutation was introduced into ApcΔ716 knockout mice (652 ± 198 polyps in ApcΔ716 knockout mice vs. 93 ± 98 polyps in ApcΔ716/ COX-2 knockout mice)[13]. Medical therapy using Sulindac or a specific COX-2 inhibitor also diminished colonic polyp formation by approximately 50% and 75% in ApcΔ716 knockout mice.

Moreover, in addition to the inhibition of prostaglandin synthesis, a direct proapoptotic and antiproliferative effect of NSAID, which is mediated by the inhibition of the transcription factor NF-κB, as well as the inhibition of the peroxisome-proliferation-associated receptors (PPAR), form a further protective mechanism against the development of colorectal cancer[14,15] (Figure 1).

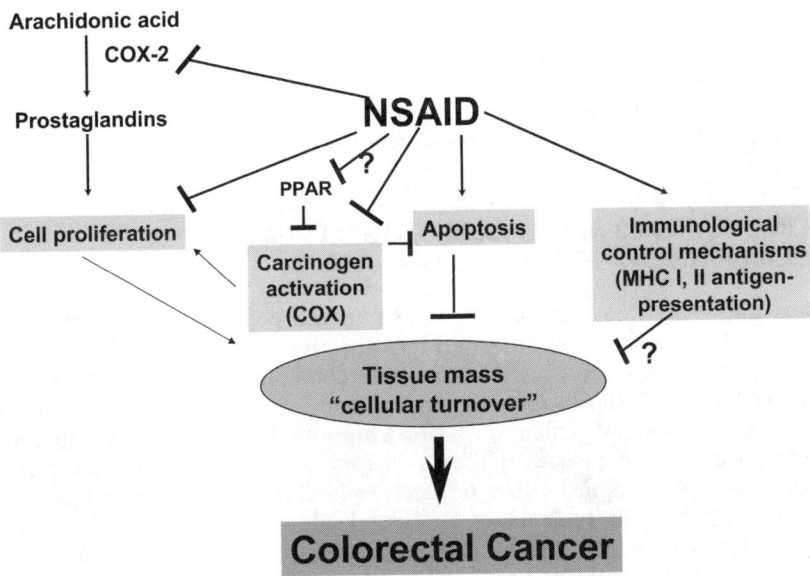

Figure 1 Effects of NSAID on colon carcinogenesis. NSAID influence the 'cellular turnover', and hence the carcinogenesis, by direct or indirect inhibition of the rate of proliferation and the activation of carcinogens, which can inhibit apoptosis-promoting genes. In addition, by suppressing the activation of the transcription factor NF-κB, NSAID lead directly to an increased rate of apoptosis. Possibly NSAID cause an increased elimination of tumour cells by up-regulating the MHCI, II antigen presentation, or may indirectly down-regulate the activation of carcinogens by the inhibition of PPAR (modified from ref. 42)

CHEMOPREVENTION WITH MESALAMINE (5-ASA)

One of the major shortcomings of aspirin is the anticipated side-effect of bleeding if this drug is applied regularly as a chemopreventive agent. Most likely severe episodes of bleeding would outweigh the protective effects for colorectal cancer[16]. Agents with a more favourable adverse event profile, such as 5-ASA, would clearly have an advantage for chemoprevention. In several retrospective analyses (see below) continuous 5-ASA therapy revealed a protective effect for the development of colorectal cancer in patients with UC. In contrast to the molecular effects of aspirin and other NSAID knowledge of the potential mechanisms of cancer prevention by 5-ASA is only barely elucidated[17]. In two mice models with colorectal cancer the administration of balsalazide, a prodrug broken down to 5-aminosalicylic acid in the colon, demonstrated a significant negative effect on the development of intestinal tumours[18]. *In-vitro* studies reveal that these effects are probably due to an increase of apoptosis by the activation of caspase 3 and to a direct DNA stabilizing effect of mesalazine, resulting in a significant reduction of spontaneous microsatellite mutations[19,20]. These experimental findings are corroborated by two observations in humans. Bus et al. were able to demonstrate, on the basis of tissue biopsy material, that there was a significant increase in the rate of apoptosis in patients with colorectal cancer after 14 days of treatment with mesalazine enemas[21]. Furthermore, the oral administration of Eudragit L-coated mesalazine pellets at a dose of 1 g/day resulted in an inhibition of the epithelial proliferation rate in the rectum with a simultaneous increase in the apoptosis rate in the region of the crypts[22].

CLINICAL TRIALS AND EPIDEMIOLOGICAL DATA ON CHEMOPREVENTIVE EFFECTS OF 5-ASA

Most data regarding the role of 5-ASA in the prevention of dysplasia or colorectal cancer have been derived retrospectively in patients with UC. The first and only prospectively performed, placebo-controlled, double-blind trial of 5-ASA prophylaxis of adenoma recurrence in patients not suffering from UC did not demonstrate efficacy of this compound in preventing adenoma recurrence[23]. Patients with a recent history of histologically documented adenomas were assigned either to receive placebo or 1 g 5-ASA daily for 3 years. A total of 241 patients were randomized and a follow-up colonoscopy was performed 3 years after the qualifying endoscopy. No significant difference could be detected between the placebo- and the 5-ASA-treated group, which could be due to the relatively small sample size or the low dose of 5-ASA employed in this study.

A recently published meta-analysis evaluating the association between 5-ASA use and colorectal cancer in patients with UC identified nine retrospective studies[24–32] with a total of 334 cases of colorectal cancer, 140 cases of dysplasia and a total of 1932 subjects[33]. The analysis demonstrated a protective association between the use of 5-ASA and either dysplasia or colorectal cancer with an odds ratio of 0.51 and a 95% confidence interval of 0.38–0.69.

Table 3 Factors negatively influencing adherence to the prescribed 5-ASA dose[36]

Independent predictors of non-compliance	OR	95% CI
Three times daily dosing	3.1	1.8–8.4
Full-time employment	2.7	1.1–6.9
Depression	10.5	1.8–79

This chemopreventive effect seems to be dose-dependent and a dose > 1.2 g of 5-ASA is probably necessary to exert the above-described chemopreventive effects[34]. Furthermore adherence to medication is another important factor[27], which could explain some of the variation in the findings in the published analyses[35], since 40–60% of the patients do not comply with the prescribed 5-ASA dosage[36–38] (Table 3).

To clearly define a role of 5-ASA for chemoprevention in patients with UC a prospective, double-blind placebo-controlled trial would be required. However, such a trial would have several obstacles, which makes it very unlikely that it will ever take place. For a trial comparing 5-ASA treatment with placebo the follow-up time required for the endpoint of a 2% cumulative incidence of colorectal cancer would be 10 years, and a total recruitment of 5260 patients would be needed[35]. Besides problems with compliance and dropouts, this trial would also ethically be almost impossible to implement, since a standard therapy for UC would be withheld in the placebo arm. Taking the above-described dose response into account, and comparing two different maintenance doses of 5-ASA for chemoprevention of colorectal cancer, the number of patients to be recruited would rise to 72 000, which clearly indicates that such a study will never be conducted.

URSODEOXYCHOLIC ACID (UDCA) AND CHEMOPREVENTION

A recently published placebo-controlled, double-blind, prospective study investigating the effects of a relatively low dose of UDCA (8–10 mg/kg of body weight per day) on the recurrence of colonic adenomas did not demonstrate an overall significant effect of this compound. However, the recurrence of high-grade dysplasia in colorectal adenomas was significantly diminished[39] (Table 4). Long-term therapy with UDCA in patients with UC and primary sclerosing cholangitis (PSC) has chemopreventive effects for the development of colorectal cancer[40,41]. Patients receiving 13–15 mg UDCA/kg of body weight per day for the treatment of the underlying PSC have a calculated risk reduction of about 70% for the development of colorectal cancer. There are at present no data available regarding the clinical value of a combination therapy of UDCA and 5-ASA preparations.

Table 4 Risk of adenoma recurrence in patients treated with either ursodeoxycholic acid or placebo

	Ursodeoxycholic acid n = 661	Placebo n = 624	OR	95% CI
Adenoma recurrence	41.0%	43.9%	0.89	0.71–1.12
Adenoma with high-grade dysplasia	5.5%*	8.7%	0.61	0.39–0.96

A total of 1285 individuals who had undergone removal of a colorectal adenoma within the past 6 months before inclusion into the study were randomized to daily treatment with UDCA (8–10 mg/kg body weight) or with placebo for 3 years[39].

*$p < 0.03$ vs. placebo.

CONCLUSIONS

Patients suffering from left-sided colitis or pancolitis have a significantly higher risk for developing colorectal cancer. On the basis of epidemiological and experimental *in-vitro* and *in-vivo* data, as well as new data derived from prospective placebo-controlled clinical trials, regular prophylactic administration of aspirin and NSAID appears to be protective against the development of colorectal cancer in non-IBD patients. Nearly all studies available in patients with UC, who regularly took 5-ASA-containing preparations at a dose of at least 1.2 g/day, reveal a significant reduction in the risk of colorectal cancer. Hence, according to current knowledge, continuous maintenance therapy of patients with UC with preparations containing 5-ASA probably represents an important option to prevent the development of colorectal cancer. Patients with concurrent PSC should also be treated with UDCA, which not only slows the progression of PSC in the liver but also most likely exerts chemopreventive effects in the colon.

References

1. Itzkowitz SH, Harpaz N. Diagnosis and management of dysplasia in patients with inflammatory bowel diseases. Gastroenterology. 2004;126:1634–48.
2. Munkholm P, Loftus EV Jr, Reinacher-Schick A, Kornbluth A, Mittmann U, Esendal B. Prevention of colorectal cancer in inflammatory bowel disease: value of screening and 5-aminosalicylates. Digestion. 2006;73:11–19.
3. Collins PD, Mpofu C, Watson AJ, Rhodes JM. Strategies for detecting colon cancer and/or dysplasia in patients with inflammatory bowel disease. Cochrane Database Syst Rev 2006: CD000279.
4. Velayos FS, Loftus EV Jr, Jess T et al. Predictive and protective factors associated with colorectal cancer in ulcerative colitis: a case–control study. Gastroenterology. 2006;130: 1941–9.
5. Jess T, Loftus EV Jr, Velayos FS et al. Risk of intestinal cancer in inflammatory bowel disease: a population-based study from olmsted county, Minnesota. Gastroenterology. 2006;130:1039–46.
6. Canavan C, Abrams KR, Mayberry J. Meta-analysis: colorectal and small bowel cancer risk in patients with Crohn's disease. Aliment Pharmacol Ther. 2006;23:1097–104.

7. Hawk ET, Levin B. Colorectal cancer prevention. J Clin Oncol. 2005;23:378–91.

8. Sandler RS, Halabi S, Baron JA et al. A randomized trial of aspirin to prevent colorectal adenomas in patients with previous colorectal cancer. N Engl J Med. 2003;348:883–90.

9. Chan AT, Giovannucci EL, Schernhammer ES et al. A prospective study of aspirin use and the risk for colorectal adenoma. Ann Intern Med. 2004;140:157–66.

10. Baron JA, Cole BF, Sandler RS et al. A randomized trial of aspirin to prevent colorectal adenomas. N Engl J Med. 2003;348:891–9.

11. Mann JR, DuBois RN. Cyclooxygenase-2 and gastrointestinal cancer. Cancer J. 2004;10: 145–52.

12. Brown JR, DuBois RN. COX-2: a molecular target for colorectal cancer prevention. J Clin Oncol. 2005;23:2840–55.

13. Oshima M, Dinchuk JE, Kargman SL et al. Suppression of intestinal polyposis in Apc delta716 knockout mice by inhibition of cyclooxygenase 2 (COX-2). Cell. 1996;87:803–9.

14. Allgayer H. Review article: Mechanisms of action of mesalazine in preventing colorectal carcinoma in inflammatory bowel disease. Aliment Pharmacol Ther. 2003;18:10–14.

15. Schottelius AJ, Dinter H. Cytokines, NF-κB, microenvironment, intestinal inflammation and cancer. Cancer Treat Res. 2006;130:67–87.

16. Imperiale TF. Aspirin and the prevention of colorectal cancer. N Engl J Med. 2003;348: 879–80.

17. Gasche C. Review article: The chemoprevention of colorectal carcinoma. Aliment Pharmacol Ther. 2004;20(Suppl. 4):31–5.

18. MacGregor DJ, Kim YS, Sleisenger MH, Johnson LK. Chemoprevention of colon cancer carcinogenesis by balsalazide: inhibition of azoxymethane-induced aberrant crypt formation in the rat colon and intestinal tumour formation in the B6-Min/+ mouse. Int J Oncol. 2000;17:173–9.

19. Reinacher-Schick A, Schoeneck A, Graeven U, Schwarte-Waldhoff I, Schmiegel W. Mesalazine causes a mitotic arrest and induces caspase-dependent apoptosis in colon carcinoma cells. Carcinogenesis. 2003;24:443–51.

20. Gasche C, Goel A, Natarajan L, Boland CR. Mesalazine improves replication fidelity in cultured colorectal cells. Cancer Res. 2005;65:3993–7.

21. Bus PJ, Nagtegaal ID, Verspaget HW et al. Mesalazine-induced apoptosis of colorectal cancer: on the verge of a new chemopreventive era? Aliment Pharmacol Ther. 1999;13: 1397–402.

22. Reinacher-Schick A, Seidensticker F, Petrasch S et al. Mesalazine changes apoptosis and proliferation in normal mucosa of patients with sporadic polyps of the large bowel. Endoscopy. 2000;32:245–54.

23. Schmiegel W, Pox C, Reiser M. Effect of 5-aminosalicylate (5-ASA) on the recurrence rate of sporadic colorectal adenomas. Gastroenterology. 2004;126:A452 (Abstract).

24. Moody GA, Jayanthi V, Probert CS, Mac Kay H, Mayberry JF. Long-term therapy with sulphasalazine protects against colorectal cancer in ulcerative colitis: a retrospective study of colorectal cancer risk and compliance with treatment in Leicestershire. Eur J Gastroenterol Hepatol. 1996;8:1179–83.

25. Rutter M, Saunders B, Wilkinson K et al. Severity of inflammation is a risk factor for colorectal neoplasia in ulcerative colitis. Gastroenterology. 2004;126:451–9.

26. Bernstein CN, Blanchard JF, Metge C, Yogendran M. Does the use of 5-aminosalicylates in inflammatory bowel disease prevent the development of colorectal cancer? Am J Gastroenterol. 2003;98:2784–8.

27. van Staa TP, Card T, Logan RF, Leufkens HG. 5-Aminosalicylate use and colorectal cancer risk in inflammatory bowel disease: a large epidemiological study. Gut. 2005;54:1573–8.

28. Rubin DT, Djordjevic A, Huo D, Yadron N, Hanauer SB. Use of 5-ASA is associated with decreased risk of dysplasia and colon cancer in ulcerative colitis. Gastroenterology. 2003;123:A36 (Abstract).

29. Eaden J, Abrams K, Ekbom A, Jackson E, Mayberry J. Colorectal cancer prevention in ulcerative colitis: a case-control study. Aliment Pharmacol Ther. 2000;14:145–53.

30. Pinczowski D, Ekbom A, Baron J, Yuen J, Adami HO. Risk factors for colorectal cancer in patients with ulcerative colitis: a case–control study. Gastroenterology. 1994;107:117–20.

31. Lindberg BU, Broome U, Persson B. Proximal colorectal dysplasia or cancer in ulcerative colitis. The impact of primary sclerosing cholangitis and sulfasalazine: results from a 20-year surveillance study. Dis Colon Rectum. 2001;44:77–85.

32. Lashner BA, Provencher KS, Seidner DL, Knesebeck A, Brzezinski A. The effect of folic acid supplementation on the risk for cancer or dysplasia in ulcerative colitis. Gastroenterology. 1997;112:29–32.

33. Velayos FS, Terdiman JP, Walsh JM. Effect of 5-aminosalicylate use on colorectal cancer and dysplasia risk: a systematic review and metaanalysis of observational studies. Am J Gastroenterol. 2005;100:1345–53.

34. Eaden JA, Abrams KR, Mayberry JF. The risk of colorectal cancer in ulcerative colitis: a meta-analysis. Gut. 2001;48:526–35.

35. Rubin DT, Lashner BA. Will a 5-ASA a day keep the cancer (and dysplasia) away? Am J Gastroenterol. 2005;100:1354–6.

36. Shale MJ, Riley SA. Studies of compliance with delayed-release mesalazine therapy in patients with inflammatory bowel disease. Aliment Pharmacol Ther. 2003;18:191–8.

37. Kane S, Huo D, Aikens J, Hanauer S. Medication nonadherence and the outcomes of patients with quiescent ulcerative colitis. Am J Med. 2003;114:39–43.

38. Kane SV. Systematic review: adherence issues in the treatment of ulcerative colitis. Aliment Pharmacol Ther. 2006;23:577-85.

39. Alberts DS, Martinez ME, Hess LM et al., for the Phoenix and Tucson Gastroenterologist N. Phase III trial of ursodeoxycholic acid to prevent colorectal adenoma recurrence. J Natl Cancer Inst. 2005;97:846–53.

40. Pardi DS, Loftus EV Jr, Kremers WK, Keach J, Lindor KD. Ursodeoxycholic acid as a chemopreventive agent in patients with ulcerative colitis and primary sclerosing cholangitis. Gastroenterology. 2003;124:889–93.

41. Tung BY, Emond MJ, Haggitt RC et al. Ursodiol use is associated with lower prevalence of colonic neoplasia in patients with ulcerative colitis and primary sclerosing cholangitis. Ann Intern Med. 2001;134:89–95.

42. Shiff SJ, Rigas B. Nonsteroidal anti-inflammatory drugs and colorectal cancer: evolving concepts of their chemopreventive actions. Gastroenterology. 1997;113:1992–8.

17
Role of antibiotics and probiotics in Crohn's disease

M. L. SCRIBANO and C. PRANTERA

In recent years a large set of experimental and clinical data have indicated that Crohn's disease (CD) is the consequence of an abnormal immune response to the intestinal flora in genetically susceptible individuals. This hypothesis justifies a therapeutic role for antibiotics, and antibiotics are often employed in clinical practice for treating CD, even though controlled studies have produced uncertain results.

The two antibiotics most widely employed in CD are metronidazole and ciprofloxacin, alone or in association.

Metronidazole is active against most anaerobic bacteria and exhibits immunomodulatory properties. It is used in treating perianal CD and open studies have shown its efficacy in closing fistulas and healing perianal abscesses, even if these lesions do often reappear when the therapy is discontinued. Randomized controlled trials of metronidazole therapy in active CD have demonstrated that this antibiotic is efficacious in patients with ileocolonic or colonic disease, but not in patients with disease confined to the small bowel. The positive results obtained with metronidazole when only the colon is involved might be due to the higher concentration of anaerobic bacteria in colitis, and the efficacy of this antibiotic seems to be correlated with luminal *Bacteroides* concentration. It is suggested that luminal flora is the main cause of recurrent lesions after an operation. Consequently, antibiotics have been employed for maintenance of remission after surgery, and two randomized placebo-controlled trials have been published. In the first study Rutgeerts et al.[1] showed that metronidazole, at a dose of 20 mg/kg per day for a 3-month period, significantly decreased the incidence of severe endoscopic recurrence and also seemed to delay symptomatic recurrence, but it was associated with a high percentage of side-effects. More recently the same authors[2] have used ornidazole in order to reduce the incidence of side-effects. This antibiotic, given for 1 year at a dosage of 1 g/day, significantly reduced the clinical recurrence of CD, but more than 30% of patients in the ornidazole group discontinued therapy because of side-effects. The side-effects of metronidazole remain of concern. Apart from short-term side-effects in around 50% of treated patients (nausea, metallic taste, reaction to alcohol), polyneuropathy secondary to metronidazole limits long-term use.

Ciprofloxacin is a quinolone that is particularly effective against *Escherichia coli* and Enterobacteriaceae, but not against anaerobic bacteria. Ciprofloxacin has been anecdotally reported[3–5] to be efficacious in the long-term treatment of 10 patients with active perianal CD, in four cases of Crohn's ileitis and, associated with metronidazole, in an uncontrolled series of 31 patients with active CD. Five randomized controlled trials[6–10] have employed ciprofloxacin in the treatment of the acute phase of CD, reporting interesting results. This antibiotic is better tolerated in the short term, but is associated with tendonitis and Achilles tendon rupture, especially with concomitant steroids. In a large series, long-term side-effects of metronidazole and ciprofloxacin caused treatment interruption in over 20% of cases and a reduced compliance in over 30% of patients .

An interesting antibiotic is rifaximin, a rifamycin derivative, characterized by a negligible intestinal absorption – less than 1% of the oral dose is excreted in the urine – conferring on it an excellent safety. Its large antimicrobial spectrum covers Gram-positive and Gram-negative bacteria, including aerobes and anaerobes. In particular rifaximin is active against *Bacteroides* and *E. coli*, two bacteria frequently found in the intestinal mucosa of CD patients.

Very recently Prantera et al.[11] have performed a multicentre, randomized, double-blind trial in which two doses of rifaximin gastroresistant granules, 800 mg once a day, and 800 mg twice a day, were compared to placebo in the treatment of 83 patients with mild to moderate active CD. This exploratory study has shown that a 12-week treatment with rifaximin, given at a dose of 800 mg twice daily, was superior to placebo in inducing clinical remission of active CD (52% vs 33%). Although this difference was not statistically significant, the number of failures in the placebo group was significantly higher than that in the rifaximin 800 mg b.i.d. group (33% vs 4%; $p = 0.01$). The best response of rifaximin 800 mg b.i.d. was obtained in the group of patients with elevated CRP values: remission and response rates were significantly higher than those of placebo and rifaximin 800 mg o.d. ($p < 0.05$). The antibiotic has shown a good safety profile, and no serious drug-related side-effects were observed during the study.

Manipulation of gut flora with probiotics is an appealing alternative to the use of antibiotics. Their therapeutic effect may include a competitive action with commensal and pathogenic flora and an influence on the immune response through various mechanisms. Some researchers have reported the success of different strains of probiotics in the treatment of ulcerative colitis. Given their potentially high safety profile, the use of probiotics for maintaining CD remission induced by drugs or surgery is particularly appealing. In a controlled study[12] 45 patients were randomized after surgical resection to receive *Lactobacillus rhamnosus* strain GG (LGG) at a dose of 12 billion/day or placebo for 1 year. Clinical recurrence rates were 16.5% for LGG patients and 10.5% for the placebo group. Endoscopic recurrence was observed in 60% and in 35.3% of patients in clinical remission with probiotic and placebo, respectively. There were no significant differences in severity of lesions between the two groups. Another trial[13], in which 98 patients were randomized after surgery to receive *Lactobacillus Johnsonii* or placebo for 6 months did not show a difference in clinical recurrence between the two groups. Endoscopic recurrence occurred in 49% of patients on probiotic and in 64% on placebo. In a trial on medically induced remission[14], 75 children were randomly allocated to receive 10^{10} of LGG bacteria or placebo for 2 years as an adjunct to standard maintenance treatment. The study did not show any differences between the active and placebo groups.

The cumulative result of these three studies[12–14] is not encouraging, and at the moment probiotics are not a therapeutic option for CD patients either in acute phase or in maintenance[15].

References

1. Rutgeerts P, Hiele M, Geboes K et al. Controlled trial of metronidazole treatment for prevention of Crohn's recurrence after ileal resection. Gastroenterology. 1995;108:1617–21.

2. Rutgeerts PJ, Van Assche G, Vermeire S et al. Ornidazole for prophylaxis of postoperative Crohn's disease recurrence: a randomised, double blind, placebo controlled trial. Gastroenterology. 2005;128:856–61.

3. Turunen U, Farkkila M, Valtonen V et al. Long-term outcome of ciprofloxacin treatment in severe perianal or fistulous Crohn's disease. Gastroenterology. 1993;104:A793.

4. Peppercorn MA. Is there a role for antibiotics as primary therapy in Crohn's ileitis? J Clin Gastroenterol. 1993;17:235–7.

5. Prantera C, Kohn A, Zannoni F et al. Metronidazole plus ciprofloxacin in the treatment of active, refractory Crohn's disease: results of an open study. J Clin Gastroenterol. 1994;19: 79–80.

6. Turunen U, Farkkila M, Hakala K et al. Ciprofloxacin treatment combined with conventional therapy in Crohn's disease: a prospective, double-blind, placebo controlled study. Gut. 1995;37:A193.

7. Prantera C, Zannoni F, Scribano ML et al. An antibiotic regimen for the treatment of active Crohn's disease: a randomized, controlled clinical trial of metronidazole plus ciprofloxacin. Am J Gastroenterol. 1996;91:328–32.

8. Colombel JF, Lemann M, Cassagnou M et al. A controlled trial comparing ciprofloxacin with mesalazine for the treatment of active Crohn's disease. Am J Gastroenterol. 1999;94: 674–8.

9. Arnold GL, Beaves MR, Pryjdun VO, Mook WJ. Preliminary study of ciprofloxacin in active Crohn's disease. Inflamm Bowel Dis. 2002;8:10–15.

10. Steinhart AH, Feagan BG, Wong CJ et al. Combined budesonide and antibiotic therapy for active Crohn's disease: a randomised controlled trial. Gastroenterology. 2002;123:33–40.

11. Prantera C, Lochs H, Campieri M et al. Antibiotic treatment of Crohn's disease: results of a multicentre, double blind, randomised, placebo-controlled trial with Rifaximin. Aliment Pharmacol Ther. 2006;23:1117–25.

12. Prantera C, Scribano ML, Falasco G et al. Ineffectiveness of probiotics in preventing recurrence after curative resection for Crohn's disease: a randomised controlled trial with *Lactobacillus* GG. Gut. 2002;51:405–9.

13. Marteau P, Lemann M, Seksik P et al. Ineffectiveness of *Lactobacillus johnsonii* LA1 for prophylaxis of postoperative recurrence in Crohn's disease: a randomised, double blind, placebo controlled GETAID trial. Gut. 2006;55:842–7.

14. Bousvaros A, Guandalini S, Baldassano RN et al. A randomized, double-blind trial of *Lactobacillus* GG versus placebo in addition to standard maintenance therapy for children with Crohn's disease. Inflamm Bowel Dis. 2005;11:833–9.

15. Prantera C. Should probiotics be given as an adjunct to standard maintenance therapy for children with Crohn's disease? Nat Clin Pract Gastroenterol Hepatol. 2006;3:130–1.

Section IV
Management of inflammatory bowel disease: 2nd session

Chair: YA SHELYGIN and SR TARGAN

18
Indications for use of infliximab in inflammatory bowel disease

G. ROGLER

INTRODUCTION

Infliximab was the first so-called 'biological' treatment that has been available for the treatment of inflammatory bowel disease (IBD). The development of this drug certainly marks an important step in the search for new and improved therapies for chronic inflammatory disorders. On the other hand only a few new drugs have caused so much discussion among physicians. Infliximab has been attributed by some gastroenterologists as 'the drug we have been waiting for in Crohn's disease[1], whereas others clearly opposed such statements[2]. There are advocates for a very early treatment with infliximab in the disease course of IBD favouring the so-called 'top-down' or 'early-hit' strategy (in my opinion the term 'top-down' is preferable, as 'early-hit' sounds more or less like a military scenario rather than the description of a medical strategy). On the other hand there are experts who never tire of warning against use of infliximab in general, and preferring a conservative treatment regime. Unfortunately facts and fantasies are sometimes mixed up in this discussion; or only certain facts and arguments are selected for the support or rejection of infliximab therapy. This chapter is an attempt to reflect an objective and neutral position for the use of infliximab in IBD – if that is at all possible.

INFLIXIMAB USE IN PATIENTS WITH CROHN'S DISEASE

Why anti-TNF treatment strategies have been developed for Crohns' disease

Crohn's disease (CD) is a transmural inflammatory disorder which can involve any part of the gastrointestinal tract. It is characterized by chronicity, recurrences, frequent extraintestinal manifestations and complications such as fistulas, abscesses, strictures and stenoses. As hitherto there is no cure for the disease any CD treatment aims at the induction of remission, maintenance of remission and – if possible – prevention or reduction of complications.

Tumour necrosis factor, TNF, which is a potent proinflammatory cytokine, can elicit a wide spectrum of responses such as fever, tissue injury, tumour necrosis, induction of other cytokines, cell proliferation, differentiation and apoptosis[3–8]. It is thought to be a key proinflammatory mediator in CD as well as in other diseases associated with chronic inflammation such as rheumatoid arthritis (RA)[9–13], spondylarthropathy[14] and psoriasis[15–17]. TNF is produced as a 26-kDa transmembrane protein with an intracellular tail[18–20], which is cleaved by a metalloproteinase (TACE; TNF-converting enzyme)[21] to be secreted as a 17-kDa soluble protein. This 17-kDa protein forms trimers that can interact with two receptors, the p55 TNF receptor 1 and the p75 TNF receptor 2[22,23]. TNF is synthesized mainly by activated macrophages and T lymphocytes among other cells. During flares of CD TNF production is increased in the intestinal mucosa[24–29]. Therefore it has been postulated that neutralization of TNF could be beneficial for the course of CD and can be a treatment option.

Infliximab is a neutralizing mouse/human immunoglobulin (Ig)G1 chimeric anti-human tumour necrosis factor monoclonal antibody. It is composed of human constant and murine variable regions. Infliximab neutralizes TNF both *in vitro* and *in vivo* by blocking soluble TNF and binding to transmembrane TNF[30,31].

Human TNF is bound by infliximab with an association constant of $10^{10}/$ M^{32}. Infliximab has a half-life of 10 days after intravenous infusion[33]. The clearance rate of infliximab from the circulation is 10 ml/h. In week 12 after application of 5 mg/kg body weight infliximab levels are no longer detectable. The exact serum level of infliximab needed to exert its therapeutic effect has not so far been determined[32].

The mechanism of action of infliximab is not well understood[32,34]. Only neutralization of soluble TNF seems to be insufficient, as soluble TNF receptors such as etanercept (p75 fusion protein)[35,36] and onercept (p55 receptor)[37,38], which bind TNF efficiently, seem to have no clinical activity in CD (on the other hand, the respective trials were relatively small and likely to be underpowered, and did not have a design comparable to the successful infliximab studies). It has been speculated that the beneficial effect of infliximab may be achieved by induction of apoptosis of T cells and monocytes/ macrophages that express membrane-bound TNF on their cell surfaces[39–42]. However, it was recently demonstrated that another antibody to TNF not inducing apoptosis (certolizumab, a pegylated Fab′ fragment of a humanized anti-TNF antibody) is also effective in the treatment of active CD[43,44]. This indicates that the induction of apoptosis cannot play a crucial role in mediating the treatment effect.

Infliximab was licensed for the treatment of CD in both North America and Europe in 2000[45]. The drug is administered intravenously, usually over a 2-h period.

When should infliximab be used in CD?

Evidence-based guidelines in many countries recommend 5-ASA derivatives such as sulphasalazine as the first-line medical therapy in CD[46]. Trials found that, with this medication, up to 43% of patients experience clinical remission compared to 30% of placebo-treated patients. This is especially the case in patients with mainly colonic disease[47]. However, due to a high NNT this result is controversial[48].

The second-line (or first-line in cases of initially moderate to severely active disease) therapy for CD is the topic or systemic administration of steroids. Steroids are effective for inducing remission in patients with CD. Several studies have shown that up to 80% of patients initially respond to steroids, and only 20–30% are steroid-refractory[47]. Certainly steroids should not be administered for maintenance therapy in CD. Up to one-third of patients finally become steroid-dependent. In these cases symptoms reoccur when the steroid medication is tapered.

On the other hand population-based epidemiological studies showed that up to one-third of CD patients never receive steroids[49,50]. This means that such patients can be effectively treated with 5-ASA or other medications, or they had initial surgery and then were in remission. There is general agreement that steroids should not be used in the long-term because of their adverse effects[51–55]. Glucocorticoids are the most common cause of drug-induced osteoporosis[56.] Avascular necrosis (osteonecrosis), most common in the femoral head, can occur in active patients on long-term, high-dose corticosteroids[57]. Over 30% of patients treated with systemic glucocorticoids over long periods develop posterior subcapsular cataracts[57]. Frequently glucocorticoid-induced hypertension, hyperglycaemia through increased gluconeogenesis or new-onset diabetes mellitus (steroid diabetes) are found. Increased serum triglyceride and cholesterol levels are also associated with glucocorticoid therapy. Glucocorticoids furthermore are a risk factor for postoperative infectious complications[58]. Supporters of infliximab therapy argue that those adverse effects can be avoided by early substitution of glucocorticoids with infliximab. On the other hand it should be kept in mind that we know those side-effects very well due to long experience with glucocorticoids and that very serious side-effects are extremely rare.

It is widely accepted that the next step in the treatment of CD is the use of immunosuppressants such as azathioprine or methotrexate when steroids fail or patients become steroid-dependent. Most national and international guidelines recommend that those immunosuppressants should be used before the use of biologicals[47,59–65]. Azathioprine, 6-mercaptopurine and methotrexate are steroid-sparing and have been shown to be effective in inducing and maintaining remission in patients with CD[66–71]. In terms of maintaining remission, patients should have had a trial of azathioprine, mercaptopurine or methotrexate before the use of biologicals. Azathioprine in the standard dose of 2 mg/kg per day will maintain remission in up to two-thirds of patients. Approximately half the patients who do not tolerate azathioprine will tolerate mercaptopurine[66,70,71]. Methotrexate may be effective in both inducing and maintaining remission if azathioprine and mercaptopurine fail.

When these traditional drug therapies have been exhausted, and the patient still has active disease, or remission cannot be maintained, what does infliximab have to offer?

Clinical efficacy of infliximab in CD

An early multicentre, double-blind study on 108 patients with moderate to severe CD refractory to 5-ASA, corticosteroids, and/or immunomodulators, showed an 81% response rate at 4 weeks after 5 mg/kg infliximab compared with 17% in patients receiving placebo[72]. Forty-eight per cent of the patients who had received 5 mg/kg body weight infliximab still had a clinical response at week 12 in this first and important study. Remarkably, there was no dose response when compared to 10 mg/kg. This early experience was later confirmed in several other studies[73,74]; therefore it seems to be clear that infliximab is able to induce a clinical response or remission in patients with CD. The question arose whether infliximab could be used for maintenance of response or remission.

In the ACCENT I trial it could be demonstrated that, with regular subsequent dosing, 28% of initial responders are in remission after 12 months[75]. It is important to take a look at the study design that has recently been adopted for several other clinical trials on anti-TNF agents in CD. Five hundred and seventy-three patients with a Crohn's disease activity index (CDAI) of at least 220 received a 5 mg/kg intravenous infusion of infliximab at week 0. After assessment of response at week 2, non-responders were excluded from the further study and published data did not refer to all initially treated patients but only to the responders that were randomized. This study design has been discussed extensively, and obviously has some shortcomings: the CD patient who receives infliximab for the first time is of course at a similar point as the initially open-label-treated patients in the ACCENT I study. It has been argued that the study was designed not to evaluate remission rates, but maintenance of remission. In the clinical situation, however, induction of remission and maintenance of remission with the same drug cannot be separated.

After excluding all non-responders from the ongoing ACCENT I study patients were randomly assigned to repeated infusions of placebo at weeks 2 and 6 and then every 8 weeks thereafter until week 46 (group I), repeated infusions of 5 mg/kg infliximab at the same time points (group II), or 5 mg/kg infliximab at weeks 2 and 6 followed by 10 mg/kg (group III). Three hundred and thirty-five (58%) patients responded to a single infusion of infliximab within 2 weeks[75]. At week 30, 23 of 110 (21%) patients in group I (placebo) were in remission, compared with 44 of 113 patients (39%) in group II, and 50 of 112 patients (45%) in group III. Patients in groups II and III combined were more likely to sustain clinical remission than patients in group I.

A recent Cochrane review on the use of TNF antibodies for the induction of remission in CD patients identified 10 randomized controlled trials[76]. Three studies[74,75,77], were excluded from the analysis as the authors state that they did not describe the use of TNF blocking agents for induction of remission. The ACCENT I trial[75] and Rutgeerts et al.[79] were excluded because they only described the use of TNF agents for maintenance of remission. The Present study[77] was excluded as it describes the effect of infliximab for the treatment of fistulas in patients with CD. A publication of D'Haens and co-workers[73] was excluded from the Cochrane review, as it is not a primary study but a subgroup analysis of an earlier study by Targan and colleagues[72]. The reviewers finally identified only four randomized controlled trials that satisfied the inclusion criteria (TNF blocking agents for the induction of remission of CD), only one of them studying the efficacy of infliximab[72]. This indicates that, despite all discussions and controversies, the number of good studies and the quality of evidence is limited with respect to the infliximab-induced remission of CD. Based on the above-mentioned analysis the Cochrane review concluded that 'infliximab may be an effective treatment for active CD among patients who no longer respond to corticosteroids or immunosuppressive drugs'[76].

In some countries, such as the UK, infliximab is limited to patients with severe active CD (Harvey Bradshaw index > 8, CDAI > 300) refractory to or intolerant of corticosteroids and immunosuppression for whom surgery is inappropriate[47]. In line with the UK guidelines a European expert panel agreed that infliximab is appropriate for corticosteroid dependence, corticosteroid refractoriness or corticosteroid intolerance, and that it can be considered after failure of either azathioprine/6-mercaptopurine (AZA/6-MP) or methotrexate (MTX)[47]. Whereas some experts argue that infliximab should be administered only after all established treatment steps including MTX have been applied, the ECCO expert panel agreed that 'there is no need to have failed both AZA/6-MP and MTX before infliximab'[47].

After the initial infusions re-treatment is usually necessary after a variable interval (most commonly 8–16 weeks)[78–83]. However, in the ACCENT I trial scheduled treatment was not superior to treatment on demand at every time point. Nevertheless, clinical experience shows that CD patients who really depend on infliximab treatment are in need of the administration every 6–10 weeks.

It has been generally recommended over recent years that all patients treated with infliximab additionally should receive an immunosuppressant such as AZA, 6-MP or MTX (if tolerated) as this reduces the development of antibodies against infliximab[84,85]. These human anti-chimeric antibodies (HACA) may reduce efficacy and may increase side-effects such as allergic reactions[84,86–88]. The development of HACA may lead to infusion reactions. Strategies to reduce the frequency of HACA formation in addition to the continuous administration of immunosuppressants as mentioned above include premedication with intravenous corticosteroids (i.e. 100 mg methylprednisolone intravenously). However, it seems doubtful whether corticosteroid premedication is of any effect. In addition there are recent concerns as to whether a combination therapy of AZA and infliximab will increase the risk of lymphoma, especially in younger patients (see below).

A regular treatment regime with infliximab also seems to reduce the risk of neutralizing antibodies or infusion reactions compared to treatment on demand[78,81,89,90].

Whereas it is clear that clinical remission is the primary goal of the medical treatment of CD, with the introduction of infliximab a new paradigm has been introduced in CD therapy: a number of investigators support the concept of mucosal healing as an important treatment goal[81,82,90–96]. This has been discussed controversially[97,98]. It seems to be reasonable that maintenance of remission will be easier if the mucosa shows complete healing. Therefore, regulatory agencies such as the FDA have adopted 'mucosal healing' as a (in all cases) secondary endpoint for most newer studies on the treatment of CD. Experience has shown that frequently what seems to be logical is not necessarily true or effective in clinical medicine. The evidence we have so far that would support the concept of mucosal healing is very limited. A recent study that provided data on the potential role of mucosal healing focused on an attempt to treat lesions in a topdown approach. One hundred and thirty patients with active, recently diagnosed CD never treated with steroids, AZA or infliximab, were randomized to either infliximab induction treatment plus AZA, or initial steroid treatment using budesonide or prednisolone, which was then tapered. The endpoint was achievement of clinical remission (a CDAI score of <150) without glucocorticosteroid medication. This endpoint was reached more often in the infliximab group at 6 months. The difference, however, was not significant at the 12-month visit; therefore it is hard to conclude that the aggressive treatment of mucosal lesions may clearly be beneficial.

When a Scottish study assessed the frequency of mucosal inflammatory activity in 30 clinically inactive CD patients (CDAI <150) with good quality-of-life index ongoing mucosal inflammation was detectable in up to two-thirds of CD patients in clinical remission[99]. Rutgeerts and co-workers found a close correlation between clinical remission and endoscopic healing under infliximab treatment in the ACCENT I trial[90]; but even in this large clinical study only a numerical trend for patients with better mucosal healing to have a lower rate of CD-related hospitalizations was observed, meaning that there was no statistically significant improvement in the clinical course of CD when mucosa healing was achieved[90]. In conclusion, evidence is lacking that the long-term outcome of patients achieving mucosal healing is better compared to patients only having clinical remission. Most of the data so far published even argue against mucosal healing as an important treatment goal. As long as no prospective studies are available clearly showing an advantage of mucosal healing it can only be concluded that: (1) mucosal healing seems possible with continued therapy using immunosuppressants; (2) current data do not provide evidence that, once mucosal healing has been achieved, the long-term prognosis changes; and (3) it is plausible, but not yet proven, that maintaining mucosal healing may change long-term outcome[98].

Infliximab treatment for CD fistulas

Fistulas are a frequent problem in patients suffering from CD. The reported incidence ranges from 17% up to 50%[100–106]. This may be due to a centre bias as fistulizing CD is seen more frequently in centres for inflammatory bowel disease (IBD), but also population-based studies show a high incidence of fistulas in CD[49,50,107]. In a recent population-based study Sandborn and co-workers reported occurrence of fistulas in up to 35% of the patients, with perianal fistulas occurring in about 20%[107,108]. The cumulative incidence of fistulizing CD in the study was 33% after 10 years and increased up to 50% after 20 years, making it a major clinical problem of disease management. Two-thirds of those patients, however, had only a single fistula episode; 34% of these patients had recurrent fistulas. Recurrent fistulas occurred less frequently in patients who received maintenance therapy with an immunosuppressive agent. If abscesses are present, drainage is first required and conservative treatment will not be successful.

The conservative, medical treatment of perianal and rectovaginal fistulas complicating CD is still unsatisfactory. Conventional treatments, such as sulphasalazine, 5-ASA and glucocorticoids, are not effective. Mostly uncontrolled studies have reported efficacy of administration of antibiotics such as metronidazole and ciprofloxacin for several weeks[104,109–111]. Furthermore, positive results have been reported with AZA, 6-MP and cyclosporine A[112–115]; however, data from prospective randomized trials are rare. Cyclosporine administered intravenously has been shown to improve drainage of 10 of 12 fistulas after a mean of 7.9 days (range 3–28 days) in five patients, with two relapses under oral therapy[116]. In a study by Present and Lichtiger 14 of 16 patients (88%) responded to intravenous cyclosporine (closure 44%, improvement 44%)[117].

Infliximab has been reported to be effective in a first randomized, multicentre, double-blind, placebo-controlled study on the use of infliximab in the treatment of fistulizing CD in 1999[77]. In this study Present et al. examined two infliximab doses, 5 mg/kg body weight and 10 mg/kg, given at weeks 0, 2 and 6, and compared the effect with placebo. The primary efficacy endpoint was an achievement of 50% or greater reduction from baseline in the number of draining fistulas for at least two consecutive evaluation visits (at least 1 month). A fistula was considered to be closed if it no longer drained despite gentle compression. Secondary efficacy endpoints were determined by a complete response (closure of all fistulas for at least two consecutive study visits), CDAI score, patients' global assessment and quality-of-life measurements. Patients were considered to be treatment failures for the study medication if any of the following three occurred: (a) an increase in dosage of their concomitant medication(s); (b) initiation of additional medication(s); (c) surgery needed to treat the fistulas during the trial. In both infliximab treatment groups a statistically greater number of patients achieved the primary endpoint (62%) compared with the control group (26%). A statistically significant dose–response effect was not observed between the 5 mg/kg and the 10 mg/kg groups. Closure of draining fistulas by infliximab treatment was characterized by rapid onset (usually within 2 weeks) and a median duration of closure of 12 weeks. However, after 22 weeks there was no difference in the proportion of patients responding between either dose of infliximab and placebo.

In the ACCENT II study, 282 patients with fistulizing CD were treated with 5 mg/kg infliximab at weeks 0, 2 and 6[118,119]. Again, as in the ACCENT I trial, only the 195 (69%) responders at week 14 were randomized to receive placebo maintenance or infliximab (5 mg/kg) maintenance every 8 weeks. The median time to loss of response was 14 weeks for placebo maintenance and more than 40 weeks for infliximab ($p < 0.001$). Overall, 62% of placebo-maintained patients had a loss of response over 54 weeks, compared with 42% in the infliximab-maintained group.

Taken together these studies indicate that reopening of fistulas is very frequent, suggesting the persistence of deep fistulous tracts despite superficial healing. This indicates that the introduction of infliximab into medical treatment of perianal CD has improved our treatment option; however, it is not a 'revolution' or 'dramatic' change of therapy.

Safety concerns for infliximab use in CD patients

In general the potential benefits of a biologic therapy need to be weighed against potential risks. The clinical safety of infliximab in CD has been evaluated in more than 1200 patients with CD included in the randomized, placebo-controlled studies mentioned above[72,74,77,120]. Clearly there have been reports of severe infections seen under anti-TNF therapy, including primary and disseminated tuberculosis, pneumonia, sepsis, urinary tract infections, abscesses and peritonitis. Systemic infections, including cytomegalovirus, coccidioidomycosis, aspergillosis, disseminated histoplasmosis, candidiasis, listeriosis, cutaneous nocardiosis and *Pneumocystis carinii* pneumonia, have been described in patients treated with infliximab.

The reactivation of latent tuberculosis occurred in 350 of more than 400 000 patients treated with infliximab[79]. This indicates that infliximab is associated with a fourfold or fivefold increase in risk of tuberculosis. Therefore, all patients are recommended to have chest radiography and a tuberculosis skin test before application. Infliximab is contraindicated if chest radiography shows signs of active tuberculosis. Unfortunately, a number of reported cases were miliary tuberculosis[121–124] without any previous sings in chest radiography. Furthermore, the reliability of a skin test monitoring an immunological reaction is of course questionable when the patient is currently being treated with immunosuppressants such as steroids or AZA. Consecutively one has to accept that there is no safe procedure for exclusion of tuberculosis or for estimating the risk of tuberculosis. It has to be taken into account that the risk of developing tuberculosis depends on the population prevalence in the patient group as well as on ethnicity and geographical location[32,124–138]. Some physicians recommend that patients with a positive tuberculosis test should have chemoprophylaxis and then can receive infliximab. However, this has to be an individual decision and no general evidence-based guideline is available for this situation. Negative tests in those taking immunomodulators are unreliable, as mentioned.

Before treating a patient with fistulizing and/or perianal disease with infliximab an abscess should certainly be excluded.

As outlined above, treatment with infliximab may result in the development of antibodies to infliximab (HACA). Patients treated episodically with infliximab develop HACA more frequently (30–61%)[84,89,139] than those with maintenance treatment (7–10%)[79,89]. It has been observed that the occurrence of HACA is lower in patients concurrently being treated with immunomodulators than in those not receiving them. If HACA develop, the risk of infusion reactions is increased and the duration of clinical response is likely to be shorter[84].

In general, infusion reactions occurred in 16–21% of infliximab-treated patients[75,119]. An acute infusion reaction generally occurs during infusion or within 2 h after infusion. Infusion reactions are usually characterized by symptoms of headache, dizziness, nausea, injection-site irritation, flushing, chest pain, dyspnoea or pruritus[75]. The infusion should either be stopped or (if the symptoms are mild) slowed down and combined with symptomatic treatment with diphenhydramine, acetaminophen, antihistamines and corticosteroids[80]. Rare and serious side-effects are anaphylactic shock, larynx oedema and stridor.

There have been reports of new-onset heart failure, worsening of existing heart failure, demyelination disorders and drug-induced lupus under infliximab therapy.

After treatment with infliximab antibodies to double-stranded DNA (anti-dsDNA) and antinuclear antibodies can occur. The maintenance trials demonstrated a higher prevalence of these antibodies in patients treated with infliximab (23.3–34% for anti-dsDNA and 46–56% for antinuclear antibodies) than placebo (6.3–11% for anti-dsDNA and 18–35% for antinuclear antibodies)[75,119]. Symptoms of drug-induced lupus reactions not involving the central nervous system or the kidneys occurred in 0.2% of patients treated with infliximab. In the same trials the incidence of infections requiring antibiotics ranged between 30% and 34% for infliximab recipients and between 27% and 37% for placebo recipients. Serious infections occurred in 3–4% of patients treated with infliximab and in 4–6% of patients treated with placebo[75,119].

Since immunosuppressed patients have an increased risk of developing lymphoproliferative disorders a relationship between treatment with infliximab and the occurrence of lymphomas in CD patients has been discussed. In addition, there is concern about an increased risk for other malignancies with the use of infliximab, because TNF may be protective against cancer development. However, hitherto no clear corroborating epidemiological data support this concern. Infliximab treatment in the controlled studies mentioned above did not show an increased incidence of any cancer[79]. This is in line with the results of the TREAT registry[140], in which no statistical difference has been observed in malignancies between patients who were treated and those who were not treated with infliximab. The TREAT registry was established to study the long-term safety of infliximab and other therapies in prospectively followed patients with Crohn's disease[140]. There were 6290 patients (3179 infliximab recipients and 3111 other therapies) enrolled in this registry by August 2004[140]. According to available data in the TREAT registry, the safety of infliximab was similar to that of conventional immunomodulators[140].

In a recent paper Colombel et al. summarized the side-effects of infliximab therapy in the first 500 patients treated at the Mayo Clinic[141]. They reported serious or severe infections in 8.2% of the patients, possibly related to infliximab, including two patients developing fatal sepsis and two developing fatal pneumonia[141]. Over all, five deaths (1%) were felt to be related to infliximab. Therefore, longer follow-up of the safety data is still necessary, as the data are in contrast to the TREAT registry.

In July 2006 Centocor Inc informed health-care professionals all over the world that hepatosplenic T-cell lymphoma, a rare entity of lymphoma primarily affecting the liver and the spleen, occurred in six children treated with infliximab. Five of these six children have so far died. All patients had received infliximab combined with AZA. Several physicians therefore argue that AZA might be responsible for the observed lymphoma in these patients, and that combination therapy should be carefully re-evaluated or even avoided (which is in contrast to what has been suggested during recent years by the same colleagues). A detailed recent review analysed all published data regarding the risk of lymphoma induced by AZA and 6-MP[142]. From a significant number of large well-designed population-based studies exploring the lymphoma risk associated with AZA and 6-MP therapy it was concluded that it is likely to be of minimal clinical significance compared to the established and more frequent risks of myelosuppression and infection, and is far outweighed by the clinical benefit of immunomodulator therapy in IBD[142].

By March 2001 it is estimated that 121 000 patients had been given infliximab for either rheumatoid arthritis or CD[143]. The reported numbers of lymphoma cases potentially associated with infliximab was calculated at 6.6/100 000 patients treated[143]. However, because of incomplete ascertainment, it has been assumed that this calculation was an underestimate of the true incidence of lymphoma in infliximab-treated patients[142]. In addition, from November 2001 to September 2002, 39 more cases of 'possible' or 'probable' infliximab-associated lymphoma were reported to the FDA. In October 2004, advised by the FDA, an amendment was added to the package insert of infliximab that malignancy, including lymphoma, could be a potential adverse reaction to infliximab treatment. This was based upon an evaluation of marketed TNF blockers by the Arthritis Advisory Committee of the FDA in March 2003[144]. The committee noted an eight-fold higher rate of lymphoma in CD patients treated with infliximab in clinical trials as compared to age-, gender- and race-matched populations[144].

From the available data it is impossible to conclude whether AZA or infliximab, or a combination of the two, could be responsible for the reported six cases of hepatosplenic T-cell lymphoma. The only possible conclusion can be that combined administration of the drugs needs to be considered with care. Side-effects should not be underestimated but also not overestimated; a careful and individual risk–benefit balance calculation is necessary.

INDICATION FOR INFLIXIMAB USE IN ULCERATIVE COLITIS

Ulcerative colitis (UC) is a chronic relapsing inflammatory disorder of the large bowel. Compared to CD the role of TNF-blocking agents in UC is less clear, and recent studies have not yielded uniform results. In 2001 and 2002 a number of uncontrolled studies[145–149] and a small randomized controlled trial[150] have suggested that there may be a role for TNF-blocking agents in patients with UC. Later a randomized controlled trial did not support the use of infliximab for the management of glucocorticoid-resistant UC[151].

In a very recent Cochrane review[52] seven randomized controlled trials were identified on infliximab use in UC[150,151,153–156]. These studies compared infliximab use in UC with either placebo or corticosteroids. Two of those studies (the ACT1 and ACT2 trials) had high patient numbers.

The ACT1 trial was conducted globally at 62 sites and evaluated 364 patients. All participants had moderately to severely active UC despite concurrent treatment with corticosteroids, and/or AZA or 6-MP[153]. Patients who previously had not responded to, or could not tolerate, corticosteroids, AZA or 6-MP were not required to be taking any concurrent therapy at enrolment. Eligible patients were randomized in a 1:1:1 ratio and received intravenous infusions of infliximab at a dose of 5 mg/kg (n = 121), 10 mg/kg (n = 122) or placebo (n = 121) at weeks 0, 2, and 6 and then every 8 weeks through week 46. The primary endpoint was clinical response at week 8. Secondary endpoints were clinical response at weeks 30 and 54 among others. The design of the ACT2 trial was very similar[153]; it was conducted globally at 55 sites and involved 364 patients. Eligible patients had moderately to severely active UC despite concurrent treatment with corticosteroids, and/or AZA or 6-MP and/or 5-ASA. This means that patients who had only failed to respond to 5-ASA therapy could be included in the study. Unfortunately no data have been given so far as to how many patients were included that only had received 5-ASA before.

Eligible patients were randomized in a 1:1:1 ratio to receive intravenous infusions of infliximab at a dose of 5 mg/kg (n = 121), 10 mg/kg (n = 120) or placebo (n = 123) at weeks 0, 2, and 6 and then every 8 weeks through week 22. Patients were followed through week 30. The primary endpoint was clinical response at week 8. Secondary endpoints were clinical response at week 30, clinical remission, and mucosal healing at weeks 8 and 30, clinical remission with discontinuation of corticosteroids at week 30, and clinical response at week 8 according to corticosteroid-refractory status.

Taken together with the trials by Jarnerot et al.[155] and Probert et al.[151] the ACT1 and ACT2 studies combined data from 816 participants (531 infliximab and 285 placebo)[152]. The ACT1 and ACT2 results both showed a statistically significant benefit for infliximab[153]. The studies by Jarnerot et al.[155] and Probert et al.[151] (n = 45 and 43) did not show a statistically significant benefit for infliximab over placebo, but both were underpowered[152]. In the ACT1 and ACT2 studies a total of 728 patients (484 infliximab and 244 placebo) were included[153]. The results of the meta-analysis showed that infliximab was effective for induction of clinical remission at 8 weeks (NNT = 5)[152]. Infliximab was also effective in producing a clinical response (NNT = 4)[152].

There is still general consent that 5-ASA, corticosteroids and immunosuppressive agents should be used prior to infliximab therapy for UC. Whether infliximab should be used prior to cyclosporine, which has been shown to be effective in severe UC[157–168], or after cyclosporine failed, is still a matter for discussion. There are so far no good studies directly comparing infliximab and cyclosporine. The question of when it is appropriate to use infliximab in clinical practice should therefore be addressed in future studies.

References

1. Rutgeerts P. Infliximab is the drug we have been waiting for in Crohn's disease. Inflamm Bowel Dis. 2000;6:132–6.
2. Shanahan F. Anti-TNF therapy for Crohn's disease: a perspective (infliximab is not the drug we have been waiting for). Inflamm Bowel Dis. 2000;6:137–9.

3. Ehlers S. Tumor necrosis factor and its blockade in granulomatous infections: differential modes of action of infliximab and etanercept? Clin Infect Dis. 2005;41(Suppl. 3):S199–203.
4. Goodsell DS. The molecular perspective: tumor necrosis factor. Oncologist. 2006;11:83–4.
5. So T, Lee SW, Croft M. Tumor necrosis factor/tumor necrosis factor receptor family members that positively regulate immunity. Int J Hematol. 2006;83:1–11.
6. Arch RH. Function of tumor necrosis factor receptor family members on regulatory T-cells. Immunol Res. 2005;32:15–29.
7. Wang J, Fu YX. Tumor necrosis factor family members and inflammatory bowel disease. Immunol Rev. 2005;204:144–55.
8. Ghezzi P, Cerami A. Tumor necrosis factor as a pharmacological target. Methods Mol Med. 2004;98:1–8.
9. Feldmann M, Brennan F, Paleolog E, Taylor P, Maini RN. Anti-tumor necrosis factor alpha therapy of rheumatoid arthritis. Mechanism of action. Eur Cytokine Netw. 1997;8: 297–300.
10. Moreland LW. Inhibitors of tumor necrosis factor: new treatment options for rheumatoid arthritis. Cleve Clin J Med. 1999;66:367–74.
11. Beutler BA. The role of tumor necrosis factor in health and disease. J Rheumatol Suppl. 1999;57:16–21.
12. Hsu HC, Wu Y, Mountz JD. Tumor necrosis factor ligand-receptor superfamily and arthritis. Curr Dir Autoimmm. 2006;9:37–54.
13. Feldmann M, Maini RN. Discovery of TNF-alpha as a therapeutic target in rheumatoid arthritis: preclinical and clinical studies. Joint Bone Spine. 2002;69:12–18.
14. Tse SM, Burgos-Vargas R, Laxer RM. Anti-tumor necrosis factor alpha blockade in the treatment of juvenile spondylarthropathy. Arthritis Rheum. 2005;52:2103–8.
15. Brandt J, Braun J. Anti-TNF-alpha agents in the treatment of psoriatic arthritis. Expert Opin Biol Ther. 2006;6:99–107.
16. Tobin AM, Kirby B. TNF alpha inhibitors in the treatment of psoriasis and psoriatic arthritis. BioDrugs. 2005;19:47–57.
17. Mease PJ. Tumour necrosis factor (TNF) in psoriatic arthritis: pathophysiology and treatment with TNF inhibitors. Ann Rheum Dis. 2002;61:298–304.
18. Liu AY, Miskovsky EP, Stanhope PE, Siliciano RF. Production of transmembrane and secreted forms of tumor necrosis factor (TNF)-alpha by HIV-1-specific CD4$^+$ cytolytic T lymphocyte clones. Evidence for a TNF-alpha-independent cytolytic mechanism. J Immunol. 1992;148:3789–98.
19. Pocsik E, Duda E, Wallach D. Phosphorylation of the 26 kDa TNF precursor in monocytic cells and in transfected HeLa cells. J Inflamm. 1995;45:152–60.
20. Domonkos A, Udvardy A, Laszlo L, Nagy T, Duda E. Receptor-like properties of the 26 kDa transmembrane form of TNF. Eur Cytokine Netw. 2001;12:411–19.
21. Moss ML, Jin SL, Becherer JD et al. Structural features and biochemical properties of TNF-alpha converting enzyme (TACE). J Neuroimmunol. 1997;72:127–9.
22. Bigda J, Holtmann H. TNF receptors – how they function and interact. Arch Immunol Ther Exp (Warsz). 1997;45:263–70.
23. Riches DW, Chan ED, Winston BW. TNF-alpha-induced regulation and signalling in macrophages. Immunobiology. 1996;195:477–90.
24. Reinecker HC, Steffen M, Witthoeft T et al. Enhanced secretion of tumour necrosis factor-alpha, IL-6, and IL-1 beta by isolated lamina propria mononuclear cells from patients with ulcerative colitis and Crohn's disease. Clin Exp Immunol. 1993;94:174–81.
25. Beil WJ, Weller PF, Peppercorn MA, Galli SJ, Dvorak AM. Ultrastructural immunogold localization of subcellular sites of TNF-alpha in colonic Crohn's disease. J Leukoc Biol. 1995;58:284–98.
26. Reimund JM, Wittersheim C, Dumont S et al. Increased production of tumour necrosis factor-alpha interleukin-1 beta, and interleukin-6 by morphologically normal intestinal biopsies from patients with Crohn's disease. Gut. 1996;39:684–9.
27. Van Deventer SJ. Tumour necrosis factor and Crohn's disease. Gut. 1997;40:443–8.
28. Plevy SE, Landers CJ, Prehn J et al. A role for TNF-alpha and T helper-1 cytokines in the pathogenesis of Crohn's disease. J Immunol. 1997;159:6276–82.
29. Schreiber S, Nikolaus S, Hampe J et al. Tumour necrosis factor alpha and interleukin 1 beta in relapse of Crohn's disease. Lancet. 1999;353:459–61.

30. Siegel SA, Shealy DJ, Nakada MT et al. The mouse/human chimeric monoclonal antibody cA2 neutralizes TNF *in vitro* and protects transgenic mice from cachexia and TNF lethality *in vivo*. Cytokine. 1995;7:15–25.

31. Scallon BJ, Moore MA, Trinh H, Knight DM, Ghrayeb J. Chimeric anti-TNF-alpha monoclonal antibody cA2 binds recombinant transmembrane TNF-alpha and activates immune effector functions. Cytokine. 1995;7:251–9.

32. Rutgeerts P, Van Assche G, Vermeire S. Infliximab therapy for inflammatory bowel disease – seven years on. Aliment Pharmacol Ther. 2006;23:451–63.

33. Cornillie F, Shealy D, D'Haens G et al. Infliximab induces potent anti-inflammatory and local immunomodulatory activity but no systemic immune suppression in patients with Crohn's disease. Aliment Pharmacol Ther. 2001;15:463–73.

34. Kirman I, Whelan RL, Nielsen OH. Infliximab: mechanism of action beyond TNF-alpha neutralization in inflammatory bowel disease. Eur J Gastroenterol Hepatol. 2004;16:639–41.

35. Sandborn WJ, Hanauer SB, Katz S et al. Etanercept for active Crohn's disease: a randomized, double-blind, placebo-controlled trial. Gastroenterology. 2001;121:1088–94.

36. Travers SB. Etanercept for Crohn's disease. N Engl J Med. 2004;350:840; author reply 840.

37. Rutgeerts P, Sandborn WJ, Fedorak RN et al. Onercept for moderate-to-severe Crohn's disease: a randomized, double-blind, placebo-controlled trial. Clin Gastroenterol Hepatol. 2006;4:888–93.

38. Rutgeerts P, Lemmens L, Van Assche G, Noman M, Borghini-Fuhrer I, Goedkoop R. Treatment of active Crohn's disease with onercept (recombinant human soluble p55 tumour necrosis factor receptor): results of a randomized, open-label, pilot study. Aliment Pharmacol Ther. 2003;17:185–92.

39. van Deventer SJ. Transmembrane TNF-alpha, induction of apoptosis, and the efficacy of TNF-targeting therapies in Crohn's disease. Gastroenterology. 2001;121:1242–6.

40. Van den Brande JM, Braat H, van den Brink GR et al. Infliximab but not etanercept induces apoptosis in lamina propria T-lymphocytes from patients with Crohn's disease. Gastroenterology. 2003;124:1774–85.

41. Ohshima S, Mima T, Sasai M et al. Tumour necrosis factor alpha (TNF-alpha) interferes with Fas-mediated apoptotic cell death on rheumatoid arthritis (RA) synovial cells: a possible mechanism of rheumatoid synovial hyperplasia and a clinical benefit of anti-TNF-alpha therapy for RA. Cytokine. 2000;12:281–8.

42. Lugering A, Schmidt M, Lugering N, Pauels HG, Domschke W, Kucharzik T. Infliximab induces apoptosis in monocytes from patients with chronic active Crohn's disease by using a caspase-dependent pathway. Gastroenterology. 2001;121:1145–57.

43. Sisson G, Harris A. Certolizumab pegol (CDP870) for treatment of Crohn's disease. Gastroenterology. 2006;130:285–6; author reply 286.

44. Schreiber S, Rutgeerts P, Fedorak RN et al. A randomized, placebo-controlled trial of certolizumab pegol (CDP870) for treatment of Crohn's disease. Gastroenterology. 2005;129:807–18.

45. Bell S, Kamm MA. Antibodies to tumour necrosis factor alpha as treatment for Crohn's disease. Lancet. 2000;355:858–60.

46. Buning C, Lochs H. Conventional therapy for Crohn's disease. World J Gastroenterol. 2006;12:4794–806.

47. Travis SP, Stange EF, Lemann M et al. European evidence-based consensus on the diagnosis and management of Crohn's disease: current management. Gut. 2006;55(Suppl. 1):i16–35.

48. Lim WC, Hanauer SB. Controversies with aminosalicylates in inflammatory bowel disease. Rev Gastroenterol Disord. 2004;4:104–17.

49. Silverstein MD, Loftus EV, Sandborn WJ et al. Clinical course and costs of care for Crohn's disease: Markov model analysis of a population-based cohort. Gastroenterology. 1999;117:49–57.

50. Loftus EV Jr, Silverstein MD, Sandborn WJ, Tremaine WJ, Harmsen WS, Zinsmeister AR. Crohn's disease in Olmsted County, Minnesota, 1940–1993: incidence, prevalence, and survival. Gastroenterology. 1998;114:1161–8.

51. Kimberly RP. Glucocorticoids. Curr Opin Rheumatol. 1994;6:273–80.

52. Adler RA, Rosen CJ. Glucocorticoids and osteoporosis. Endocrinol Metab Clin N Am. 1994;23:641–54.

53. Umland SP, Schleimer RP, Johnston SL. Review of the molecular and cellular mechanisms of action of glucocorticoids for use in asthma. Pulm Pharmacol Ther. 2002;15:35–50.

54. Franchimont D. Overview of the actions of glucocorticoids on the immune response: a good model to characterize new pathways of immunosuppression for new treatment strategies. Ann NY Acad Sci. 2004;1024:124–37.

55. Czock D, Keller F, Rasche FM, Haussler U. Pharmacokinetics and pharmacodynamics of systemically administered glucocorticoids. Clin Pharmacokinet. 2005;44:61–98.

56. Recommendations for the prevention and treatment of glucocorticoid-induced osteoporosis. American College of Rheumatology Task Force on Osteoporosis Guidelines. Arthritis Rheum. 1996;39:1791–801.

57. Lester RS, Knowles SR, Shear NH. The risks of systemic corticosteroid use. Dermatol Clin. 1998;16:277–88.

58. Aberra FN, Lewis JD, Hass D, Rombeau JL, Osborne B, Lichtenstein GR. Corticosteroids and immunomodulators: postoperative infectious complication risk in inflammatory bowel disease patients. Gastroenterology. 2003;125:320–7.

59. van Berge Henegouwen GP. [Consensus for infliximab treatment of patients with Crohn's disease]. Ned Tijdschr Geneeskd. 2000;144:1844–5.

60. Schreiber S, Campieri M, Colombel JF et al. Use of anti-tumour necrosis factor agents in inflammatory bowel disease. European guidelines for 2001–2003. Int J Colorectal Dis. 2001;16:1–11; discussion 12–13.

61. Reissmann A, Fleig W. [Therapy of Crohn disease according to the guidelines of the German Society for the treatment of digestive and metabolic diseases]. Z Arztl Fortbild Qualitatssich. 2002;96:233–8.

62. Panaccione R, Fedorak RN, Aumais G et al. Canadian Association of Gastroenterology Clinical Practice Guidelines: the use of infliximab in Crohn's disease. Can J Gastroenterol. 2004;18:503–8.

63. Fedorak RN. Canadian Association of Gastroenterology Clinical Practice Guidelines: the use of infliximab in Crohn's disease. Can J Gastroenterol. 2001;15:367–70.

64. Bauerfeind P, Beglinger C, Beltinger J et al. [Infliximab–practical guidelines for the treatment of Crohn's disease]. Rev Med Suisse. 2006;2:1807–15.

65. Lichtenstein GR, Abreu MT, Cohen R, Tremaine W. American Gastroenterological Association Institute medical position statement on corticosteroids, immunomodulators, and infliximab in inflammatory bowel disease. Gastroenterology. 2006;130:935–9.

66. Pearson DC, May GR, Fick G, Sutherland LR. Azathioprine for maintaining remission of Crohn's disease. Cochrane Database Syst Rev. 2000:CD000067.

67. Sandborn W, Sutherland L, Pearson D, May G, Modigliani R, Prantera C. Azathioprine or 6-mercaptopurine for inducing remission of Crohn's disease. Cochrane Database Syst Rev. 2000:CD000545.

68. Mate-Jimenez J, Hermida C, Cantero-Perona J, Moreno-Otero R. 6-mercaptopurine or methotrexate added to prednisone induces and maintains remission in steroid-dependent inflammatory bowel disease. Eur J Gastroenterol Hepatol. 2000;12:1227–33.

69. Chong RY, Hanauer SB, Cohen RD. Efficacy of parenteral methotrexate in refractory Crohn's disease. Aliment Pharmacol Ther. 2001;15:35–44.

70. Plevy SE. Corticosteroid-sparing treatments in patients with Crohn's disease. Am J Gastroenterol. 2002;97:1607–17.

71. Markowitz JF. Therapeutic efficacy and safety of 6-mercaptopurine and azathioprine in patients with Crohn's disease. Rev Gastroenterol Disord. 2003;3(Suppl. 1):S23–9.

72. Targan SR, Hanauer SB, van Deventer SJ et al. A short-term study of chimeric monoclonal antibody cA2 to tumor necrosis factor alpha for Crohn's disease. Crohn's Disease cA2 Study Group. N Engl J Med. 1997;337:1029–35.

73. D'Haens G, Van Deventer S, Van Hogezand R et al. Endoscopic and histological healing with infliximab anti-tumor necrosis factor antibodies in Crohn's disease: A European multicenter trial. Gastroenterology. 1999;116:1029–34.

74. Rutgeerts P, D'Haens G, Targan S et al. Efficacy and safety of retreatment with anti-tumor necrosis factor antibody (infliximab) to maintain remission in Crohn's disease. Gastroenterology. 1999;117:761–9.

75. Hanauer SB, Feagan BG, Lichtenstein GR et al. Maintenance infliximab for Crohn's disease: the ACCENT I randomised trial. Lancet. 2002;359:1541–9.

76. Akobeng AK, Zachos M. Tumor necrosis factor-alpha antibody for induction of remission in Crohn's disease. Cochrane Database Syst Rev. 2004:CD003574.
77. Present DH, Rutgeerts P, Targan S et al. Infliximab for the treatment of fistulas in patients with Crohn's disease. N Engl J Med. 1999;340:1398–405.
78. Mendoza JL, Garcia-Paredes J, Cruz Santamaria DM et al. Infliximab treatment and prognostic factors for response in patients with Crohn's disease. Rev Esp Enferm Dig. 2002;94:269–79.
79. Rutgeerts P, Van Assche G, Vermeire S. Optimizing anti-TNF treatment in inflammatory bowel disease. Gastroenterology. 2004;126:1593–610.
80. Sandborn WJ, Hanauer SB. Infliximab in the treatment of Crohn's disease: a user's guide for clinicians. Am J Gastroenterol. 2002;97:2962–72.
81. Rutgeerts P, Feagan BG, Lichtenstein GR et al. Comparison of scheduled and episodic treatment strategies of infliximab in Crohn's disease. Gastroenterology. 2004;126:402–13.
82. Geboes K, Rutgeerts P, Opdenakker G et al. Endoscopic and histologic evidence of persistent mucosal healing and correlation with clinical improvement following sustained infliximab treatment for Crohn's disease. Curr Med Res Opin. 2005;21:1741–54.
83. Sands BE, Blank MA, Diamond RH, Barrett JP, Van Deventer SJ. Maintenance infliximab does not result in increased abscess development in fistulizing Crohn's disease: results from the ACCENT II study. Aliment Pharmacol Ther. 2006;23:1127–36.
84. Baert F, Noman M, Vermeire S et al. Influence of immunogenicity on the long-term efficacy of infliximab in Crohn's disease. N Engl J Med. 2003;348:601–8.
85. Lemann M, Mary JY, Duclos B et al. Infliximab plus azathioprine for steroid-dependent Crohn's disease patients: a randomized placebo-controlled trial. Gastroenterology. 2006; 130:1054–61.
86. Sandborn WJ, Hanauer SB. Antitumor necrosis factor therapy for inflammatory bowel disease: a review of agents, pharmacology, clinical results, and safety. Inflamm Bowel Dis. 1999;5:119–33.
87. Wagner CL, Schantz A, Barnathan E et al. Consequences of immunogenicity to the therapeutic monoclonal antibodies ReoPro and Remicade. Dev Biol (Basel). 2003;112:37–53.
88. Sandborn WJ. Optimizing anti-tumor necrosis factor strategies in inflammatory bowel disease. Curr Gastroenterol Rep. 2003;5:501–5.
89. Hanauer SB, Wagner CL, Bala M et al. Incidence and importance of antibody responses to infliximab after maintenance or episodic treatment in Crohn's disease. Clin Gastroenterol Hepatol. 2004;2:542–53.
90. Rutgeerts P, Diamond RH, Bala M et al. Scheduled maintenance treatment with infliximab is superior to episodic treatment for the healing of mucosal ulceration associated with Crohn's disease. Gastrointest Endosc. 2006;63:433–42; quiz 464.
91. Arnott ID, Watts D, Ghosh S. Review article: Is clinical remission the optimum therapeutic goal in the treatment of Crohn's disease? Aliment Pharmacol Ther. 2002;16:857–67.
92. D'Haens G. Mucosal healing in pediatric Crohn's disease: the goal of medical treatment. Inflamm Bowel Dis. 2004;10:479–80.
93. Hanauer SB. Crohn's disease: step up or top down therapy. Best Pract Res Clin Gastroenterol. 2003;17:131–7.
94. Mahadevan U. Mucosal healing in Crohn's disease: what you see is what you get? Gastrointest Endosc. 2006;63:443–4.
95. Rutgeerts PJ. An historical overview of the treatment of Crohn's disease: why do we need biological therapies? Rev Gastroenterol Disord. 2004;4(Suppl. 3):S3–9.
96. Walker-Smith JA. Mucosal healing in Crohn's disease. Gastroenterology. 1998;114:419–20.
97. Bousvaros A. Mucosal healing in children with Crohn's disease: appropriate therapeutic goal or medical overkill? Inflamm Bowel Dis. 2004;10:481–3.
98. Scholmerich J. Review article: Should we treat symptoms or lesions in Crohn's disease? The case for treating symptoms. Aliment Pharmacol Ther. 2006;24(Suppl. 3):33–6.
99. Arnott ID, Drummond HE, Ghosh S. Frequency of continuing mucosal inflammation in clinically inactive Crohn's disease. Scott Med J. 2001;46:136–9.
100. Hellers G, Bergstrand O, Ewerth S, Holmstrom B. Occurrence and outcome after primary treatment of anal fistulae in Crohn's disease. Gut. 1980;21:525–7.

101. Michelassi F, Stella M, Balestracci T, Giuliante F, Marogna P, Block GE. Incidence, diagnosis, and treatment of enteric and colorectal fistulae in patients with Crohn's disease. Ann Surg. 1993;218:660–6.
102. Solomon MJ. Fistulae and abscesses in symptomatic perianal Crohn's disease. Int J Colorectal Dis. 1996;11:222–6.
103. Hobbiss JH, Schofield PF. Management of perianal Crohn's disease. J R Soc Med. 1982;75: 414–17.
104. Person B, Wexner SD. Management of perianal Crohn's disease. Curr Treat Options Gastroenterol. 2005;8:197–209.
105. Basu A, Wexner SD. Perianal Crohn's disease. Curr Treat Options Gastroenterol. 2002;5:197–206.
106. Bell SJ, Williams AB, Wiesel P, Wilkinson K, Cohen RC, Kamm MA. The clinical course of fistulating Crohn's disease. Aliment Pharmacol Ther. 2003;17:1145–51.
107. Loftus EV Jr, Schoenfeld P, Sandborn WJ. The epidemiology and natural history of Crohn's disease in population-based patient cohorts from North America: a systematic review. Aliment Pharmacol Ther. 2002;16:51–60.
108. Schwartz DA, Loftus EV Jr, Tremaine WJ et al. The natural history of fistulizing Crohn's disease in Olmsted County, Minnesota. Gastroenterology. 2002;122:875–80.
109. Rutgeerts P. Review article: Treatment of perianal fistulizing Crohn's disease. Aliment Pharmacol Ther. 2004;20(Suppl. 4):106–10.
110. Arseneau KO, Cohn SM, Cominelli F, Connors AF Jr. Cost–utility of initial medical management for Crohn's disease perianal fistulae. Gastroenterology. 2001;120:1640–56.
111. Rutgeerts P. Management of perianal Crohn's disease. Can J Gastroenterol. 2000;14(Suppl. C):7–12C.
112. Lowry PW, Weaver AL, Tremaine WJ, Sandborn WJ. Combination therapy with oral tacrolimus (FK506) and azathioprine or 6-mercaptopurine for treatment-refractory Crohn's disease perianal fistulae. Inflamm Bowel Dis. 1999;5:239–45.
113. Pearson DC, May GR, Fick GH, Sutherland LR. Azathioprine and 6-mercaptopurine in Crohn disease. A meta-analysis. Ann Intern Med. 1995;123:132–42.
114. Hoffmann JC, Zeitz M. Treatment of Crohn's disease. Hepatogastroenterology. 2000;47: 90–100.
115. Zboril V, Prokopova L, Dite P, Pokorny A, Dastych M Jr, Pazourkova M. Immunosuppressive treatment of Crohn's disease with fistulae. Bratisl Lek Listy. 2002; 103:127–30.
116. Hanauer SB, Smith MB. Rapid closure of Crohn's disease fistulas with continuous intravenous cyclosporin A. Am J Gastroenterol. 1993;88:646–9.
117. Present DH, Lichtiger S. Efficacy of cyclosporine in treatment of fistula of Crohn's disease. Dig Dis Sci. 1994;39:374–80.
118. Sands BE, Blank MA, Patel K, van Deventer SJ. Long-term treatment of rectovaginal fistulas in Crohn's disease: response to infliximab in the ACCENT II Study. Clin Gastroenterol Hepatol. 2004;2:912–20.
119. Sands BE, Anderson FH, Bernstein CN et al. Infliximab maintenance therapy for fistulizing Crohn's disease. N Engl J Med. 2004;350:876–85.
120. Kam LY, Targan SR. TNF-alpha antagonists for the treatment of Crohn's disease. Expert Opin Pharmacother. 2000;1:615–22.
121. Contini S, Raimondi G, Graziano P, Saltini C, Bocchino M. Difficult diagnosis of infliximab-related miliary tuberculosis. Monaldi Arch Chest Dis. 2004;61:128–30.
122. Rovere Querini P, Vecellio M, Sabbadini MG, Ciboddo G. Miliary tuberculosis after biological therapy for rheumatoid arthritis. Rheumatology (Oxford). 2002;41:231.
123. Mayordomo L, Marenco JL, Gomez-Mateos J, Rejon E. Pulmonary miliary tuberculosis in a patient with anti-TNF-alpha treatment. Scand J Rheumatol. 2002;31:44–5.
124. Stas P, D'Hoore A, Van Assche G et al. Miliary tuberculosis following infliximab therapy for Crohn disease: a case report and review of the literature. Acta Gastroenterol Belg. 2006; 69:217–20.
125. Arend SM, Breedveld FC, van Dissel JT. TNF-alpha blockade and tuberculosis: better look before you leap. Neth J Med. 2003;61:111–19.
126. Hochberg MC, Lebwohl MG, Plevy SE, Hobbs KF, Yocum DE. The benefit/risk profile of TNF-blocking agents: findings of a consensus panel. Semin Arthritis Rheum. 2005;34:819–36.

127. Rychly DJ, DiPiro JT. Infections associated with tumor necrosis factor-alpha antagonists. Pharmacotherapy. 2005;25:1181–92.
128. Belknap R, Reves R, Burman W. Immune reconstitution to *Mycobacterium tuberculosis* after discontinuing infliximab. Int J Tuberc Lung Dis. 2005;9:1057–8.
129. Calabrese L. The yin and yang of tumor necrosis factor inhibitors. Cleve Clin J Med. 2006; 73:251–6.
130. Crum NF, Lederman ER, Wallace MR. Infections associated with tumor necrosis factor-alpha antagonists. Medicine (Baltimore). 2005;84:291–302.
131. Dimakou K, Papaioannides D, Latsi P, Katsimboula S, Korantzopoulos P, Orphanidou D. Disseminated tuberculosis complicating anti-TNF-alpha treatment. Int J Clin Pract. 2004; 58:1052–5.
132. Dunlop H. Infliximab (Remicade) and etanercept (Enbrel): serious infections and tuberculosis. CMAJ. 2004;171:992–3.
133. Hommes DW, van Deventer SJ. Infliximab therapy in Crohn's disease: safety issues. Neth J Med. 2003;61:100–4.
134. Keane J. Tumor necrosis factor blockers and reactivation of latent tuberculosis. Clin Infect Dis. 2004;39:300–2.
135. Lim WS, Powell RJ, Johnston ID. Tuberculosis and treatment with infliximab. N Engl J Med. 2002;346:623–6.
136. Ormerod LP. Tuberculosis and anti-TNF-alpha treatment. Thorax. 2004;59:921.
137. Riminton S, Pearce N, Antony B. Tuberculosis and treatment with infliximab. N Engl J Med. 2002;346:623–6.
138. Uthman I, Sharara A. The usefulness of PPD testing in inflammatory bowel disease patients before infliximab therapy. Clin Gastroenterol Hepatol. 2004;2:xxii.
139. Vermeire S, Noman M, Van Assche G et al. Autoimmunity associated with anti-tumor necrosis factor alpha treatment in Crohn's disease: a prospective cohort study. Gastroenterology. 2003;125:32–9.
140. Lichtenstein GR, Feagan BG, Cohen RD et al. Serious infections and mortality in association with therapies for Crohn's disease: TREAT registry. Clin Gastroenterol Hepatol. 2006;4:621–30.
141. Colombel JF, Loftus EV Jr, Tremaine WJ et al. The safety profile of infliximab in patients with Crohn's disease: the Mayo Clinic experience in 500 patients. Gastroenterology. 2004; 126:19–31.
142. Kwon JH, Farrell RJ. The risk of lymphoma in the treatment of inflammatory bowel disease with immunosuppressive agents. Crit Rev Oncol Hematol. 2005;56:169–78.
143. Brown SL, Greene MH, Gershon SK, Edwards ET, Braun MM. Tumor necrosis factor antagonist therapy and lymphoma development: twenty-six cases reported to the Food and Drug Administration. Arthritis Rheum. 2002;46:3151–8.
144. Agents FBDUotT-ab. [available from URL: http://www.fda.gov/ohrms/dockets/ac/03/briefing/3930b1.htm]. 2003.
145. Chey WY, Hussain A, Ryan C, Potter GD, Shah A. Infliximab for refractory ulcerative colitis. Am J Gastroenterol. 2001;96:2373–81.
146. Chey WY. Infliximab for patients with refractory ulcerative colitis. Inflamm Bowel Dis. 2001;7(Suppl. 1):S30–3.
147. Kohn A, Prantera C, Pera A, Cosintino R, Sostegni R, Daperno M. Anti-tumour necrosis factor alpha (infliximab) in the treatment of severe ulcerative colitis: result of an open study on 13 patients. Dig Liver Dis. 2002;34:626–30.
148. Mamula P, Markowitz JE, Brown KA, Hurd LB, Piccoli DA, Baldassano RN. Infliximab as a novel therapy for pediatric ulcerative colitis. J Pediatr Gastroenterol Nutr. 2002;34:307–11.
149. Su C, Salzberg BA, Lewis JD et al. Efficacy of anti-tumor necrosis factor therapy in patients with ulcerative colitis. Am J Gastroenterol. 2002;97:2577–84.
150. Sands BE, Tremaine WJ, Sandborn WJ et al. Infliximab in the treatment of severe, steroid-refractory ulcerative colitis: a pilot study. Inflamm Bowel Dis. 2001;7:83–8.
151. Probert CS, Hearing SD, Schreiber S et al. Infliximab in moderately severe glucocorticoid resistant ulcerative colitis: a randomised controlled trial. Gut. 2003;52:998–1002.
152. Lawson M, Thomas A, Akobeng A. Tumour necrosis factor alpha blocking agents for induction of remission in ulcerative colitis. Cochrane Database Syst Rev. 2006;3: CD005112.

153. Rutgeerts P, Sandborn WJ, Feagan BG et al. Infliximab for induction and maintenance therapy for ulcerative colitis. N Engl J Med. 2005;353:2462–76.
154. Armuzzi A, De Pascalis B, Lupascu A et al. Infliximab in the treatment of steroid-dependent ulcerative colitis. Eur Rev Med Pharmacol Sci. 2004;8:231–3.
155. Jarnerot G, Hertervig E, Friis-Liby I et al. Infliximab as rescue therapy in severe to moderately severe ulcerative colitis: a randomized, placebo-controlled study. Gastroenterology. 2005;128:1805–11.
156. Ochsenkuhn T, Sackmann M, Goke B. Infliximab for acute, not steroid-refractory ulcerative colitis: a randomized pilot study. Eur J Gastroenterol Hepatol. 2004;16:1167–71.
157. Sood A, Midha V, Sood N. Oral cyclosporine in patients with active severe ulcerative colitis not responding to steroids. Indian J Gastroenterol. 2002;21:155–6.
158. McCormack G, McCormick PA, Hyland JM, O'Donoghue DP. Cyclosporin therapy in severe ulcerative colitis: is it worth the effort? Dis Colon Rectum. 2002;45:1200–5.
159. Gionchetti P, Rizzello F, Habal F et al. Standard treatment of ulcerative colitis. Dig Dis. 2003;21:157–67.
160. Arts J, D'Haens G, Zeegers M et al. Long-term outcome of treatment with intravenous cyclosporin in patients with severe ulcerative colitis. Inflamm Bowel Dis. 2004;10:73–8.
161. Regueiro M. Intravenous cyclosporine in severe ulcerative colitis: how low can you go? Inflamm Bowel Dis. 2004;10:170.
162. Danalioglu A, Kaymakoglu S, Mungan Z et al. Cyclosporin for severe ulcerative colitis attacks. Hepatogastroenterology. 2003;50(Suppl. 2):ccxcviii–ccc.
163. Campbell S, Travis S, Jewell D. Ciclosporin use in acute ulcerative colitis: a long-term experience. Eur J Gastroenterol Hepatol. 2005;17:79–84.
164. Shibolet O, Regushevskaya E, Brezis M, Soares-Weiser K. Cyclosporine A for induction of remission in severe ulcerative colitis. Cochrane Database Syst Rev. 2005:CD004277.
165. Garcia-Lopez S, Gomollon-Garcia F, Perez-Gisbert J. Cyclosporine in the treatment of severe attack of ulcerative colitis: a systematic review. Gastroenterol Hepatol. 2005;28:607–14.
166. Pham CQ, Efros CB, Berardi RR. Cyclosporine for severe ulcerative colitis. Ann Pharmacother. 2006;40:96–101.
167. Regueiro M, Curtis J, Plevy S. Infliximab for hospitalized patients with severe ulcerative colitis. J Clin Gastroenterol. 2006;40:476–81.
168. Castro M, Papadatou B, Ceriati E et al. Role of cyclosporin in preventing or delaying colectomy in children with severe ulcerative colitis. Langenbecks Arch Surg. 2006 (In press).

19
Therapy of inflammatory bowel disease: step-up or top-down?

H. HERFARTH

INTRODUCTION

Inflammatory bowel diseases are chronic inflammatory disorders, often characterized by disease courses with multiple complications such as strictures, fistulas and abscesses. Whereas ulcerative colitis is generally 'curable' by resecting the colon, Crohn's disease (CD) can be reverted neither medically nor surgically. Therefore, the overall therapeutic aim for CD is modulation of the disease course. Besides therapeutic interventions using different drugs or surgery, one has to keep in mind that smoking also has a significant negative impact on the course of CD[1].

It was first suggested by rheumatologists that the conservative medical approach for rheumatoid arthritis (RA) of adapting therapies according to the clinical severity of the disease might not be the optimal approach, since it does not prevent irreversible damage, thus significantly hampering the chances of long-term remission. The therapy should rather reflect an oncological approach, which nearly always applies a maximal dose of very potent (and toxic) drugs at the beginning and then, if this is successful, continues maintenance therapy with the least toxic compound. Recently two studies have demonstrated that aggressive intervention in early-onset RA using a combination of a biological (anti-TNF antibodies) and an immunosuppressive (methotrexate or steroid) therapy is superior than either of the two regimens alone in preventing or slowing down joint destruction and attenuating the clinical course of the disease[2,3] (Figure 1). This so-called top-down approach might work in early-onset RA, but there are still several questions to be answered, which are also of importance for the feasibility of a top-down therapy in patients with CD[4]. Is there a window of opportunity to treat early RA? Is this very aggressive treatment more beneficial than the established step-up therapy with regard to side-effects (infections, tumours) in the long run? Should corticosteroids still be part of an early aggressive approach or do they harm more than help? Does the radiographic improvement reflect the overall improvement of inflammatory activity or does it reflect only a unique mechanism of action of the employed biologic agents?

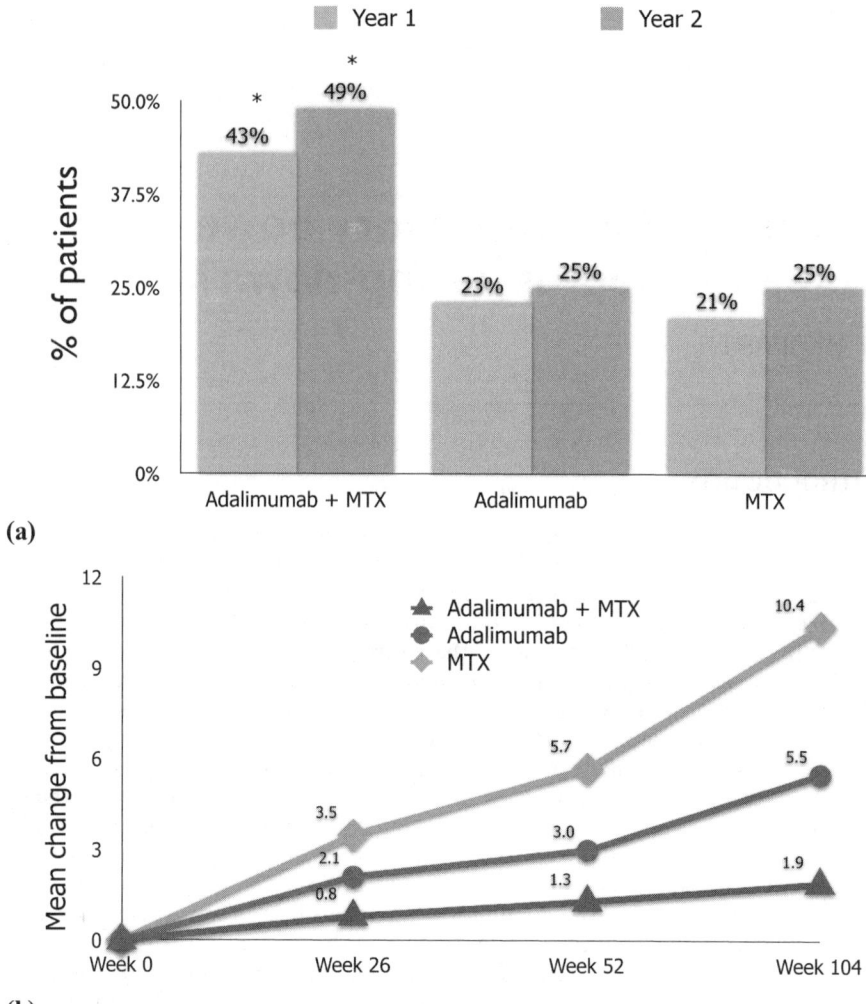

(a)

(b)

Figure 1 (a) Clinical remission (28-joint disease activity score <2.6) at year 1 and year 2 in patients with active RA <3 years duration (and no previous treatment with immunosuppressive therapy)[2]. Treatments included adalimumab 40 mg subcutaneously every other week plus oral methotrexate (MTX), adalimumab 40 mg subcutaneously every other week or weekly oral MTX. Adalimumab + MTX n = 268; adalimumab monotherapy n = 274; MTX monotherapy n = 257; *$p < 0.001$ vs adalimumab alone and MTX alone. (b) Mean change from baseline in total Sharp scores (a Sharp score is an X-ray measurement of changes in total joint damage as assessed by bone erosions and joint space narrowing) over time by treatment group[2]. Combination adalimumab + MTX $p < 0.001$ vs MTX alone and $p < 0.002$ vs adalimumab alone year 1; $p < 0.001$ vs MTX alone or adalimumab alone year 2; $p < 0.001$ adalimumab vs MTX alone year 1 and 2

One of these questions has recently been partially answered. Anti-TNF antibody therapy in RA seems to increase the risk of serious infections and malignancies significantly[5]. In a meta-analysis of nine clinical trials of anti-TNF therapy including 3493 patients treated either with infliximab or adalimumab and 1512 control patients, Bongartz et al.[5] detected a significantly higher odds ratio for patients undergoing anti-TNF therapy for developing one or more malignancies or serious infections compared to control patients (Table 1). The number needed to harm for one additional malignancy within a treatment period of 6–12 months of anti-TNF antibody therapy was 154 (95% confidence interval (CI) 91–500) and 59 (95% CI 39–125) for a serious infection within a treatment period of 2–12 months. There are some limitations of the study, but the results nevertheless indicate severe risks associated with anti-TNF therapy and overall with the aggressive top-down approach in RA.

Table 1 Effect of anti-TNF antibody therapy on occurrence of one or more malignancies or serious infections in patients with rheumatoid arthritis[5]

	Odds ratio (95% CI)			
Adverse event	*All doses anti-TNF vs placebo*	*Low-dose anti-TNF vs placebo*	*High-dose anti-TNF vs placebo*	*High-dose vs low-dose anti-TNF*
≥1 malignancy	3.3 (1.2–9.1)	1.4 (0.3–5.7)	4.3 (1.6–11.8)	3.4 (1.4–8.2)
≥1 serious infection	2.0 (1.3–3.1)	1.8 (1.1–3.1)	2.3 (1.5–3.6)	1.4 (1.0–2.0)

Low dose: ≤3 mg/kg infliximab every 4 weeks or 20 mg adalimumab every week; high dose: ≥6 mg/kg infliximab every 8 weeks or 40 mg adalimumab every 2 weeks.

Compared to patients with RA those patients with CD face similar disease perspectives. Despite intensive medical therapy CD is not well controlled and the cumulative risk of intestinal resections is 44%, 61%, and 71% at 1, 5, and 10 years, respectively, after diagnosis[6]. Clinical (symptomatic) relapses occur cumulatively in 34% of the patients 3 years after surgery[7] and in about 40–50% of the patients 5–10 years after surgery[6,8]. Re-operation rates are also high and vary between 30% and 60% after 10 years[8–10]. Therefore an early aggressive approach might alter the natural history of the disease. In children with Crohn's disease an early aggressive therapy might alter the subsequent disease course, as demonstrated by Markowitz et al. in a placebo-controlled trial of 6-mercaptopurine (6-MP) in newly diagnosed CD[11]. Fifty-five children were randomized to treatment with 6-MP (1.5 mg/kg per day) or placebo. Both groups initially received prednisone. Remission was induced in nearly 90% in both groups. However, nearly five times as many children relapsed during this 18-month trial in the placebo compared to the 6-MP group (47% vs 9%). The long-term remission was 89% (6-MP) vs 39% (placebo). In the placebo group 50% of the children became steroid dependent vs none in the 6-MP group. This approach has not yet been studied in the adult population.

TOP-DOWN VS STEP-UP IN CD

The standard therapeutic approach to CD comprises several steps taking into account the disease severity and/or concurrent medication. The initial therapy of a patient presenting with mild–moderate CD is either with mesalazine (5-ASA) compounds or steroids (including budesonide)[12,13]. The latest clinical trials data of 5-ASA therapies in CD patients indicate that the therapeutic effects of 5-ASA in inducing and maintaining remission are negligible in most patients[14,15]. Steroids, and in the case of ileocolonic CD budesonide, are very potent in inducing, but fail to maintain, remission[16–19] (Table 2). Three reports concerning the natural history and steroid therapy of CD patients also reveal that not all patients by far require steroids, and that approximately one-third of the patients requiring steroid therapy are off steroids and in remission after 1 year[20–22]. Only for patients with steroid-dependent or refractory disease initiation with immunosuppressive agents such as azathioprine, is 6-MP or methotrexate recommended, and in case of therapy failure infliximab should be considered as an additional therapeutic option[12,13]. At each stage of the therapeutic decision a surgical approach ought to be discussed, which is definitely indicated in case of fibrostenotic strictures, abscesses or complicated fistulas. In contrast to the above-mentioned therapy Hommes et al. have recently investigated the top-down approach in a prospective open-label trial including 129 patients[29]. Whereas the conventional therapy was initiated with steroids in active CD patients and then escalated to azathioprine therapy followed by the addition of infliximab at each step of therapy failure, the top-down group started initially with a combination therapy of infliximab (week 0, 2, 6) and azathioprine, which was continued as maintenance therapy. In case of therapy failure of the azathioprine regimen, regular maintenance therapy with infliximab was started. The data demonstrate a significantly higher percentage of patients being in remission (defined as CDAI <150 points and no steroids and no surgery) in the top-down compared to the step-up group after 6 and 12 months (Figure 2). However, the differences lost significance after 18 and 24 months. In the top-down group 100% and 95% and in the step-up group 74% and 77% of the patients were treated with immunosuppressive agents after 12 and 24 months, respectively. A trend was also observed for the need of surgery (4.6% and 9.2% vs 12.5% and 12.5% of the patients undergoing surgery after 12

Table 2 Need for steroid therapy and short-term response of patients with Crohn's disease in three patient cohorts in England[21], the United States[20] and Denmark[22]

	No. of patients	No. of steroids (%)		Response to therapy day 30; n (%)		
		Yes	No	Full	Partial	response
Edinburgh[21]	80	60 (75)	20 (25)	24 (40)	21 (35)	15 (25)
Olmstedt County[20]	171	74 (43)	97 (57)	43 (58)	19 (26)	12 (16)
Copenhagen[22]	196	109 (56)	87 (44)	52 (48)	35 (32)	22 (20)

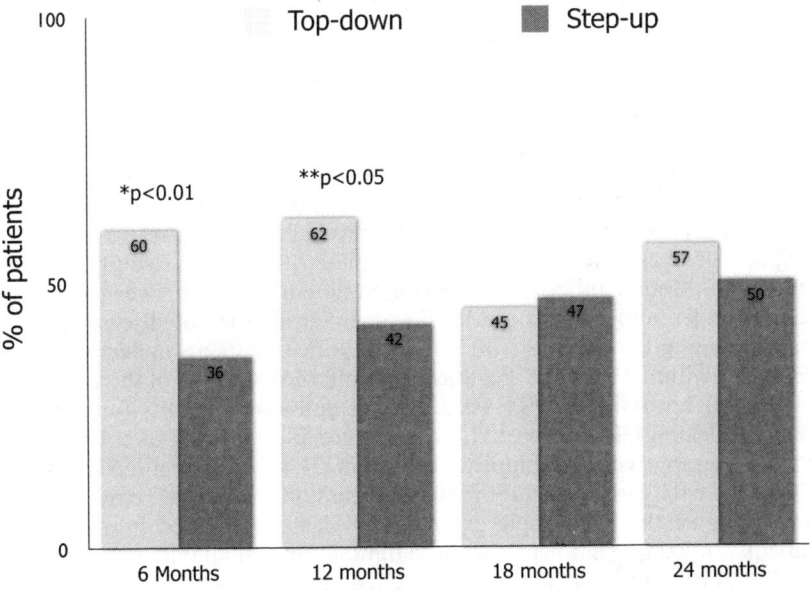

Figure 2 Remission defined as Crohn's disease activity index (CDAI) < 150, no steroids and no surgery in the top-down vs step-up trial (published so far only in abstract format)

and 24 months in the step-down and the step-up group). A significant difference was found in the mean number of days of steroid treatment (mean number of days after 24 months: 6 top-down group vs 80 step-up group). This difference is also due to the trial design. However, despite the difference in the duration of the therapy with steroids and immunosuppressive agents no significant difference in the adverse events was observed. Nevertheless in the oral presentation at the Digestive Disease Week in Los Angeles 2006 one patient with newly diagnosed stomach cancer in the top-down group was mentioned (which should be kept in mind with regard to the above-described increased risk of malignancies with anti-TNF therapy). Despite the TREAT registry, which is a prospective, observational multicentre, long-term registry of North American patients with CD, sponsored by the manufacturer of infliximab (Centocor), not reporting an increased risk of malignancies in this cohort[23], recent reports concerning T-cell lymphomas in six CD patients treated with infliximab and concomitant 6-MP or azathioprine (Remicade for intravenous injection. Package Insert. Centocor, Malvern, Pennsylvania, USA, 2006; revised May 2006), underline the urgency for further studies investigating possible effects of aggressive immunosuppressive therapy in patients with inflammatory bowel disease.

PREVENTION OF STRUCTURAL DAMAGE – MUCOSAL HEALING

Mucosal healing might be an early indicator of clinical relapse, as demonstrated by the postoperative study by Rutgeerts et al. in 1990. Recurrent lesions were observed in 73% and 85% of the patients in the neoterminal ileum within 1 and 3 years after surgery, respectively[7]. The severity of these lesions predicted the clinical outcome in the following years (Figure 3). Therefore mucosal healing in the setting of medical therapy might influence the duration of remission or prevent later complications. Mucosal healing has been investigated after therapies with steroids, azathioprine and infliximab. Modigliani et al. demonstrated no correlation between the clinical activity index and endoscopically documented severity of disease[24]. In this trial, including 131 patients with active CD, 92% of patients underwent clinical remission within 7 weeks of treatment with steroids. Only 38 of the 131 patients in clinical remission (29%) were also in endoscopic remission (complete mucosal healing). D'Haens et al. observed complete healing of colonic lesions after a therapy with azathioprine (duration 24.4 ± 13.7 months) in 14 of 20 (70%) patients with medically induced remission[25]. Clinical remission at the time point of the endoscopic examination was documented in all of the 20 patients. Infliximab has been shown to diminish intestinal inflammation, which correlates with an improvement of the CDAI ($r = 0.56$; $n = 30$)[26].

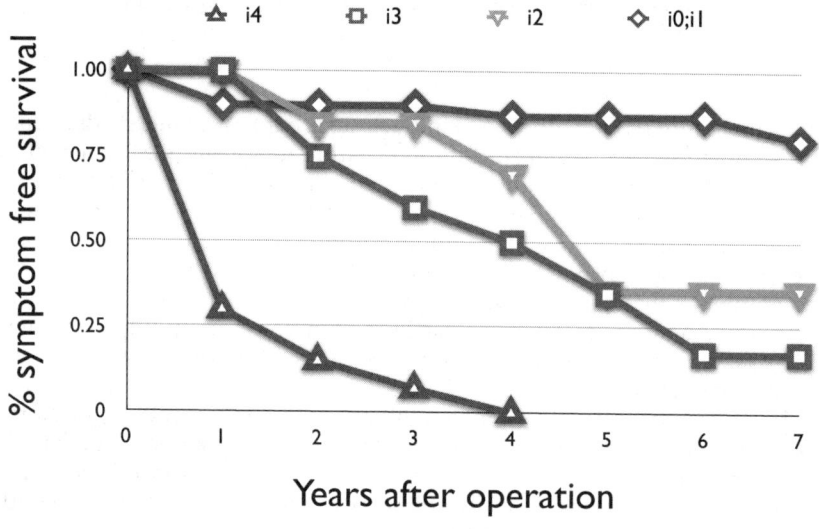

Years after operation

Figure 3 Symptomatic clinical recurrence in patients stratified according to the severity of endoscopic lesions at 1 year ileocolonoscopy after operation[7]. $n = 89$ patients; i0 = no lesions; i1 = less than five aphthous lesions; i2 = more than five aphthous lesions with normal mucosa between the lesions, or skip areas of larger lesions or lesions confined to the ileocolonic anastomosis; i3 = diffuse aphthous ileitis with diffusely inflamed mucosa; i4 = diffuse inflammation with already larger ulcers, nodules, and/or narrowing

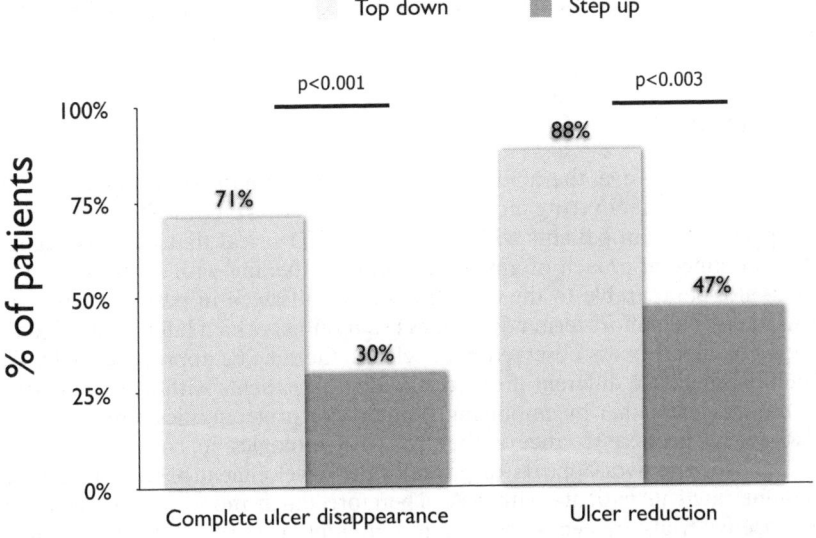

Figure 4 Mucosal healing in the top-down vs step-up trial; 44 patients underwent repeated ileocolonoscopy 24 months after inclusion into the study; 24 patients received top-down and 20 step-up therapy

Mucosal healing was also investigated in a subgroup of patients in the top-down vs step-up study[27]. Mucosal healing was significantly more pronounced in the top-down compared to the step-up group (Figure 4). This may be reflected in the lower clinical relapse rate in the top-down group compared to the step-up group after 24 months (14% vs 42%). Since these results are currently available only in abstract format one has to await the full article for the results for further analysis. As far as mucosal healing with infliximab is concerned, the results of a substudy of ACCENT I did not demonstrate an association of mucosal healing and clinical remission[28] (Table 3). Only a trend

Table 3 Correlation of mucosal healing and clinical remission in a subgroup study of ACCENT I[28]

	Week 10		Week 54	
Clinical remission	Mucosal healing (n = 14)	No mucosal healing (n = 59)	Mucosal healing (n = 18)	No mucosal healing (n = 34)
Yes	36%	41%	67%	56%
No	64%	59%	33%	44%

No relationship exists between clinical remission and complete mucosal healing. Ileocolonoscopic examinations were performed at weeks 0, 10, and 54. Infliximab was administered as induction therapy 5 mg/kg body weight at week 0. Infliximab or placebo was given at week 2 and 6 and every 8 weeks thereafter until week 46.

towards fewer hospital stays in patients treated with scheduled infliximab was observed.

CONCLUSION

An early aggressive therapeutic approach to patients suffering from CD represents a fascinating concept. However, first data from the only prospective trial in patients with early, active CD reveal that the effectiveness of a combined approach of anti-TNF antibody therapy with azathioprine: (a) seems not comparable to the overall better results seen in patients with early RA, and (b) has short-term advantages (12 months), which later level off to the degree of effectiveness observed in the classic therapeutic approach in CD. The outcome might be different if one could identify patients with a severe disease course *a priori*, either by employing genomics or proteonomics screening. This also seems necessary, since a therapy with biologics in combination with immunosuppressives appears to promote the development of malignancies as demonstrated in patients with RA. Therefore much more data generated in prospective trials are necessary. A continuing intensive search for new drugs is also mandatory, considering the moderate effects observed when two of the most potent immunosuppressive drugs in the treatment arsenal of CD are combined.

References

1. Cosnes J, Beaugerie L, Carbonnel F, Gendre JP. Smoking cessation and the course of Crohn's disease: an intervention study. Gastroenterology. 2001;120:1093–9.
2. Breedveld FC, Weisman MH, Kavanaugh AF et al. The PREMIER study: a multicenter, randomized, double-blind clinical trial of combination therapy with adalimumab plus methotrexate versus methotrexate alone or adalimumab alone in patients with early, aggressive rheumatoid arthritis who had not had previous methotrexate treatment. Arthritis Rheum. 2006;54:26–37.
3. Goekoop-Ruiterman YP, de Vries-Bouwstra JK, Allaart CF et al. Clinical and radiographic outcomes of four different treatment strategies in patients with early rheumatoid arthritis (the BeSt study): a randomized, controlled trial. Arthritis Rheum. 2005;52:3381–90.
4. Weisman MH. Progress toward the cure of rheumatoid arthritis? The BeSt study. Arthritis Rheum. 2005;52:3326–32.
5. Bongartz T, Sutton AJ, Sweeting MJ, Buchan I, Matteson EL, Montori V. Anti-TNF antibody therapy in rheumatoid arthritis and the risk of serious infections and malignancies: systematic review and meta-analysis of rare harmful effects in randomized controlled trials. J Am Med Assoc. 2006;295:2275–85.
6. Bernell O, Lapidus A, Hellers G. Risk factors for surgery and postoperative recurrence in Crohn's disease. Ann Surg. 2000;231:38–45.
7. Rutgeerts P, Geboes K, Vantrappen G, Beyls J, Kerremans R, Hiele M. Predictability of the postoperative course of Crohn's disease. Gastroenterology. 1990;99:956–63.
8. Post S, Herfarth C, Bohm E et al. The impact of disease pattern, surgical management, and individual surgeons on the risk for relaparotomy for recurrent Crohn's disease. Ann Surg. 1996;223:253–60.
9. Borley NR, Mortensen NJ, Chaudry MA et al. Recurrence after abdominal surgery for Crohn's disease: relationship to disease site and surgical procedure. Dis Colon Rectum. 2002;45:377–83.
10. Fearnhead NS, Chowdhury R, Box B, George BD, Jewell DP, Mortensen NJ. Long-term follow-up of strictureplasty for Crohn's disease. Br J Surg. 2006;93:475–82.

11. Markowitz J, Grancher K, Kohn N, Lesser M, Daum F. A multicenter trial of 6-mercaptopurine and prednisone in children with newly diagnosed Crohn's disease. Gastroenterology. 2000;119:895–902.
12. Lichtenstein GR, Abreu MT, Cohen R, Tremaine W. American Gastroenterological Association Institute Technical Review on Corticosteroids, Immunomodulators, and Infliximab in Inflammatory Bowel Disease. Gastroenterology. 2006;130:940–87.
13. Travis SPL, Stange EF, Lemann M et al., for the European Crohn's and Colitis Organization. European evidence based consensus on the diagnosis and management of Crohn's disease: current management. Gut. 2006;55:i16–35.
14. Hanauer SB, Stromberg U. Oral Pentasa in the treatment of active Crohn's disease: a meta-analysis of double-blind, placebo-controlled trials. Clin Gastroenterol Hepatol. 2004;2:379–88.
15. Akobeng AK, Gardener E. Oral 5-aminosalicylic acid for maintenance of medically-induced remission in Crohn's disease. Cochrane Database Syst Rev. 2005:CD003715.
16. Papi C, Luchetti R, Gili L, Montanti S, Koch M, Capurso L. Budesonide in the treatment of Crohn's disease: a meta-analysis. Aliment Pharmacol Ther. 2000;14:1419–28.
17. Schölmerich J. Review article: Systemic and topical steroids in inflammatory bowel disease. Aliment Pharmacol Ther. 2004;20(Suppl. 4):66–74.
18. Otley A, Steinhart AH. Budesonide for induction of remission in Crohn's disease. Cochrane Database Syst Rev. 2005:CD000296.
19. Simms L, Steinhart AH. Budesonide for maintenance of remission in Crohn's disease. Cochrane Database Syst Rev. 2001:CD002913.
20. Faubion WA Jr, Loftus EV Jr, Harmsen WS, Zinsmeister AR, Sandborn WJ. The natural history of corticosteroid therapy for inflammatory bowel disease: a population-based study. Gastroenterology. 2001;121:255–60.
21. Ho GT, Chiam P, Drummond H, Loane J, Arnott IDR, Satsangi J. The efficacy of corticosteroid therapy in inflammatory bowel disease: analysis of a 5-year UK inception cohort. Aliment Pharmacol Ther. 2006;24:319–30.
22. Munkholm P, Langholz E, Davidsen M, Binder V. Frequency of glucocorticoid resistance and dependency in Crohn's disease. Gut. 1994;35:360–2.
23. Lichtenstein GR, Feagan BG, Cohen RD et al. Serious infections and mortality in association with therapies for Crohn's disease: TREAT registry. Clin Gastroenterol Hepatol. 2006;4:621–30.
24. Modigliani R, Mary JY, Simon JF et al. Endoscopic severity index for Crohn's disease. Clinical, biological, and endoscopic picture of attacks of Crohn's disease. Evolution on prednisolone. Groupe d'Etude Therapeutique des Affections Inflammatoires Digestives. Gastrointest Endosc. 1990;36:637.
25. D'Haens G, Geboes K, Rutgeerts P. Endoscopic and histologic healing of Crohn's (ileo-) colitis with azathioprine. Gastrointest Endosc. 1999;50:667–71.
26. D'Haens G, Van Deventer S, Van Hogezand R et al. Endoscopic and histological healing with infliximab anti-tumor necrosis factor antibodies in Crohn's disease: a European multicenter trial. Gastroenterology. 1999;116:1029–34.
27. D'Haens G, Hommes DW, Baert F et al. A combined regimen of infliximab and azathioprine induces better endoscopic healing than classic step-up therapy in newly diagnosed Crohn's disease. Gastroenterology. 2006;130:A110 (Abstract).
28. Rutgeerts P, Diamond RH, Bala M et al. Scheduled maintenance treatment with infliximab is superior to episodic treatment for the healing of mucosal ulceration associated with Crohn's disease. Gastrointest Endosc. 2006;63:433–42.
29. Hommes DW, Baert F, Van Assche G et al. The ideal management of Crohn's disease: top down versus step up strategies, a randomized controlled trial. Gastroenterology. 2006;130: A108 (Abstract).

20
State-of-the-Art Lecture: Emerging biologic therapies

W. J. SANDBORN

INTRODUCTION

There are a number of emerging biologic therapies for the treatment of inflammatory bowel disease including anti-tumour necrosis factor (TNF) agents (adalimumab, certolizumab, pegol, CDP571, etanercept, onercept), anti-selective adhesion molecule agents (natalizumab, MLN-02), and miscellaneous agents such as ABT-874 (anti-interleukin 12 antibody), sargramonstim (GMCSF), and visilizumab (anti-CD3 antibody). This chapter will review the results of clinical trials with these agents in patients with Crohn's disease (CD) and ulcerative colitis (UC).

ANTI-TNF-α AGENTS

Bioengineering and construction of anti-TNF agents

The bioengineering and construction of anti-TNF-α agents have evolved from murine monoclonal antibodies. The first generation agent was infliximab, a chimeric IgG1 monoclonal antibody that is approximately 75% human and 25% murine protein. The second-generation agents were humanized monoclonal antibodies and human recombinant soluble TNF receptors. CDP571 is a humanized IgG$_4$ monoclonal antibody that is approximately 95% human and 5% murine protein, with the murine component limited to the complementarity determining regions (CDR). Etanercept is a recombinant human fusion protein consisting of a monoclonal antibody Fc receptor and two p75 soluble TNF receptors that is 100% human protein. Onercept is a recombinant human p55 soluble TNF receptor monomer that is 100% human protein. The third-generation agents were adalimumab and golimumab. Adalimumab (formerly know as D2E7) and golimumab (CNTO 148) are human IgG$_1$ monoclonal antibodies that are 100% human protein. The fourth generation of agent was a pegylated humanized monoclonal antibody FAb' fragment called certolizumab pegol. The FAb' fragment of certolizumab pegol is approximately 95% human protein.

Mechanism of action and other characteristics of the anti-TNF agents

Three anti-TNF agents, infliximab, adalimumab, and certolizumab pegol, have been demonstrated to be effective in patients with CD. All three agents neutralize TNF-α. The two IgG₁ monoclonal antibodies infliximab and adalimumab induce apoptosis in T lymphocytes *in vitro*[1–4]. In addition, these agents mediate antibody-dependent cellular cytotoxicity, and complement fixation[5,6]. In contrast, certolizumab pegol does not induce apoptosis of T cells, and does not mediate antibody-dependent cellular cytotoxicity or compliment fixation *in vitro*[6,7].

Infliximab is administered intravenously whereas adalimumab and certolizumab pegol are administered subcutaneously. The half-life for infliximab is approximately 10 days; for adalimumab 12–14 days; and for certolizumab pegol 14 days[8,9]. Using the doses and dosing regimens that have been demonstrated to be effective in patients with CD, the interval between intravenous infusions is 8 weeks for infliximab, and the interval between subcutaneous injections is 1–2 weeks for adalimumab, and 4 weeks for certolizumab pegol.

Clinical trial designs for anti-TNF trials for CD

When considering the comparative efficacy of various biologics for the treatment of CD, it is important to consider the various clinical trials designs that have been employed.

Induction of response and remission is demonstrated with a short-term trial of 4–12 weeks duration (typically 4 weeks) in patients with active disease. Such trials usually have two or three doses of active drug in addition to a placebo arm. Endpoints can be response or remission. Response-70 is defined as a 70-point reduction in the CD activity index (CDAI) score from baseline. Response-100 is defined as a 100-point reduction in the CDAI score from baseline. Remission is defined as a CDAI score <150 points. Examples of short-term induction studies would include the Targan study of infliximab and the Classic I study of adalimumab[10,11].

Maintenance of response and remission is demonstrated with a drug withdrawal trial of 26–56 weeks duration in patients who previously had active disease that responded to open-label induction therapy with the same agent. Such trials usually have one or two doses of active drug in addition to a placebo arm. Endpoints can be maintenance of 70-point response, 100-point response, or remission in responding patients. Examples of maintenance trials include the ACCENT I trial with infliximab, the CHARM trial with adalimumab, and the PRECISE II trial with certolizumab pegol[12–14].

Combined induction and maintenance is demonstrated with a placebo-controlled trial of 26–56 weeks duration in patients with active disease. Such trials usually have one or two doses of active drug in addition to a placebo arm. Endpoints can be induction of 70-point response, 100-point response, or remission at an early time point (4–6 weeks) and maintenance of response or remission at week 26 (or later) defined as a 70-point response, a 100-point response, or remission at both week 6 and week 26 (or other analogous early and late time points). This trial design, which does not really reflect clinical practice, is more of a study design to satisfy regulatory authorities. An example of a combined induction and maintenance trial is the PRECISE 1 trial with certolizumab pegol[15].

Induction therapy with anti-TNF agents

A relatively small phase II trial (Targan trial) in 108 patients with active CD demonstrated that infliximab was effective for inducing response and remission at 4 weeks[10]. The placebo remission rate at 4 weeks was 4%, compared with 48%, 25%, and 25% in the infliximab 5 mg/kg, 10 mg/kg and 20 mg/kg groups. Likewise, a moderate size phase II/III trial (Classic 1) in 299 patients with active CD demonstrated that adalimumab was effective for inducing response and remission at 4 weeks[11]. The placebo remission rate at 4 weeks was 12%, compared with 18%, 24% and 36% in the adalimumab loading dose groups of 40 mg at week 0 and 20 mg at week 2, 80 mg at week 2 and 40 mg at week 2, and 160 mg at week 0 and 80 mg at week 2. Only the 160 mg/80 mg loading dose was significantly different from placebo. Response-70 was also assessed, and at 4 weeks all three adalimumab dose groups had significantly greater response rates than patients treated with placebo. A moderate size phase II study in 292 patients with active CD demonstrated that certolizumab pegol might be effective for inducing response and remission at 12 weeks[16]. At week 4, response-100 occurred more frequently in patients who had received certolizumab pegol 200 mg and 400 mg at week 0 compared with patients who received placebo. At week 12 the rates of response-100 and remission in the patients treated with certolizumab pegol 100 mg, 200 mg and 400 mg at weeks 0, 4 and 8 were similar to those treated with placebo (primary endpoint). However, there was a high placebo rate at week 12 which made interpretation of these data difficult. Subsequently, a large phase III study (PRECISE 1) in 662 patients with active CD demonstrated that certolizumab pegol was effective for induction of response-100 at week 4 and at week 6[15]. At week 4, response-100 occurred in 29% of patients treated with certolizumab pegol 400 mg at weeks 0 and 2, compared to 22% of patients treated with placebo. At week 6, response-100 occurred in 35% of patients treated with certolizumab pegol 400 mg at weeks 0, 2 and 4, compared to 27% of patients treated with placebo. The data from these four trials demonstrate that infliximab, adalimumab and certolizumab pegol are all effective for induction treatment in patients with active CD, and that the efficacy of the three agents compared to placebo is broadly similar.

Maintenance therapy with anti-TNF agents

A large phase III trial (ACCENT I) evaluated infliximab as a maintenance therapy in patients with CD[12]. Five hundred and seventy-five patients with active CD received open-label therapy with infliximab 5 mg/kg at week 2. Three hundred and thirty-five patients who had a response-70 at week 2 were randomized to treatment with infliximab 5 mg/kg or 10 mg/kg or placebo at weeks 2 and 6 and then every 8 weeks beginning at week 14. At week 30 maintenance of response-70 occurred in 51% and 59% of patients treated with infliximab 5 mg/kg and 10 mg/kg compared to 27% of patients treated with placebo. At week 54 maintenance of response-70 occurred in 43% and 53% of patients treated with infliximab 5 mg/kg and 10 mg/kg compared to 17% of patients treated with placebo. Maintenance of remission occurred at week 30, in 39% and 45% of patients treated with infliximab 5 mg/kg and 10 mg/kg compared to 21% of patients treated with placebo, and at week 54 maintenance of remission occurred in 28% and 38% of patients treated with infliximab 5 mg/kg and 10 mg/kg compared to 14% of patients treated with placebo.

A large phase III trial (CHARM) evaluated adalimumab as a maintenance therapy in patients with CD[13]. Eight hundred and fifty-four patients with active CD received open-label therapy with adalimumab 80 mg at week 0 and 40 mg at week 2. Four hundred and ninety-nine patients had a response-70 at week 4 and were randomized to treatment with adalimumab 40 mg every other week or weekly or placebo. At week 26 response-70 occurred in 52% and 52% of patients who received adalimumab 40 mg every other week and weekly compared to 27% of patients treated with placebo. At week 56 response-70 occurred in 41% and 48% of patients receiving adalimumab 40 mg every other week and weekly compared to 17% of patients treated with placebo. Maintenance of remission occurred at week 26 in 40% and 47% of patients treated with adalimumab 40 mg every other week and weekly compared to 17% of patients treated with placebo, and at week 56 maintenance of remission occurred in 36% and 41% of patients treated with adalimumab 40 mg every other week and weekly compared to 12% of patients treated with placebo. Steroid sparing was also demonstrated[17]. At week 26 35% and 30% of patients treated with adalimumab 40 mg every other week and weekly were in remission off steroids compared to 3% of placebo-treated patients, and at week 56 29% and 23% of patients receiving adalimumab 40 mg every other week and weekly were in remission off steroids compared to 6% of patients receiving placebo. Finally, treatment of fistulas was demonstrated[13,18]. At week 26 33% and 28% of patients receiving adalimumab 40 mg every other week and weekly had complete closure of all fistulas that were draining at baseline compared to 13% of patients treated with placebo. In a combination endpoint composed of fistula closure at week 26 and week 56, 33% and 28% of patients receiving adalimumab 40 mg every other week and weekly had complete closure of fistulas that were draining at baseline compared to 13% of patients treated with placebo.

A large phase III trial (PRECISE-2) evaluated certolizumab pegol as a maintenance therapy in patients with CD[14]. Six hundred and sixty-eight patients with active CD received open-label therapy with certolizumab pegol at weeks 0, 2 and 4. Four hundred and twenty-eight patients had a response-100 and were randomized to treatment with certolizumab pegol 400 mg every 4 weeks or placebo. At week 26 response-100 occurred in 65% of patients who received certolizumab pegol compared to 36% of patients treated with placebo. Maintenance of remission occurred in 48% of patients treated with certolizumab pegol compared to 29% of patients treated with placebo. A second large phase III trial (PRECISE-1) evaluated certolizumab pegol as induction and maintenance therapy in patients with CD[15]. Six hundred and sixty-two patients with active CD were randomized to treatment with certolizumab pegol 400 mg at weeks 0, 2 and 4 and then every 4 weeks or placebo. At week 6 response-100 occurred in 35% of patient treated with certolizumab pegol compared to 27% of patients treated with placebo. At week 6 and 26 response-100 occurred in 23% of patients treated with certolizumab pegol compared to 16% of patients treated with placebo.

In order to compare the results of the ACCENT I trial with infliximab, the CHARM trial with adalimumab and the PRECISE-1 and PRECISE-2 trials with certolizumab pegol, it is necessary to perform a calculation of overall remission rates which equals the initial induction of response rate multiplied by the subsequent maintenance of remission rate. In the ACCENT I trial 59% of patients responded at week 2 and the week 30 remission rates were 39% in the infliximab 5 mg/kg group and 21% in the placebo group, yielding an overall remission rate at week 30 of 23% for infliximab and 12% for placebo. In the CHARM trial 58% of patients responded at week 4 and the week 26 remission rates were 40% in the adalimumab 40 mg every other week group and 17% in the placebo group, yielding an overall remission rate at week 26 of 23% for adalimumab and 10% for placebo. In the PRECISE-2 trial 64% of patients responded at week 6 and the week 26 remission rates were 48% in the certolizmab pegol group and 29% in the placebo group, yielding an overall remission rate at week 26 of 31% for the certolizumab pegol group and 18% for placebo. Finally, in the PRECISE-1 trial the overall remission rate at week 26 was 30% in the certolizumab pegol group and 18% in the placebo group. These data indicate that the infliximab, adalimumab and certolizumab pegol are broadly comparable for maintenance of response and remission in patients with active CD that respond to induction therapy with the same agent.

Toxicity with anti-TNF therapy in patients with CD

In addition to efficacy, the toxicity that occurs in patients with CD treated with anti-TNF antibodies must be considered. Infliximab, adalimumab and certolizumab pegol are all immunogenic to some degree and can lead to the formation of antibodies to infliximab, antibodies to adalimumab and antibodies to certolizumab pegol[9,19,20]. Monotherapy with a biologic agent administered episodically is the most immunogenic regimen and leads to the highest rates of antibody formation. Both systematic maintenance therapy with the biologic agent and concomitant immunosuppressive therapy with azathioprine, 6-mercaptopurine and methotrexate are protective against antibody formation[9,19,20].

Acute infusion reactions and delayed hypersensitivity reactions can both be seen with infliximab[21]. Injection site reactions can be seen with adalimumab and certolizumab pegol. The formation of new autoantibodies such as antinuclear antibodies and double-stranded DNA antibodies can occur with infliximab, and to a lesser degree with adalimumab, but are uncommon with certolizumab pegol[22]. A new clinical diagnosis of drug-induced lupus is uncommon with all three agents. Non-Hodgkin's lymphoma has been associated with anti-TNF therapy[8,9,23]. More recently, six children, adolescents and young adults treated with a combination therapy with infliximab and azathioprine or 6-mercaptopurine have been reported to develop gamma delta hepatosplenic T-cell lymphoma[8]. There also appears to be an association between anti-TNF therapy and skin cancers (squamous cell carcinoma and basal cell carcinoma)[8,9,23]. There is not a clear association between anti-TNF therapy and solid tumours. Patients who receive anti-TNF therapy are at increased risk for serious infections and for opportunistic infections including reactivation of latent tuberculosis, primary infections with histoplasmosis and coccidiomyocosis, etc.[24]. Finally, demyelination disorders including multiple sclerosis and optic neuritis have been reported with anti-TNF therapy, and these agents are contra-indicated in patients with concomitant multiple sclerosis.

ANTI-SELECTIVE ADHESION MOLECULE THERAPY

Natalizumab

Natalizumab is a humanized IgG_4 monoclonal antibody antibody against alpha-4 integrin that is approximately 95% human and 5% murine protein.

A moderate size phase II study in 248 patients with active CD demonstrated that natalizumab 3 mg/kg and 6 mg/kg at weeks 0 and 4 might be effective for inducing response and remission over 12 weeks[25]. No apparent dose response was observed. On this basis a large phase III study (ENACT-1) was undertaken in 905 patients with active CD that demonstrated that natalizumab might be effective for induction of response and remission[26]. At week 10 response-70 occurred in 56% of patients treated with natalizumab 300 mg at weeks 0, 4 and 8, compared to 49% of patients treated with placebo, $p = 0.51$. Similarly, at week 10, remission occurred in 37% of patient treated with natalizumab 300 mg at weeks 0, 4 and 8, compared to 30% of patients treated with placebo, p-value not significant. Subgroup analyses were conducted in patients with elevated C-reactive protein at baseline. Significant differences between the natalizumab and placebo treatment groups were observed in the rates of response-70 and remission was observed at weeks 2, 4, 6, 8, 10 and 12 among patients who had elevated C-reactive protein at baseline (approximately 75% of all the randomized patients). Based on these subgroup analyses an additional phase III induction study called the ENCORE trial was conducted in 509 patients with active CD and a C-reactive protein concentration above the upper limit of normal[27]. Patients were randomized to natalizumab 300 mg at weeks 0, 4 and 8 or placebo. At weeks 8 and 12 response-70 occurred in 48% of patients treated with natalizumab compared to 32% of patients treated with placebo,. Similarly, at weeks 8 and 12, remission occurred in 26% of patients treated with natalizumab compared to 16% of patients treated with placebo. Taking the results of the phase II natalizumab study, the subgroup analysis of the ENACT-1 trial among patients with elevated C-reactive protein, and the ENCORE trial, it seems clear that natalizumab is effective for induction of response and remission in patients with active CD.

A large phase III trial (ENACT-2) evaluated natalizumab as a maintenance therapy in patients with CD[26]. Seven hundred and twenty-four patients with active CD received therapy with natalizumab 300 mg at weeks 0, 4 and 8. Three hundred and thirty-nine patients had a response-70 at week 12 and were randomized to treatment with natalizumab 300 mg every 4 weeks or placebo. At week 36 response-70 occurred in 67% of patients who received natalizumab compared to 37% of patients treated with placebo. At week 60 response-70 occurred in 59% of patients receiving natalizumab compared to 25% of patients treated with placebo. Maintenance of remission occurred at week 36 in 55% of patients treated with natalizumab compared to 30% of patients treated with placebo, and at week 60 maintenance of remission occurred in 55% of patients treated with natalizumab compared to 22% of patients treated with placebo. Sustained response was maintained at every time point from week 12 through week 60 in 54% of patients treated with natalizumab compared to 20% of patients treated with placebo. Sustained remission at every point from week 12 through week 60 was achieved in 39% of patients treated with natalizumab compared to 15% of patients treated with placebo. Steroid sparing was also demonstrated. At week 60 42% of patients treated with natalizumab were in steroid-free remission compared to 15% of patients treated with placebo.

Natalizumab was approved by the United States Food and Drug Administration in December 2004 for the treatment of multiple sclerosis. The drug was subsequently withdrawn from the market in February 2005 after three cases of progressive multifocal leukoencephalopathy (PML) were reported[28–30]. Two of these three patients died. PML is caused by the JC polyoma virus. Primary infection with the JC virus is typically asymptomatic and occurs in childhood. The virus remains latent. Reactivation of the virus may result in PML in immunocompromised individuals. The clinical presentation is a sub-acute progression of focal neurological deficits which can include visual (retro-chiasmal) deficits, motor deficits, sensory deficits, and cerebellar deficits. Eventually cognitive impairment and behavioural abnormalities occur. The diagnosis begins with a clinical impression, followed by an MRI of the brain followed by cerebral spinal fluid analysis for the JC virus DNA by PCR. Analysis of the cerebrospinal fluid has replaced brain biopsy, which was the previous gold standard. A large safety study involving more than 3000 patients treated with natalizumab for the indications of multiple sclerosis, CD and rheumatoid arthritis was conducted[31]. This study demonstrated that the risk of PML was approximately 1:1000 (95% confidence intervals 1:200 to 1:2800) after a mean of 18 months treatment. The drug was re-approved by the United States Food and Drug Administration in the summer of 2006 and was also approved by the EMEA in Europe on a similar time-frame. It is now currently being used to treat patients with multiple sclerosis in both the United States and Europe. Regulatory review for natalizumab for the indication of CD is currently under way in Europe and it is anticipated that the manufacturers, Elan Pharmaceuticals and BiogenIdec, will file for regulatory approval in the United States in late 2006.

MLN-02

MLN-02 (previously called LDP-02) is a humanized IgG_1 monoclonal antibody against $\alpha4\beta7$ integrin that is approximately 95% human and 5%

murine protein. The FC receptor recognition and binding was deleted, thus eliminating complement fixation and cytokine release. MLN-02 is administered intravenously every 4 weeks.

A moderate size phase II trial in 181 patients with active UC demonstrated that MLN-02 was effective for inducing response and remission at 6 weeks[32]. The placebo clinical remission rate at 6 weeks was 15%, compared with 33% and 34% in the MLN-02 dose groups of 0.5 mg/kg and 2 mg/kg. Endoscopic remission and clinical response were also assessed, and at 6 weeks both MLN-02 dose groups had significantly greater endoscopic remission and clinical response rates than patients treated with placebo. Serious adverse events occurred in 8% of patients treated with MLN-02 and 5% of patients treated with placebo.

ABT-874 (anti-interleukin 12 antibody)

ABT-874 (previously called J695) is a humanized IgG_1 monoclonal antibody antibody against interleukin 12 that is approximately 95% human and 5% murine protein. ABT-874 is administered subcutaneously weekly.

A relatively small phase II trial in 79 patients with active CD demonstrated that ABT-874 was effective for inducing response and remission at 7 weeks[33]. Patients were treated with subcutaneous injections of placebo or ABT-874 at doses of 1 mg/kg or 3 mg/kg at week 0 and then weeks 4 through 9 (cohort 1) or at weeks 1–7 (cohort 2). In cohort 2 there were highly significant differences in the proportion of patients achieving response-100 and remission in patients treated with ABT-874 at the 3 mg/kg dose cohort 2 compared to placebo.

Sargramostim

Sargramostim is a recombinant growth factor, granulocyte macrophage colony stimulating factor (GMCSF) that stimulates the innate immune system. Gut inflammation, which is phenotypically similar to CD, occurs in chronic granulomatous disease, glycogen storage disease 1b and Chediak-Higashi syndrome, which are all disorders characterized by neutrophil dysfunction[34,35].

A relatively small phase II trial in 124 patients with active CD demonstrated that sargramostim might be effective for inducing response and remission[36]. Patients receiving concomitant immunosuppressive treatment with steroids, azathioprine, 6-mercaptopurine, methotrexate, or infliximab were excluded. Patients were randomized to treatment with sargramostim 6 µg/kg or placebo administered subcutaneously on a daily basis for 8 weeks. At 8 weeks the rates of response-70 were not significantly different in the sargramostim and placebo groups. However, there were significant differences in response-70 at weeks 2, 4 and 12, and there were significant differences in response-100 and remission at all time points. Taken in total these phase II data suggest that sargramostim may be effective for the treatment of CD.

Visilizumab (anti-CD3 antibody)

Murine anti-CD3 antibody (OKT3) is a highly potent immunosuppressive agent. It exerts its immunosuppressive effects both through inhibition of CD3 and through cytokine release syndrome mediated through blockade of the CD3 receptor and stimulation of the Fc receptor on T cells. OKT3 stimulation of the Fc receptor contributes significantly to the cytokine release syndrome associated with this agent that can include fevers, chills, and sometimes pulmonary distress. Visilizumab is a humanized IgG$_1$ monoclonal antibody to the CD3 receptor in which the FC receptor has been inactivated. Visilizumab has the potential to reduce the degree of immunosuppression and the cytokine release syndrome associated with OKT3.

A dose-ranging phase I trial of visilizumab 5 µg/kg, 7.5 µg/kg, 10 µg/kg and 12/5 µg/kg administered at days 0 and 1 in patients with severe steroid-refractory UC has been reported[37]. Clinical response at day 30 as measured by the modified Truelove and Witts score (Lichtiger score) occurred in approximately 60% of patients in all four dose groups, and clinical response at day 90 occurred in 35–55% of patients in the four dose groups. The rates of clinical remission, defined as a modified Truelove and Witts score of $\leqslant 3$ points at day 30, ranged from 15% to 30% in the four dose groups and then slightly declined by day 90. These preliminary phase I data suggest that visilizumab may be effective for the treatment of severe steroid-refractory UC.

CONCLUSIONS

Based on the demonstrated efficacy of infliximab, adalimumab, certolizumab pegol and natalizumab for CD and infliximab, and MLN-02 for UC, it seems certain that biologic therapies will play an important role in the future treatment of inflammatory bowel disease.

References

1. Lugering A, Schmidt M, Lugering N, Pauels HG, Domschke W, Kucharzik T. Infliximab induces apoptosis in monocytes from patients with chronic active Crohn's disease by using a caspase-dependent pathway. Gastroenterology. 2001;121:1145–57.
2. van den Brande JMH, Braat H, van den Brink GR et al. Infliximab but not etanercept induces apopotosis in lamina propria T-lymphocytes from patients with Crohn's diseease. Gastroenterology. 2003;124:1774–85.
3. Shen C, Maerten P, Van Assche G, Geboes K, Rutgeerts P, Ceuppens J. A fully human anti-TNF mAb adalimumab (D2E7) induces caspase-dependent apoptosis of human peripheral blood monocytes and T cells. Gastroenterology. 2004.
4. Shen C, Van Assche G, Rutgeerts P, Ceuppens JL. Caspase activation and apoptosis induction by adalimumab: demonstration *in vitro* and *in vivo* in a chimeric mouse model. Inflamm Bowel Dis. 2006;12:22–8.
5. Scallon BJ, Moore MA, Trinh H, Knight DM, Ghrayeb J. Chimeric anti-TNF-alpha monoclonal antibody cA2 binds recombinant transmembrane TNF-alpha and activates immune effector functions. Cytokine. 1995;7:251–9.
6. Fossati G, Nesbitt A. *In vitro* complement-dependent cytotoxicity and antibody-dependent cellular cytotoxicity by the anti-TNF agents adalimumab, etanercept, infliximab, and certolizumab pegol (CDP870). Am J Gastroenterol. 2005;100(Suppl.):S299.

7. Fossati G, Nesbitt A. Effect of the anti-TNF agents, adalimumab, etanercept, infliximab, and certolizumab PEGOL (CDP870) on the induction of apoptosis in activated peripheral blood lymphocytes and monocytes. Am J Gastroenterol. 2005;100(Suppl.):S298–9.
8. Prescribing information for Remicade (infliximab). Package Insert 2006.
9. Prescribing information for Humira (adalimumab). Package Insert 2004.
10. Targan SR, Hanauer SB, van Deventer SJ et al. A short-term study of chimeric monoclonal antibody cA2 to tumor necrosis factor alpha for Crohn's disease. Crohn's Disease cA2 Study Group. N Engl J Med. 1997;337:1029–35.
11. Hanauer SB, Sandborn WJ, Rutgeerts P et al. Human anti-tumor necrosis factor monoclonal antibody (adalimumab) in Crohn's disease: the CLASSIC I trial. Gastroenterology. 2006;130:323–33.
12. Hanauer SB, Feagan BG, Lichtenstein GR et al. Maintenance infliximab for Crohn's disease: the ACCENT I randomised trial. Lancet. 2002;359:1541–9.
13. Colombel J, Sandborn WJ, Rutgeerts P et al. Adalimumab induces and maintains clinical response and remission in patients with active Crohn's disease: results of the CHARM trial. Gastroenterology. 2006;131:950.
14. Schreiber S, Khaliq-Kareemi M, Lawrance I et al. Certolizumab pegol, a humanised anti-TNF pegylated FAb' fragment, is safe and effective in the maintenance of response and remission following induction in active Crohn's disease: a phase III study (PRECISE). Gut. 2005;54(Suppl. VII):A82.
15. Sandborn WJ, Feagan BG, Stoinov S et al. Certolizumab pegol administered subcutaneously is effective and well tolerated in patients with active Crohn's disease: results from a 26-week, placebo-controlled phase III study (PRECISE 1). Gastroenterology. 2006;130:A107 (Abstract 743).
16. Schreiber S, Rutgeerts P, Fedorak RN et al., for the CCsDSG. A randomized, placebo-controlled trial of certolizumab pegol (CDP870) for treatment of Crohn's disease. Gastroenterology. 2005;129:807–18.
17. Hanauer SB, Kamm MA, Colombel JF et al. Sustained steroid-free clinical remission in patients with moderate to severe Crohn's disease treated with adalimumab. Am J Gastroenterol. 2006;101:S460 (Abstract 1181).
18. Schwartz D, Rutgeerts P, Colombel JF et al. Induction, maintenance, and sustainability of the healing of draining fistulas in patients with Crohn's disease treated with adalimumab: results of the CHARM study. Am J Gastroenterol. 2006;101:S458–9 (Abstract 1177).
19. Baert F, Noman M, Vermeire S et al. Influence of immunogenicity on the long-term efficacy of infliximab in Crohn's disease. N Engl J Med. 2003;348:601–8.
20. Hanauer SB, Wagner CL, Bala M et al. Incidence and importance of antibody responses to infliximab after maintenance or episodic treatment in Crohn's disease. Clin Gastroenterol Hepatol. 2004;2:542–53.
21. Cheifetz A, Smedley M, Martin S et al. The incidence and management of infusion reactions to infliximab: a large center experience. Am J Gastroenterol. 2003;98:1315–24.
22. Vermeire S, Noman M, Van Assche G et al. Autoimmunity associated with anti-tumor necrosis factor alpha treatment in Crohn's disease: a prospective cohort study. Gastroenterology. 2003;125:32–9.
23. Bongartz T, Sutton AJ, Sweeting MJ, Buchan I, Matteson EL, Montori V. Anti-TNF antibody therapy in rheumatoid arthritis and the risk of serious infections and malignancies: systematic review and meta-analysis of rare harmful effects in randomized controlled trials. J Am Med Assoc. 2006;295:2275–85.
24. Keane J, Gershon S, Wise RP et al. Tuberculosis associated with infliximab, a tumor necrosis factor alpha neutralizing agent. N Engl J Med. 2001;345:1098–104.
25. Ghosh S, Goldin E, Gordon FH et al. Natalizumab for active Crohn's disease. N Engl J Med. 2003;348:24–32.
26. Sandborn WJ, Colombel JF, Enns R et al. Natalizumab induction and maintenance therapy for Crohn's disease. N Engl J Med. 2005;353:1912–25.
27. Targan SR, Feagan B, Fedorak R et al. Natalizumab induces sustained response and remission in patients with active Crohn's disease: results from the ENCORE trial. Gastroenterology. 2006;130:A108 (Abstract 747).
28. Kleinschmidt-DeMasters BK, Tyler KL. Progressive multifocal leukoencephalopathy complicating treatment with natalizumab and interferon beta-1a for multiple sclerosis [see comment]. N Engl J Med. 2005;353:369–74.

29. Langer-Gould A, Atlas SW, Green AJ, Bollen AW, Pelletier D. Progressive multifocal leukoencephalopathy in a patient treated with natalizumab [see comment]. N Engl J Med. 2005;353:375–81.

30. Van Assche G, Van Ranst M, Sciot R et al. Progressive multifocal leukoencephalopathy after natalizumab therapy for Crohn's disease [see comment]. N Engl J Med. 2005;353:362–8.

31. Yousry TA, Major EO, Rysckewitsch C et al. Evaluation of patients treated with natalizumab for progressive multifocal leukoencephaolopathy. N Engl J Med. 2006;354: 924–33.

32. Feagan BG, Greenberg GR, Wild G et al. Treatment of ulcerative colitis with a humanized antibody to the a4b7 integrin. N Engl J Med. 2005;352:2499–507.

33. Mannon PJ, Fuss IJ, Mayer L et al. Group A-I-CsDS. Anti-interleukin-12 antibody for active Crohn's disease. N Engl J Med. 2004;351:2069–79.

34. Korzenik JR, Dieckgraefe BK. Is Crohn's disease an immunodeficiency? A hypothesis suggesting possible early events in the pathogenesis of Crohn's disease. Dig Dis Sci. 2000; 45:1121–9.

35. Dieckgraefe BK, Korzenik JR, Husain A, Dieruf L. Association of glycogen storage disease 1b and Crohn disease: results of a North American survey. Eur J Pediatr. 2002;161 (Suppl. 1):S88–92.

36. Korzenik JR, Dieckgraefe BK, Valentine JF, Hausman DF, Gilbert MJ. Sargramostim in Crohn's Disease Study G. Sargramostim for active Crohn's disease. N Engl J Med. 2005; 352:2193–201.

37. Targan SR, Salzberg BA, Mayer L et al. A phase I-II study: multiple dose levels of visilizumab are well tolerated and produce rapid and sustained improvement in ulcerative colitis patients refractory to treatment with IV steroids (IVSR-UC). Gastroenterology. 2005;128(Suppl. 2).

21
Surgical treatment of complications of Crohn's disease

G. I. VOROBIEV, N. V. KOSTENKO, T. L. MIKHAILOVA and
R. I. ROMANOV

TOPICALITY

Irrespective of the development and application of new regimens of conservative therapy of Crohn's disease (CD), the majority of patients at various periods of their lives need to undergo surgical treatment. If during the 5-year anamnesis of the disease only 40% of patients are subjected to operation, the 10-year anamnesis increases this figure up to 70%[1]. Indications for the operation are the complications of the disease, that worsen the forecast and lower the lifestyle quality of patients. On the one hand complications have a local character which is associated with disorder of gastrointestinal tract function, and on the other hand they are related to severe systemic reactions on inflammation in a bowel: intoxication, metabolic imbalance, thrombosis, or embolism. These systemic complications are the main reasons for lethality, which in this group of patients during recent decades has proved to be lower than 6%[2].

Problems are connected with treatment strategy, indications for surgery, necessity of bowel resection in patients with abdominal mass. Proctocolectomy in patients with acute severe Crohn's colitis is dangerous because of metabolic disturbances, anaemia and coagulopathy. Up to this time, perianal complications, such as extrasphincter fistulas and anal canal destruction have a high rate of recurrence and in fact are impossible to cure surgically.

Finally, a high rate of recurrence of the disease, reaching 50–70%, and the necessity of small bowel reoperation, can lead to the development of the 'short intestine syndrome', which is no less dangerous to the life of a patient than the disease itself.

The aim of this study was to develop a specific surgical procedure for different complications of CD, such as infiltration, stricture, intestinal fistulas, severe colitis, or perianal lesions.

The study aimed to minimize the number of postoperational complications and lethality; to reduce the number of relapses that necessitate reoperation, and to avoid the development of the 'short intestine syndrome'.

CHARACTERISTICS OF CLINICAL MATERIAL

Between the years 2000 and 2005 a total of 83 CD patients were operated on at the Centre of Coloproctology, Moscow; these comprised 39 men and 44 women. The average age of patients was 34.6 ± 2.9 years. The duration of CD anamnesis was from 3 months to 8 years (23.8 months on average). A jejunum lesion was found in three patients, ileocaecal localization in 43 patients, and a large intestine lesion in 37 patients.

In accordance with the Crohn's Disease Activity Index (CDAI) a high activity was observed in 45 patients and a moderate level of activity in 32 patients. Despite complications in six patients systemic and local manifestations of the disease corresponded to the mild form of CD.

The frequency rate of CD complications was: infiltration, 45% of cases; strictures, 38%; intestinal fistulas, 41%; severe colitis, 23%; and perianal lesions, 42% of cases. Moreover there could be from one to four types of complication in one patient. Simultaneous combination of two types of complication was observed in 25 patients, 14 patients had three types of complication, and five patients simultaneously had four different types of complication. There was a total of 151 complications in 83 patients.

TREATMENT REGIME FOR COMPLICATIONS OF CD

Abdominal mass

A total of 37 patients had abdominal mass (45% of all operated patients). Abdominal mass was caused by terminal ileitis in 33 cases and by colitis only in four patients.

During hospitalization infiltration in four patients was accompanied by clinical manifestations of growing ileus, which necessitated urgent surgery – excision of the affected section in two cases and intestinal stoma construction in the other two cases.

The remainder of patients received intensive conservative therapy which included glucocorticoids, antibiotics, infusion therapy, hypoproteinaemia correction, and enteral feeding. Such therapy was effective in the majority of cases – 24 patients (64.8%) had a regression of infiltration, which permitted us to carry out a planned operation.

Besides four urgently operated patients, medical treatment in nine patients had no results: intoxication remained and the size of abdominal mass remained the same.

Indications for urgent surgery were: excision of the affected section in four cases, and in five cases – due to a large area of infiltration that occupied three or more anatomical sections of the stomach – the construction of a divided ileostoma as the first stage of surgical treatment.

During the period between 4 and 8 months all patients who had an intestinal stoma were operated on again. During the second stage of the surgical procedure excision of their affected section and removal of the intestinal stoma were carried out.

Strictures

Strictures comprised complications in all three cases of jejunum CD, in 22 cases of terminal ileitis, and were the indications for operation on nine patients with Crohn's colitis. There was also a combination of strictures with other types of complication, such as intraintestinal fistulas and infiltration of the abdominal cavity, when the inflammatory process was localized to the terminal section of the ileum.

In 30 cases (88.2% of all patients with strictures) the length of the strictured area was more than 3 cm and perifocal inflammation was observed. This did not permit us to execute strictureplasty and was the indication for resection of the affected segment. In the presence of enteric permeability subcompensation and prestricture distension the operation was carried out for the excision of the segment with the lesion and the construction of a temporary divided intestinal stoma (18 patients). In 10 cases the operation included simultaneous formation of an intraintestinal anastomosis; in six cases proctocolectomy was necessary on account of extensive strictures of the large intestine. In the remaining patients strictureplasty was carried out.

Intestinal fistula

In a total of 32 (38%) patients 45 intestinal fistulas were observed. The fistula internal opening was in the majority of cases (84.4%) located in the terminal section of the ileum. The topography of fistulas was as follows: external intestinal fistula, 12; intraintestinal fistulas of small intestine, 7; intraintestinal fistulas of large intestine, 11; enteric–urinary bladder fistula, 4; ileovaginal fistula, 1; internal incomplete intestinal fistula, 10.

The most difficult to diagnose were incomplete internal fistulas that were combined with the development of infiltration of the abdominal cavity. A complex multiple-view scanning and ultrasonic examination was used. In cases of manifested abdominal inflammation and non-drained cavities two- and three-stage operations were performed with a deferred construction of an anastomosis.

Severe colitis

Severe complications of Crohn's colitis led to systemic manifestations associated with severe metabolic imbalances and intoxication, which were observed in 25 patients. In all of these cases the disease activity corresponded to the severe rate of CDAI. The body weight index of patients was less than 18 (a marked body weight deficit) and in 12 patients clinical and laboratory manifestations of bacteraemia were observed.

The difficulty in choosing the appropriate treatment regime was in making the diagnosis, as it was impossible to use invasive methods of examination on account of the danger of perforation of the large intestine. When ulcerative colitis is excluded we consider it expedient to carry out the surgical procedure of 'switching off' – formation of a temporary divided ileostoma sparing laparoscopic access. Such a surgical procedure was carried out in all patients with Crohn's colitis.

Ileostomy made it possible to arrest intoxication and bring the condition to normal, and to compensate metabolic imbalances in 23 out of 25 patients (92%). Later, on account of irreversibility of the disease of the large intestine and perianal complications, 14 patients had proctocolectomy as the second stage of surgical procedure after the compensation of metabolic imbalances, and in 11 patients the surgical procedure included segmentary resection of the colon with the restoration of anal defaecation.

As a variant of reconstruction in the absence of the large intestine lesion we consider it possible to form a pouch ileorectal anastomosis ($n = 4$). Such a procedure permits us to achieve satisfactory dynamics of the disease (frequency of defaecation two to four times per 24 h), and to lower the rate of complications. Moreover no relapse of the disease was observed in the small intestine after colectomy surgery.

Perianal complications

Perianal manifestations in the form of extensive destructive lesions of the anal canal and perianal cutis in some patients form a condition that condemns patients to a permanent stoma.

In the trialled group a total of 35 patients (42.2%) had perianal lesions; in 28 cases this was combined with CD; and in seven cases with terminal ileitis. Pararectal fistulas were observed in 18 patients, including rectovaginal fistulas in six patients. Anal ulcerative fissures were observed in 22 patients including circular destruction of the anal canal as the most vivid manifestation of the local ulcerative colitis – in seven patients.

There were multiple fistulas in the area of the rectum in seven patients (18 patients had a total of 25 fistulas), including intrasphincter fistulas in four cases, trans-sphincter, seven cases; extrasphincter, eight; rectovaginal, six patients.

With the aim of creating conditions for cicatrization of perianal manifestations the treatment was carried out after the switching off of the passage along the rectum. After bypass surgery for the formation of intestinal stoma and local conservative therapy, healing of anal ulcers and fissures was achieved in 15 patients, and of intrasphincter fistulas in four patients. Surgical procedures were carried out in 15 patients with complex types of fistula (trans-sphincter, extrasphincter, rectovaginal). It was noted that in 11 cases, where there were extrasphincter and rectovaginal fistulas, the interior opening was located proximal to the anorectal line, and fistulas were of a cryptogenic character.

In seven patients with extensive loop lesions of the anal canal and manifested ulcerative proctitis the healing process led to scarring of the low ampullar section of the rectum, which did not permit restoration of anal defaecation. Three patients with extrasphincter fistulas and two patients with rectovaginal fistulas had to be subjected to two to four successive operations on the account of fistula recurrence. In one case with steady relapse it was also impossible to restore anal defaecation.

RESULTS OF SURGICAL TREATMENT

A total of 146 surgical procedures were carried out in 83 patients; these are listed in Table 1. With the aim of performing organ-preserving surgery the surgical treatment of 49 (59%) patients was divided into several stages (two, three and more) A one-stage surgical procedure was carried out in 34 patients, two-stage treatment in 35 patients, and three- and more-stage surgical treatment in 14 patients.

Table 1   Surgical procedures carried out for CD

Surgical procedure	Number of operations
Small intestine excision	3
Ileocaecal section excision	43
Large intestine segmentary excision	17
Proctocolectomy	14
Large intestine bypass operation (ileostoma)	32
Restoration surgery	15
Excision of pararectal fistulas	22

The indications for combined surgical procedures carried out in 12 patients were internal intestinal fistulas communicating with other anatomical sections of the intestine or other hollow organs. In seven patients we used comprised resection of terminal ileum and resection of sigmoid colon with internal fistula.

Multi-stage surgery with the deferred formation of intestinal anastomosis was given preference in cases of extensive inflammatory processes. In severe cases of colitis or perianal lesions bypass surgery ('switching off') was performed.

The initial severe condition of patients with serious metabolic imbalances was the main background for the development of postoperative complications of the disease, which were observed in 15.7% of cases. A total of 23 complications were observed in 13 patients; these are listed in Table 2. Three patients died after the operation (3.6%); these deaths were caused by sepsis; multiple lung, liver and kidney abscesses; superior vena cava thrombosis; or peritonitis.

Taking into consideration the possibility of disease recurrence after the operation, we consider it expedient to carry out prolonged antirecurring therapy, together with dynamic monitoring of the condition of the intestine, especially of the interintestinal anastomosis area.

After surgical treatment all patients received antirecurring therapy for 2–4 years (5-ASA 2 g per day, AZA 150 mg/day).

The control examination included colonoscopy every 3 months for 2 years following surgery, and then once every 6 months. For more than 2 years after the operation 56 patients (67.5%) were followed up. Relapses were reported in 12 patients (21.4%); in four cases the recurrence of Crohn's colitis after segmentary resection of the large intestine was the indication for reoperation.

Table 2 Postoperative complications

Postoperative complications	Number of cases
Small intestine adhesive obstruction	3
Eventration	3
Small intestine perforation	4
Peritonitis	2
Ostomy sutures failure	1
Residual cavity formation	3
Sepsis	3
Superior vena cava thrombosis	1

Table 3 Frequency of CD recurrence depending on the localization of the primary lesion and the surgical procedure performed

Primary lesion localization	Surgical procedure	No of relapses (%)	No. of reoperations (%)
Jejunum ($n = 3$)	Jejunum resection ($n = 3$)	–	–
Terminal ileitis ($n = 29$)	Ileocaecal section resection ($n = 29$)	7 (16.3%)	–
Large intestine ($n = 24$)	Large intestine segmentary resection ($n = 11$)	5 (45.4%)	4 (36.4%)
	Proctocolectomy ($n = 13$)	–	–

DISCUSSION

CD complications are the consequences of transmural inflammatory processes in the intestinal wall, which, in case of inadequate therapy and resistance to treatment, leads to irreversible after-effects – ulcerative destruction of the intestinal wall; formation of fistulas, strictures, or infiltrations.

Infiltration developed in patients due to the formation of interior incomplete or insufficiently drained fistulas. This is why we consider it unacceptable to divide abdominal mass without resection of segment with internal fistula. Exterior intestinal fistulas have the very same genesis, they develop after appendectomy as the result of the poor diagnosis of CD.

It is of interest that, in combination of strictures and fistulas, the interior opening of the latter was located as a rule on the proximal border of the constriction. This confirms the fact that one of the pathogenetic mechanisms of fistula development in CD is intraintestinal hypertension in the inflamed section, which is observed particularly in the prestricture part of the affected segment.

First attacks of severe Crohn's colitis in more than half of patients led to irreversible changes in the large intestine wall, and serve as an indication for its total excision. The long follow-up of patients shows a high probability of disease reccurrence (36.4%) also after segmentary resections. At the same time there are no reports on cases of CD relapses in the small intestine after excision of the large intestine. It is possible that this proves the heterogeneity of Crohn's colitis and CD ileocaecal localization.

Perianal lesions in the form of destructive changes of the anal canal mucosa, development of ulcerative fissures and pararectal fistulas were observed in no more than 40% of CD patients. Most frequently the perianal lesions were combined with severe colitis. Taking into consideration the development of perianal manifestations as a local inflammatory reaction, we consider it as having no future in treating these lesions prior to the decrease of inflammation in the area of ulcerative blemishes. Alongside local and systemic conservative therapy switching off the intestino-rectal passage was also an effective method of treatment. In these conditions regeneration was achieved in 17 patients (48%), and in nine (26%) patients it was possible to carry out satisfactory plastic surgery on excision of fistulas. Irreversible loss of anal canal function on account of cicatrization and fistula recurrence was observed in nine (26%) patients.

In the majority of patients (59%) the multistage regime of surgical treatment was applied. Such tactics were used with the aim of reducing surgical risks in patients with severe metabolic imbalances and septic conditions. In patients with perifocal reactive inflammation this also, in our opinion, avoids unjustified resection of those sections of the intestine which are not affected by granulomatous inflammation.

CONCLUSIONS

1. The selected surgical treatment regime of CD led to postoperative complications in 15.7% of cases and to lethality in 3.6% of cases.

2. The number of relapses of CD with prolonged therapy constituted 21.4%, and the necessity for repeat surgery occurred in 7.3% of cases.

3. Two- and three-stage surgical procedures in patients with extensive inflammation made it possible to avoid the development of 'short intestine syndrome' and to retain anal defaecation in 83.1% of cases of complicated forms of CD.

Reference

1. Adler G. Morbus Crohn – Colitis ulcerosa. Berlin: Springer-Verlag, 1996.
2. Lashner BA. Clinical features, laboratory findings and course of Crohn's disease. In: Kirsner JB (ed.), Inflammatory Bowel Disease, Saunders, 2000:305–14.

Bibliography

Bernell O, Lapidus A, Helleris G. Risk factors for surgery and recurrence in 907 patients with primary ileocaecal Crohn's disease. Br J Surg. 2000;87:1697–701.

Duepree HJ, Senagore AJ, Delaney CP, Brady KM, Fazio VW. Advantages of laparoscopic resection for ileocecal Crohn's disease. Dis Colon Rectum. 2000;45:605–10.

Oliver M, Neill J, Mortensen C. Surgical treatment of Crohn's disease. In: Satsangi J, Sutherland LR (eds). Inflammatory Bowel Diseases. Churchill Livingstone, 2003:513–14.

Parente F, Maconi G, Bollani S et al. Bowel ultrasound in assessment of Crohn's disease and detection of related small bowel strictures: a prospective comparative study versus X-ray and intraoperative findings. Gut. 2002;50:p.490–5.

Vorobiov GI. Osnovy koloproktologii. Feniks, 2001.

Yamamoto T, Keighley MR. Enterovesical fistulae complicating Crohn's disease: clinicopathological features and management. Int J Colorectal Dis. 2000;15:-211–15.

22
Surgical treatment of ulcerative colitis

G. I. VOROBIEV, T. L. MIKHAILIVA and N. V. KOSTENKO

INTRODUCTION

Surgical treatment of ulcerative colitis (UC) up to this time can be considered as one of the dramatic pages of surgical gastroenterology. Speedy development of the disease, re-estimation of the possibilities of conservative therapy, and the absence of precise indications for surgery very often lead to delaying the time of operation. At the same time, extensive resection of the large intestine in the terminal phase of intoxication and metabolic derangements are accompanied by unsatisfactory results of surgical treatment – postoperative complications amount to 50–90% and lethality up to 12.5–60%[1,2]. Even if a patient with UC has recovered after the operation, in most cases his or her future may involve end-ileostomy, invalidity and insufficient social rehabilitation.

Among UC patients the necessity for surgical treatment amounts to 10–15%, and two-thirds of patients are operated on in connection with the inefficiency of conservative therapy[3,4]. At the same time the criteria of inefficient therapy, especially in the severe hormone-resistant form of UC, are considered individually, depending on the set of human factors, specialization and experience of a clinician, the extent of therapy received, and differences in national public health programmes[5].

It is worth mentioning that, even if clinical and endoscopic remission is achieved in 55–70% of cases, it is not accompanied by 'morphological remission', or by the absence of pathomorphological changes of the colon mucosa characteristic of UC[6,7]. Modern genetic research proved the high risk of cancer mutations in the colon mucosa after a lengthy course of inflammation. Chromosomal abnormalities and the development of colorectal cancer occur in approximately 3% of cases at the beginning of the second decade of the course of illness[8].

The possibility of overcoming invalidity and improving the lifestyle of patients after extensive resections of the large intestine is connected with the development of reconstructive operations in UC, and attempts to preserve or restore anal defaecation. In the opinion of many authors[9] the standard surgical treatment of UC was total resection of the large intestine and the introduction of ileal pouch–anal anastomosis (ileoanal pouch). However, with the growth in the number of operated patients and of the length of the follow-up period, analysis of the remote results demonstrated a high rate (up to 30%) of late postoperative complications[10,11].

An important role in improvement of the surgical procedure results, in the decrease of the number of postoperative complications and lethality is played by timely determination of indications for surgery, development of surgical techniques, and intensive pathogenetic therapy in pre- and postoperative periods. For successful reconstruction surgery it is necessary to take into consideration individual characteristics of the patient, and use different kinds of reconstructive surgery, which is carried out when a patient's condition is favourable for the operation.

PATIENT CHARACTERISTICS

For the period 1990–2005 a total of 1086 patients with UC were seen at the Center of Coloproctology in Moscow; the severe form of the disease was observed in 491 (45.2%) cases, 220 patients underwent surgical treatment, which constituted 20.3% of all the UC patients and 44.8% of the severe forms of the UC. A total of 129 patients were operated on with UC forms resistant to conservative therapy. Inefficiency of conservative therapy was determined by hormone therapy resistance in 91 patients, and by hormone dependency in 38 patients. Complications were observed in 50 patients: melaena, 26 patients; toxic dilation, 13; perforation of the large intestine, 11; 41 patients had cancer.

Table 1 Distribution of patients depending on sex and age

	Sex		Age (years)					
Group of patients	F	M	Under 20	20–29	30–39	40–49	50–59	60+
Hormone-resistant form (n = 91)	42	49	12 (13%)	19 (21%)	25 (27%)	16 (18%)	7 (8%)	12 (13%)
Hormone-dependent form (n = 38)	18	20	2 (5%)	10 (27%)	12 (32%)	8 (21%)	4 (10%)	2 (5%)
UC complications (n = 50)	21	29	3 (6%)	11 (22%)	17 (34%)	10 (20%)	6 (12%)	3 (6%)
Colorectal cancer (n = 41)	19	22	–	6 15%	9 (22%)	12 (29%)	6 (15%)	8 (19%)

Among operated patients women prevailed (male/female = 100/120), the average age of patients was 34.2 ± 3.4 years. Table 1 shows the distribution of patients depending on sex and age.

The cases were classified depending on the course of illness and the extension of the lesion of the large intestine. In groups with hormone resistance and malignancy the total form of colitis prevailed; in cases with UC complications

Table 2 Distribution of patients depending on UC clinical course

	Clinical course		
Groups of patients	Acute	Recurrent	Continuous
Hormone-resistant form (n = 91)	25 (27.5%)	48 (52.7%)	18 (19.8%)
Hormone-dependent form (n = 38)	–	5 (13.2%)	33 (86.8%)
Complications of UC (n = 50)	17 (34.0%)	26 (52.0%)	7 (14.0%)
Colorectal cancer (n = 41)	–	33 (80.5%)	8 (19.5%)

more than a half of patients had left-sided and subtotal lesion of the large intestine (Tables 2 and 3). The development of cancer was more often observed (in 80.5%) in cases with the chronic course of the inflammatory process with rare relapses.

The age of patients with UC who developed tumours of the large intestine varied from 20 to 78 years (43.8 ± 4.7 years on average). The length of the UC anamnesis prior to the time cancer was diagnosed was on average 18.5 ± 4.6 years. The neoplastic process in eight patients had a multicentric character with the development of from two to nine focuses of adenocarcinoma, which had different levels of differentiation. At the time when cancer was diagnosed 14 patients (34.1%) had remote metastasis.

Table 3 Distribution of patients depending on the extension of lesion of the large intestine

	Extension of lesion		
Groups of patients	Left-side	Subtotal	Total
Hormone-resistant form (n = 91)	12 (13.2%)	25 (27.5%)	54 (59.3%)
Hormone-dependent form (n = 38)	2 (5.3%)	9 (23.7%)	27 (71.0%)
Complications of UC (n = 50)	8 (16.0%)	18 (36.0%)	24 (48.0%)
Colorectal cancer (n = 41)	2 (4.9%)	14 (34.1%)	25 (61.0%)

In cases of UC surgery is necessary in 10–30% of cases, when the inflammatory process cannot be corrected by preparations available at present. The absence of effect from conservative therapy becomes apparent in the severe condition of a patient against the background of local and systemic toxic reactions, destructive inflammation in the large intestine wall and metabolic stress manifestations. Therefore direct results of surgery are connected with the conservative treatment regime, severity of the disease prior to the surgical procedure and the development of complications in the abdominal cavity.

SURGICAL TREATMENT OF UC COMPLICATIONS

The most severe contingent of UC patients comprises cases of intestinal complications of the disease that can have a blitzkrieg and fatal character. Melaena, toxic dilation of the colon and perforation of the large intestine develop as manifestations of the hormone resistance (inefficiency of treatment with high doses of corticosteroids)[5,12], and probably due to some iatrogenic factors: not a timely determination of indications for surgery, inadequacy of course of conservative therapy undertaken, use of invasive methods of examination of the large intestine due to severe forms of exacerbation of colitis and others. Intestinal complications were observed in 50 patients.

INDICATIONS FOR OPERATION

Melaena

This group was formed by the following clinical and radiological criteria:

1. Frequency of defaecation is 12 times and more during 24 h with macroscopically manifested blood, while having complex therapy with introduction of steroid preparations.

2. The volume of faeces with intensive blood – 1000 ml and more in 24 h.

3. The volume of blood loss as confirmed by (radionuclide) scintigraphy is 150 ml and more during 24 h.

The aforementioned symptoms were observed in 26 UC patients.

Toxic dilation of the colon

This is diagnosed when the diameter of one or several colon sections is dilated for 9 cm and more. This was observed in 13 patients. Patients of this group, besides having a clinical picture of severe UC, also had such features as bloating, and percussionary tympanitis in the projection of the colon. An alarming symptom was that in six patients the frequency of stool during 24 h abruptly decreased by twofold.

Radiography showed that in nine cases the biggest dilation (9–15 cm) was observed in the projection of the transversal colon, in four cases – of sigmoid intestine (9–13 cm). All patients received endoscopic decompression via colonoscope, with gas and liquid intestinal content aspiration; however, within 24 h a relapse of dilation was observed, which was an indication for urgent surgery.

Perforation

Perforation of the large intestine is found in the most serious group of patients with UC complications; it was diagnosed in 11 patients. Eight patients had this diagnosis at the time of hospitalization into this centre, three patients developed this complication while having conservative therapy treatment at the centre.

There was no typical picture of the acute perforation of a hollow organ. Clinical features were: increase of the intoxication symptoms, bloating (seven patients), and appearance of peritoneal symptoms (six patients). An absolute symptom of perforation was the presence of intraperitoneal gas, which was observed during radiological tests only in seven patients.

At the first stage of surgical treatment of severe and complicated UC forms we give preference to subtotal resection of the colon, while keeping the whole large intestine and distal part of sigmoid intestine with the ileostoma and sigmostoma formation. This operation was performed on 43 patients.

During the surgical procedure for UC subtotal resection combines the benefits of easier endurance as compared to proctocolectomy, the possibility of future rehabilitation, with the preservation of the large intestine, and at the same time the seat of the complication is excised.

In six cases with voluminous intestinal bleeding one-stage surgery was performed – colectomy with abdominoanal resection (AAR) of the rectum, ileostomy. Due to the concurrent serious heart failure of one male patient, aged 81, with the perforation of sigmoid intestine he was operated on with the minimal possible resection – left-sided hemiolectomy by Mikulitch and the formation of divided colostoma.

Postoperative complications were observed in 24 patients (48%); these are listed in Table 4. Lethality occurred in 11 patients (22%); however, in the past 5 years this figure decreased to 6.7%. For the period 2000–2005 one patient died of general peritonitis, related to the large intestine perforation prior to his hospitalization to the Centre of Coloproctology.

Table 4 Postoperative complications in patients with complicated forms of UC

Complications	Quantity
Bleeding from the defunctioned bowel	2
Abdominal bleeding	2
Eventation	5
Laparotomy wound suppuration	7
Failure of sigmostoma sutures	3
Heart failure	5
Small intestine fistula	1
Exudative pleurisy	2
Pneumonia	4
Pulmonary arteries thrombosis	2
Dissimilated intravessel coagulation-syndrome	1

SURGICAL TREATMENT OF RESISTANT UC FORMS

Hormone-resistant form

To date, glucocorticoids remain the main preparation for treating severe froms of UC. Their high doses (2 mg/kg per 24 h) permits us to achieve clinical and endoscopic remission in 70–80% of patients[4,12]; however, in 20–30% of patients inflammatory processes are resistant to hormone therapy, and in this case the disease grows progressively worse, which demands timely surgery[5,12].

Complex conservative therapy consisted of: infusion therapy, glucocorticoid hormones, antibacterial therapy, or symptomatic treatment.

It is a very complicated task to determine the inefficiency of the conservative therapy of a severe attack of UC due to the patient's grave condition and the polymorphism of clinical manifestations of metabolic disorders. Several different systems of appraising the severity of UC have been developed, but none of them specifies a group of patients who need surgical treatment. We have determined a set of clinical, laboratory and instrumental data that in our opinion are sufficiently informative for the estimation of the efficacy of UC treatment (defaecation frequency, volume of faeces, frequency of heart beat, average blood pressure, temperature of body, pain in the abdominal area, haemoglobin and leucocyte rates, ESR, levels of albumen, plasma potassium, and colon dilation as per radiography analysis). Those parameters were determined at the time of hospitalization and in the dynamics not less than once in 2–3 days. Not only the improvement of condition, but also the absence of positive dynamics as estimated by the aforementioned parameters during 2 weeks after the beginning of the treatment, was considered as resistance to the relevant treatment.

As regards hormone resistance alongside a serious general condition, 91 patients were operated. The following procedures were carried out: subtotal resection of the colon, 73 patients; colectomy by Hartman, two patients; colectomy and AAR of the rectum, ileostomy, 15 patients; hemiolectomy, one patient.

For the total follow-up period postoperative complications constituted 16.5%, lethality 3.3%, and during the past 5 years there have been no lethal cases.

Hormone-dependent form

The phenomenon of hormone dependency occurs under different autoimmune conditions. The constant necessity for hormone medication in UC is in our opinion an indication for surgical treatment. Clinical and endoscopic remission among 38 patients was maintained only by continuous intake of prednisolone, 15–30 mg/day. As it was impossible to stop the hormone therapy during 4–6 and more months it served as an indication for the surgical procedure due to the developed osteoporosis and pathological spine fracture (three patients, 7.9%), steroid diabetes (nine patients, 23.7%), pyoderma (15 patients, 39.5%). This group of patients also showed intolerance and inefficiency of immunosuppressive therapy (azathioprine).

When determining the treatment regime of such patients the possibility of primary reconstructive operations should be taken into consideration, i.e. restoration of anal defaecation by forming a direct or pouch ileorectal anastomosis ($n = 10$), and also formation of a pelvic ileoanal pouch ($n = 6$). It becomes possible, due to subsidence of inflammation in the large intestine at the intake of glucocorticoids, to achieve clinical and even endoscopic remission, and correction of metabolic imbalances.

A total of 38 patients were operated on for hormone-dependent forms of the disease. The following surgical procedures were carried out: colectomy by Hartman, one patient; colectomy and AAR of the rectum, ileostomy, three patients; colectomy with ileorectal anastomosis, 10 patients; colectomy with abdominoanal resection of the rectum, and pelvic ileal pouch, six patients.

Postoperative complications constituted 15.8%, which was connected during the first years of follow-up with technical complications of one-stage reconstructive surgery. There was one lethal case during the first years of follow-up.

SURGICAL TREATMENT OF COLORECTAL UC CANCER

Colonic cancer was diagnosed in the majority of cases during colonoscopy made during the prophylactic medical examination or during the examination of patients with manifested tumour complications (ileus, intoxication, metastasis).

Total excision of the large intestine was carried out for rectal cancer, as malignization is the outcome of local genetic transformations, which can recur in any part of the large bowel mucosa affected by a continuous inflammatory process.

There were 41 patients operated on; the surgical procedures are listed in Table 5.

Table 5 Surgical procedures used

Subtotal colon excision	3
Colectomy and AAR of rectum, ileostomy	16
Proctocolectomy	9
Hemicolectomy	1
Symptomatic ileostomy	12

The results of the study of 29 resected bowel samples are interesting. The endorphite forms of tumour prevailed (72.4%); they were of loop character and were up to 17 cm long, and in one case the length approached 70 cm. It was difficult not only to detect the tumour limits macroscopically, but even to detect its presence in three patients, as it was manifested by slight thickening similar to inflammatory polypus.

Microscopy showed tumours of mixed morphological structure represented by several focuses (low-grade differentiation cancer and adenocarcinoma of different grades of differentiation). The following data were obtained when the tumour was differentiated in accordance to the most malignant component:

Low-grade differentiation adenocarcinoma	8 (27.6%)
Average-grade differentiation adenocarcinoma	9 (31.0%)
High-grade differentiation adenocarcinoma	5 (17.3%)

Among operated patients 28 (68.3%) were followed up for 5 years, and only six (21.4%) patients lived through that period.

CHOICE OF THE EXTENT AND TECHNIQUES OF SURGERY

During the past 10 years it has been shown that the minimal extent of surgery for UC is subtotal colon resection. The autoimmune component of the systemic inflammatory process leads to severe recurrence of inflammation in the preserved after-segmentary excisions sections of the colon, which makes the future of such operations doubtful.

Surgical treatment of weak patients with severe forms was divided into two stages with reconstruction procedures after the normalization of homeostasis.

In surgical procedures of severe forms of UC such features as the development of coagulopathy against the background of haemorrhagic syndrome, the decrease of elasticity of the intestinal wall, the risk of damage to it due to manipulations during the operation, and decrease of the regenerative activity of tissues were taken into consideration. Reanimation and anaesthetic maintenance corresponded to the severity of cases and the risk of surgery; moreover, the possibilities of postoperative problems were forecast: peridural anaesthesia was used, and transfusion of protein preparations and therapy with respect to hypovolaemia and hypoxia were undertaken.

Surgical techniques included:

- Precise haemostasis at every stage of the operation, including ligation of dilated vessels of the parietal peritoneum.

- Microbiological study of the abdominal cavity axudation.

- Observance of the principle of 'not touching' the affected large intestine wall, to avoid trauma.

- Ligation of great vessels immediately before the removal of a bowel.

- Precise fixation of intestinal stomas, suture of defaected abdominal cavity.

- Long-term (3–5 days) catchment of the abdominal cavity.

During the past 7 years we have also used such technologies as laparoscopic techniques (14 patients), and intestinal mobilization with the help of an ultrasonic scalpel (54 patients). These technologies helped to reduce blood loss during the operation and the pain sydrome, to speed up the rehabilitation period and to shorten the time of inpatient treatment.

POSTOPERATIVE FOLLOW-UP

To bring homeostasis to normal in patients with severe UC during the postoperative period it was necessary to carry out intensive therapy for not less than 10–14 days, and the prescribed outpatient therapy should last not less than 2–3 months. In the immediate postoperative period a complex treatment was executed when the daily dynamics of clinical changes, and laboratory data on homeostasis systems were reported. The following procedure was carried out:

1. Hormone therapy: (a) introduction of adequate doses of glucocorticoids (prednisolone 2 mg/kg or hydrocortisone 10 mg/kg parenterally; (b) anabolic steroids once (1) a week; (c) mineral corticoids in adrenal gland deficiency; (d) adiuretin.

2. Infusion therapy (crystalloids 50 ml/kg per day, colloids (polyglucin, helophusin) 20 ml/kg per day under the control of total blood volume, diuresis.

3. Correction of hypoproteinaemia (fresh-frozen plasma, albumen, protein).

4. Correction of electrolytic disorders (potassium, calcium, magnesium).

5. Antibacterial therapy (1, metronidadazole + cephalosporins; 2, fluorinequinolone).

6. Adequate anaesthesia of the postoperative period (mainly peridural).

7. Intestinal forcing, Vaseline oil.

8. Enteral feeding – 200–400 g of dry powder per day.

9. Sedative therapy.

10. Ultrasound monitoring of the abdominal cavity.

This scheme, alongside surgery techniques, permitted us to show no complications in the post-operative period in 87.2% of patients operated on for UC.

SURGICAL REHABILITATION

Radical excision of the large intestine for UC, the necessity in the majority of patients to construct an ileostoma after the excision, alongside the serious condition of such patients, constitute a serious task of the rehabilitation of operated patients. Several variants of reconstructive operations of UC cases have been used:

1. Colectomy with the formation of a 'direct' ileorectal anastomosis.

2. Colectomy with front resection of the rectum and construction of a 'low' pouch ileorectal anastomosis.

3. Total excision of the large intestine and construction of an ileoanal pouch.

We considered it possible to preserve the rectum for reconstruction in the following cases:

- Absence of active ulcerative proctitis and malignization (in accordance with morphological data).

- Absence of rectal stricture.

- Preservation of the obturative function of the rectum.

- Absence of inflammatory perianal complications.

Operations with a primary reconstructive stage were carried out in 15 patients, who were operated on in satisfactory somatic condition for the hormone-dependent form of UC (nine patients, colectomy with the construction of a 'direct' ileorectal anastomosis; six patients, colectomy with abdominoanal resection and construction of an ileoanal pouch).

The majority of patients ($n = 141$, 78.8%) were operated on during the severe condition of the disease, determined by active inflammatory process in the large intestine; however, the absence of melaena and the rectum stricture made it possible to preserve the rectum. At the first stage of surgical treatment in the total of 118 patients the rectum was preserved; the necessity for total excision of the large intestine occurred in 21 patients.

The question of the possibility of the second-stage reconstructive operation was considered during 6–24 months after the excision of the large intestine when local therapy was undertaked aimed at subsidence of proctitis. In this group 93 out 118 patients (78.8%) were followed up. Reconstructive operations were carried out in 49 patients, which were 'low' pouch ileorectal anastomosis, 12 patients; excision of the rectum with the formation of an ileoanal pouch (social indications), 8 patients.

In the remaining 44 patients, irrespective of local therapy, proctitis remained, and the rectal stricture developed, which was an indication for its excision – thus an abdominoanal resection with ileostoma was carried out.

In the group of 29 patients with the constructed ileorectal anastomosis (including all patients after the construction of a pouch ileorectal anastomosis), the reconstructive stage was supplemented with the formation of a preventive divided ileostoma, which was closed within 6 weeks–4 months (the third stage of surgical treatment) Such an ileorectal anastomosis in 21 patients was immediately included into the intestinal passage. Postoperative complications were observed in 14.3% of cases without the formation of the ileostoma, and in 6.9% of cases with a preventive ileostoma. There were no lethal cases.

Analysis of the late results of the reconstructive operations showed that five patients had a severe relapse of proctitis after the formation of an ileorectal anastomosis, one patient with ileoanal pouch had pouchitis with an ileovaginal fistula. In view of the above there were indications for the rectum and the reservoir excision, with the subsequent construction of a permanent ileostoma in these six cases (12.2% among those operated with reconstructive surgery stage).

Thus, 108 patients were followed up, 15 of them had a one-stage operation with the reconstruction of anal defaecation, 93 had a two-stage operation. It is worth mentioning that in 58 (53.7%) patients anal defaecation was restored, and 50 patients (46.3%) were adapted to a permanent ileostoma.

All patients with preserved rectal mucosa after reconstructive surgery should undergo outpatient observation, and those with 10 years anamnesis should have annual biopsy tests.

CONCLUSION

During recent years (1999–2005) the use of new medical regimes, including the joint follow-up of patients by gastroenterologists and proctologists, made it possible to clearly and in a timely way to determine the indications for surgery and subsequently to influence the results of surgical treatment (Table 6). Thus during this period (as long as 7 years) there were no lethal cases after operations for severe UC hormone-resistant and hormone-dependent forms. The number of postoperative complications was also reduced. Such a tendency is also observed in treating complicated UC forms, where the number of lethal cases decreased threefold.

Table 6 Postoperative complications and lethality

Groups of patients	Years of observation	Postoperative complications	Lethality
Hormone-resistant form (n = 91)	1990–1998 (n = 48)	9 (18.7%)	3 (6.3%)
	1999–2005 (n = 43)	6 (13.9%)	0
Hormone-dependent form (n = 38)	1990–1998 (n = 21)	4 (19.0%)	1 (4.8%)
	1999–2005 (n = 17)	2 (11.7%)	0
UC complications (n = 50)	1990–1998 (n = 27)	16 (59.3%)	9 (33.3%)
	1999–2005 (n = 23)	8 (34.8%)	2 (8.7%)
Colorectal cancer (n = 41)	1990–1998 (n = 21)	6 (28.6%)	3 (14.3%)
	1999–2005 (n = 20)	4 (20.0%)	2 (10.0%)

Indications for operation in UC

At present indications for operation in UC can be divided into several groups:

1. Intestinal complications of UC: (a) melaena; (b) colon toxic dilation; (c) perforation of the large intestine.

2. Inefficiency of the conservative therapy of UC: (a) hormone resistance; (b) hormone dependence.

3. Malignization of UC (colorectal cancer).

At present the succession of therapeutic and surgical methods of treatment, the timely determination of indications for surgery, the expedient selection of the type and techniques of surgical operation, postoperative complex therapy, and individual choice of methods of surgical rehabilitation help solve the problem of achieving satisfactory results in UC surgery.

References

1. Greenstein AJ, Sachar DB, Gibas A. Outcome of toxic dilatation in ulcerative and Crohn colitis. J Clin Gastroenterol. 1985;7:137.
2. Hurst RD, Finco C, Rubin M. Prospective analysis of perioperative morbidity in one hundred consecutive colectomies for ulcerative colitis. Surgery. 1995;118:748.
3. Vorobiev GI. Aspects of Coloproctology. Feniks, Rostov-on-Don, 2001:414.
4. Dozois RR, Kelly KA. The surgical management of ulcerative colitis. In: Kirshner JB, editor. Inflammatory Bowel Disease, 5th edn. Saunders, 2000:411–45.
5. Picco MF, Bayless T. Prognostic considerations in idiopatic inflammatory bowel disease. In: Kirshner JB, editor. Inflammatory Bowel Disease, 5th edn. Saunders, 2000:765–80.
6. Aruin LI, Kapuller LL, Isakov VA. Morfologicheskaya diagnostika bolesney jeludka i kishechnika. Triada-Kh. 1998:496.
7. Riddell RH, Path FRC. Pathology of idiopathic inflammatory bowel disease. In: Kirshner JB, editor. Inflammatory Bowel Disease, 5th edn. Saunders, 2000:427–47.
8. Butt JH, Lennard-Jones JE, Ritchie JA. A practical approach to the risk of cancer in inflammatory bowel disease: reassure, watch, or act? Med Clin N Am. 1980;64:1203–20.
9. Williams NS. Restorative proctocolectomy is the first choice elective surgical procedure for ulcerative colitis. Br J Surg. 1989;76:1109–10.
10. Breen EM, Schoetz DJ, Marcello PW. Functional results after perineal complications of ileal pouch–anal anastomosis. Dis Colon Rectum, 1998:41:691–5.
11. Fazio VW, Ziv Y, Church JM et al. Ileal pouch–anal anastomoses complications and function in 1005 patients. Ann Surg. 1995;222:120.
12. Pinna-Pintor M, Ares P, Bona R. Severe steroid unresponsive ulcerative colitis: outcome of restorative proctocolectomy in patients undergoing cyclosporin treatment. Dis Colon Rectum. 2000;43:609–13.

Index

Falk Symposium Series

43. Reutter W, Popper H, Arias IM, Heinrich PC, Keppler D, Landmann L, eds.: *Modulation of Liver Cell Expression*. Falk Symposium No. 43. 1987
ISBN: 0-85200-677-2*
44. Boyer JL, Bianchi L, eds.: *Liver Cirrhosis*. Falk Symposium No. 44. 1987
ISBN: 0-85200-993-3*
45. Paumgartner G, Stiehl A, Gerok W, eds.: *Bile Acids and the Liver*. Falk Symposium No. 45. 1987
ISBN: 0-85200-675-6*
46. Goebell H, Peskar BM, Malchow H, eds.: *Inflammatory Bowel Diseases – Basic Research & Clinical Implications*. Falk Symposium No. 46. 1988
ISBN: 0-7462-0067-6*
47. Bianchi L, Holt P, James OFW, Butler RN, eds.: *Aging in Liver and Gastrointestinal Tract*. Falk Symposium No. 47. 1988
ISBN: 0-7462-0066-8*
48. Heilmann C, ed.: *Calcium-Dependent Processes in the Liver*. Falk Symposium No. 48. 1988
ISBN: 0-7462-0075-7*
50. Singer MV, Goebell H, eds.: *Nerves and the Gastrointestinal Tract*. Falk Symposium No. 50. 1989
ISBN: 0-7462-0114-1
51. Bannasch P, Keppler D, Weber G, eds.: *Liver Cell Carcinoma*. Falk Symposium No. 51. 1989
ISBN: 0-7462-0111-7
52. Paumgartner G, Stiehl A, Gerok W, eds.: *Trends in Bile Acid Research*. Falk Symposium No. 52. 1989
ISBN: 0-7462-0112-5
53. Paumgartner G, Stiehl A, Barbara L, Roda E, eds.: *Strategies for the Treatment of Hepatobiliary Diseases*. Falk Symposium No. 53. 1990   ISBN: 0-7923-8903-4
54. Bianchi L, Gerok W, Maier K-P, Deinhardt F, eds.: *Infectious Diseases of the Liver*. Falk Symposium No. 54. 1990   ISBN: 0-7923-8902-6
55. Falk Symposium No. 55 not published
55B. Hadziselimovic F, Herzog B, Bürgin-Wolff A, eds.: *Inflammatory Bowel Disease and Coeliac Disease in Children*. International Falk Symposium. 1990
ISBN 0-7462-0125-7
56. Williams CN, eds.: *Trends in Inflammatory Bowel Disease Therapy*. Falk Symposium No. 56. 1990   ISBN: 0-7923-8952-2
57. Bock KW, Gerok W, Matern S, Schmid R, eds.: *Hepatic Metabolism and Disposition of Endo- and Xenobiotics*. Falk Symposium No. 57. 1991   ISBN: 0-7923-8953-0
58. Paumgartner G, Stiehl A, Gerok W, eds.: *Bile Acids as Therapeutic Agents: From Basic Science to Clinical Practice*. Falk Symposium No. 58. 1991   ISBN: 0-7923-8954-9
59. Halter F, Garner A, Tytgat GNJ, eds.: *Mechanisms of Peptic Ulcer Healing*. Falk Symposium No. 59. 1991   ISBN: 0-7923-8955-7
60. Goebell H, Ewe K, Malchow H, Koelbel Ch, eds.: *Inflammatory Bowel Diseases – Progress in Basic Research and Clinical Implications*. Falk Symposium No. 60. 1991
ISBN: 0-7923-8956-5
61. Falk Symposium No. 61 not published
62. Dowling RH, Folsch UR, Löser Ch, eds.: *Polyamines in the Gastrointestinal Tract*. Falk Symposium No. 62. 1992   ISBN: 0-7923-8976-X
63. Lentze MJ, Reichen J, eds.: *Paediatric Cholestasis: Novel Approaches to Treatment*. Falk Symposium No. 63. 1992   ISBN: 0-7923-8977-8
64. Demling L, Frühmorgen P, eds.: *Non-Neoplastic Diseases of the Anorectum*. Falk Symposium No. 64. 1992   ISBN: 0-7923-8979-4
64B. Gressner AM, Ramadori G, eds.: *Molecular and Cell Biology of Liver Fibrogenesis*. International Falk Symposium. 1992   ISBN: 0-7923-8980-8

*These titles were published under the MTP Press imprint.

Falk Symposium Series

65. Hadziselimovic F, Herzog B, eds.: *Inflammatory Bowel Diseases and Morbus Hirschprung.* Falk Symposium No. 65. 1992   ISBN: 0-7923-8995-6
66. Martin F, McLeod RS, Sutherland LR, Williams CN, eds.: *Trends in Inflammatory Bowel Disease Therapy.* Falk Symposium No. 66. 1993   ISBN: 0-7923-8827-5
67. Schölmerich J, Kruis W, Goebell H, Hohenberger W, Gross V, eds.: *Inflammatory Bowel Diseases – Pathophysiology as Basis of Treatment.* Falk Symposium No. 67. 1993   ISBN: 0-7923-8996-4
68. Paumgartner G, Stiehl A, Gerok W, eds.: *Bile Acids and The Hepatobiliary System: From Basic Science to Clinical Practice.* Falk Symposium No. 68. 1993   ISBN: 0-7923-8829-1
69. Schmid R, Bianchi L, Gerok W, Maier K-P, eds.: *Extrahepatic Manifestations in Liver Diseases.* Falk Symposium No. 69. 1993   ISBN: 0-7923-8821-6
70. Meyer zum Büschenfelde K-H, Hoofnagle J, Manns M, eds.: *Immunology and Liver.* Falk Symposium No. 70. 1993   ISBN: 0-7923-8830-5
71. Surrenti C, Casini A, Milani S, Pinzani M , eds.: *Fat-Storing Cells and Liver Fibrosis.* Falk Symposium No. 71. 1994   ISBN: 0-7923-8842-9
72. Rachmilewitz D, ed.: *Inflammatory Bowel Diseases – 1994.* Falk Symposium No. 72. 1994   ISBN: 0-7923-8845-3
73. Binder HJ, Cummings J, Soergel KH, eds.: *Short Chain Fatty Acids.* Falk Symposium No. 73. 1994   ISBN: 0-7923-8849-6
73B. Möllmann HW, May B, eds.: *Glucocorticoid Therapy in Chronic Inflammatory Bowel Disease: from basic principles to rational therapy.* International Falk Workshop. 1996   ISBN 0-7923-8708-2
74. Keppler D, Jungermann K, eds.: *Transport in the Liver.* Falk Symposium No. 74. 1994   ISBN: 0-7923-8858-5
74B. Stange EF, ed.: *Chronic Inflammatory Bowel Disease.* Falk Symposium. 1995   ISBN: 0-7923-8876-3
75. van Berge Henegouwen GP, van Hoek B, De Groote J, Matern S, Stockbrügger RW, eds.: *Cholestatic Liver Diseases: New Strategies for Prevention and Treatment of Hepatobiliary and Cholestatic Liver Diseases.* Falk Symposium 75. 1994.   ISBN: 0-7923-8867-4
76. Monteiro E, Tavarela Veloso F, eds.: *Inflammatory Bowel Diseases: New Insights into Mechanisms of Inflammation and Challenges in Diagnosis and Treatment.* Falk Symposium 76. 1995.   ISBN 0-7923-8884-4
77. Singer MV, Ziegler R, Rohr G, eds.: *Gastrointestinal Tract and Endocrine System.* Falk Symposium 77. 1995.   ISBN 0-7923-8877-1
78. Decker K, Gerok W, Andus T, Gross V, eds.: *Cytokines and the Liver.* Falk Symposium 78. 1995.   ISBN 0-7923-8878-X
79. Holstege A, Schölmerich J, Hahn EG, eds.: *Portal Hypertension.* Falk Symposium 79. 1995.   ISBN 0-7923-8879-8
80. Hofmann AF, Paumgartner G, Stiehl A, eds.: *Bile Acids in Gastroenterology: Basic and Clinical Aspects.* Falk Symposium 80. 1995   ISBN 0-7923-8880-1
81. Riecken EO, Stallmach A, Zeitz M, Heise W, eds.: *Malignancy and Chronic Inflammation in the Gastrointestinal Tract – New Concepts.* Falk Symposium 81. 1995 ISBN 0-7923-8889-5
82. Fleig WE, ed.: *Inflammatory Bowel Diseases: New Developments and Standards.* Falk Symposium 82. 1995   ISBN 0-7923-8890-6

Falk Symposium Series

Falk Symposium Series

100. Blum HE, Bode Ch, Bode JCh, Sartor RB, eds. *Gut and the Liver.* Falk Symposium 100. 1998   ISBN 0-7923-8736-8
101. Rachmilewitz D, ed. *V International Symposium on Inflammatory Bowel Diseases.* Falk Symposium 101. 1998   ISBN 0-7923-8743-0
102. Manns MP, Boyer JL, Jansen PLM, Reichen J, eds. *Cholestatic Liver Diseases.* Falk Symposium 102. 1998   ISBN 0-7923-8746-5
102B. Manns MP, Chapman RW, Stiehl A, Wiesner R, eds. *Primary Sclerosing Cholangitis.* International Falk Workshop. 1998.   ISBN 0-7923-8745-7
103. Häussinger D, Jungermann K, eds. *Liver and Nervous System.* Falk Symposium 102. 1998   ISBN 0-7924-8742-2
103B. Häussinger D, Heinrich PC, eds. *Signalling in the Liver.* International Falk Workshop. 1998   ISBN 0-7923-8744-9
103C. Fleig W, ed. *Normal and Malignant Liver Cell Growth.* International Falk Workshop. 1998   ISBN 0-7923-8748-1
104. Stallmach A, Zeitz M, Strober W, MacDonald TT, Lochs H, eds. *Induction and Modulation of Gastrointestinal Inflammation.* Falk Symposium 104. 1998   ISBN 0-7923-8747-3
105. Emmrich J, Liebe S, Stange EF, eds. *Innovative Concepts in Inflammatory Bowel Diseases.* Falk Symposium 105. 1999   ISBN 0-7923-8749-X
106. Rutgeerts P, Colombel J-F, Hanauer SB, Schölmerich J, Tytgat GNJ, van Gossum A, eds. *Advances in Inflammatory Bowel Diseases.* Falk Symposium 106. 1999   ISBN 0-7923-8750-3
107. Špičák J, Boyer J, Gilat T, Kotrlik K, Mareček Z, Paumgartner G, eds. *Diseases of the Liver and the Bile Ducts – New Aspects and Clinical Implications.* Falk Symposium 107. 1999   ISBN 0-7923-8751-1
108. Paumgartner G, Stiehl A, Gerok W, Keppler D, Leuschner U, eds. *Bile Acids and Cholestasis.* Falk Symposium 108. 1999   ISBN 0-7923-8752-X
109. Schmiegel W, Schölmerich J, eds. *Colorectal Cancer – Molecular Mechanisms, Premalignant State and its Prevention.* Falk Symposium 109. 1999   ISBN 0-7923-8753-8
110. Domschke W, Stoll R, Brasitus TA, Kagnoff MF, eds. *Intestinal Mucosa and its Diseases – Pathophysiology and Clinics.* Falk Symposium 110. 1999   ISBN 0-7923-8754-6
110B. Northfield TC, Ahmed HA, Jazwari RP, Zentler-Munro PL, eds. *Bile Acids in Hepatobiliary Disease.* Falk Workshop. 2000   ISBN 0-7923-8755-4
111. Rogler G, Kullmann F, Rutgeerts P, Sartor RB, Schölmerich J, eds. *IBD at the End of its First Century.* Falk Symposium 111. 2000   ISBN 0-7923-8756-2
112. Krammer HJ, Singer MV, eds. *Neurogastroenterology: From the Basics to the Clinics.* Falk Symposium 112. 2000   ISBN 0-7923-8757-0
113. Andus T, Rogler G, Schlottmann K, Frick E, Adler G, Schmiegel W, Zeitz M, Schölmerich J, eds. *Cytokines and Cell Homeostasis in the Gastrointestinal Tract.* Falk Symposium 113. 2000   ISBN 0-7923-8758-9
114. Manns MP, Paumgartner G, Leuschner U, eds. *Immunology and Liver.* Falk Symposium 114. 2000   ISBN 0-7923-8759-7
115. Boyer JL, Blum HE, Maier K-P, Sauerbruch T, Stalder GA, eds. *Liver Cirrhosis and its Development.* Falk Symposium 115. 2000   ISBN 0-7923-8760-0
116. Riemann JF, Neuhaus H, eds. *Interventional Endoscopy in Hepatology.* Falk Symposium 116. 2000   ISBN 0-7923-8761-9

Falk Symposium Series

116A. Dienes HP, Schirmacher P, Brechot C, Okuda K, eds. *Chronic Hepatitis: New Concepts of Pathogenesis, Diagnosis and Treatment.* Falk Workshop. 2000
ISBN 0-7923-8763-5

117. Gerbes AL, Beuers U, Jüngst D, Pape GR, Sackmann M, Sauerbruch T, eds. *Hepatology 2000 – Symposium in Honour of Gustav Paumgartner.* Falk Symposium 117. 2000 ISBN 0-7923-8765-1

117A. Acalovschi M, Paumgartner G, eds. *Hepatobiliary Diseases: Cholestasis and Gallstones.* Falk Workshop. 2000 ISBN 0-7923-8770-8

118. Frühmorgen P, Bruch H-P, eds. *Non-Neoplastic Diseases of the Anorectum.* Falk Symposium 118. 2001 ISBN 0-7923-8766-X

119. Fellermann K, Jewell DP, Sandborn WJ, Schölmerich J, Stange EF, eds. *Immunosuppression in Inflammatory Bowel Diseases – Standards, New Developments, Future Trends.* Falk Symposium 119. 2001 ISBN 0-7923-8767-8

120. van Berge Henegouwen GP, Keppler D, Leuschner U, Paumgartner G, Stiehl A, eds. *Biology of Bile Acids in Health and Disease.* Falk Symposium 120. 2001
ISBN 0-7923-8768-6

121. Leuschner U, James OFW, Dancygier H, eds. *Steatohepatitis (NASH and ASH).* Falk Symposium 121. 2001 ISBN 0-7923-8769-4

121A. Matern S, Boyer JL, Keppler D, Meier-Abt PJ, eds. *Hepatobiliary Transport: From Bench to Bedside.* Falk Workshop. 2001 ISBN 0-7923-8771-6

122. Campieri M, Fiocchi C, Hanauer SB, Jewell DP, Rachmilewitz R, Schölmerich J, eds. *Inflammatory Bowel Disease – A Clinical Case Approach to Pathophysiology, Diagnosis, and Treatment.* Falk Symposium 122. 2002 ISBN 0-7923-8772-4

123. Rachmilewitz D, Modigliani R, Podolsky DK, Sachar DB, Tozun N, eds. *VI International Symposium on Inflammatory Bowel Diseases.* Falk Symposium 123. 2002 ISBN 0-7923-8773-2

124. Hagenmüller F, Manns MP, Musmann H-G, Riemann JF, eds. *Medical Imaging in Gastroenterology and Hepatology.* Falk Symposium 124. 2002 ISBN 0-7923-8774-0

125. Gressner AM, Heinrich PC, Matern S, eds. *Cytokines in Liver Injury and Repair.* Falk Symposium 125. 2002 ISBN 0-7923-8775-9

126. Gupta S, Jansen PLM, Klempnauer J, Manns MP, eds. *Hepatocyte Transplantation.* Falk Symposium 126. 2002 ISBN 0-7923-8776-7

127. Hadziselimovic F, ed. *Autoimmune Diseases in Paediatric Gastroenterology.* Falk Symposium 127. 2002 ISBN 0-7923-8778-3

127A. Berr F, Bruix J, Hauss J, Wands J, Wittekind Ch, eds. *Malignant Liver Tumours: Basic Concepts and Clinical Management.* Falk Workshop. 2002
ISBN 0-7923-8779-1

128. Scheppach W, Scheurlen M, eds. *Exogenous Factors in Colonic Carcinogenesis.* Falk Symposium 128. 2002 ISBN 0-7923-8780-5

129. Paumgartner G, Keppler D, Leuschner U, Stiehl A, eds. *Bile Acids: From Genomics to Disease and Therapy.* Falk Symposium 129. 2002 ISBN 0-7923-8781-3

129A. Leuschner U, Berg PA, Holtmeier J, eds. *Bile Acids and Pregnancy.* Falk Workshop. 2002 ISBN 0-7923-8782-1

130. Holtmann G, Talley NJ, eds. *Gastrointestinal Inflammation and Disturbed Gut Function: The Challenge of New Concepts.* Falk Symposium 130. 2003
ISBN 0-7923-8783-X

131. Herfarth H, Feagan BJ, Folsch UR, Schölmerich J, Vatn MH, Zeitz M, eds. *Targets of Treatment in Chronic Inflammatory Bowel Diseases.* Falk Symposium 131. 2003
ISBN 0-7923-8784-8

Falk Symposium Series

132. Galle PR, Gerken G, Schmidt WE, Wiedenmann B, eds. *Disease Progression and Carcinogenesis in the Gastrointestinal Tract.* Falk Symposium 132. 2003
ISBN 0-7923-8785-6

132A. Staritz M, Adler G, Knuth A, Schmiegel W, Schmoll H-J, eds. *Side-effects of Chemotherapy on the Gastrointestinal Tract.* Falk Workshop. 2003
ISBN 0-7923-8791-0

132B. Reutter W, Schuppan D, Tauber R, Zeitz M, eds. *Cell Adhesion Molecules in Health and Disease.* Falk Workshop. 2003   ISBN 0-7923-8786-4

133. Duchmann R, Blumberg R, Neurath M, Schölmerich J, Strober W, Zeitz M. *Mechanisms of Intestinal Inflammation: Implications for Therapeutic Intervention in IBD.* Falk Symposium 133. 2004   ISBN 0-7923-8787-2

134. Dignass A, Lochs H, Stange E. *Trends and Controversies in IBD – Evidence-Based Approach or Individual Management?* Falk Symposium 134. 2004
ISBN 0-7923-8788-0

134A. Dignass A, Gross HJ, Buhr V, James OFW. *Topical Steroids in Gastroenterology and Hepatology.* Falk Workshop. 2004   ISBN 0-7923-8789-9

135. Lukáš M, Manns MP, Špičák J, Stange EF, eds. *Immunological Diseases of Liver and Gut.* Falk Symposium 135. 2004   ISBN 0-7923-8792-9

136. Leuschner U, Broomé U, Stiehl A, eds. *Cholestatic Liver Diseases: Therapeutic Options and Perspectives.* Falk Symposium 136. 2004   ISBN 0-7923-8793-7

137. Blum HE, Maier KP, Rodés J, Sauerbruch T, eds. *Liver Diseases: Advances in Treatment and Prevention.* Falk Symposium 137. 2004   ISBN 0-7923-8794-5

138. Blum HE, Manns MP, eds. *State of the Art of Hepatology: Molecular and Cell Biology.* Falk Symposium 138. 2004   ISBN 0-7923-8795-3

138A. Hayashi N, Manns MP, eds. *Prevention of Progression in Chronic Liver Disease: An Update on SNMC (Stronger Neo-Minophagen C).* Falk Workshop. 2004
ISBN 0-7923-8796-1

139. Adler G, Blum HE, Fuchs M, Stange EF, eds. *Gallstones: Pathogenesis and Treatment.* Falk Symposium 139. 2004   ISBN 0-7923-8798-8

140. Colombel J-F, Gasché C, Schölmerich J, Vucelic C, eds. *Inflammatory Bowel Disease: Translation from Basic Research to Clinical Practice.* Falk Symposium 140. 2005.   ISBN 1-4020-2847-4

141. Paumgartner G, Keppler D, Leuschner U, Stiehl A, eds. *Bile Acid Biology and its Therapeutic Implications.* Falk Symposium 141. 2005   ISBN 1-4020-2893-8

142. Dienes H-P, Leuschner U, Lohse AW, Manns MP, eds. *Autoimmune Liver Disease.* Falk Symposium 142. 2005   ISBN 1-4020-2894-6

143. Ammann RW, Büchler MW, Adler G, DiMagno EP, Sarner M, eds. *Pancreatitis: Advances in Pathobiology, Diagnosis and Treatment.* Falk Symposium 143. 2005
ISBN 1-4020-2895-4

144. Adler G, Blum AL, Blum HE, Leuschner U, Manns MP, Mössner J, Sartor RB, Schölmerich J, eds. *Gastroenterology Yesterday – Today – Tomorrow: A Review and Preview.* Falk Symposium 144. 2005   ISBN 1-4020-2896-2

145. Henne-Bruns D, Buttenschön K, Fuchs M, Lohse AW, eds. *Artificial Liver Support.* Falk Symposium 145. 2005   ISBN 1-4020-3239-0

146. Blumberg RS, Gangl A, Manns MP, Tilg H, Zeitz M, eds. *Gut–Liver Interactions: Basic and Clinical Concepts.* Falk Symposium 146. 2005   ISBN 1-4020-4143-8

147. Jewell DP, Colombel JF, Peña AS, Tromm A, Warren BS, eds. *Colitis: Diagnosis and Therapeutic Strategies.* Falk Symposium 147. 2006   ISBN 1-4020-4315-5

Falk Symposium Series

148. Kruis W, Forbes A, Jauch K-W, Kreis ME, Wexner SD, eds. *Diverticular Disease: Emerging Evidence in a Common Condition.* Falk Symposium 148. 2006
ISBN 1-4020- 4317-1

149. van Cutsem E, Rustgi AK, Schmiegel W, Zeitz M, eds. *Highlights in Gastrointestinal Oncology.* Falk Symposium 149. 2006.   ISBN 1-4020-5108-5

150. Galle PR, Gerken G, Schmidt WE, Wiedenmann B, eds. *Disease Progression and Disease Prevention in Hepatology and Gastroenterology.* Falk Symposium 150. 2006
ISBN 1-4020-5109-3

151. Fraser A, Gibson PR, Hibi T, Qian J-M, Schölmerich, eds. *Emerging Issues in Inflammatory Bowel Disease.* Falk Symposium 151. 2006
ISBN-13 978-1-4020-5701-4

152. Not published.

153. Dignass A, Rachmilewitz D, Stange E-F, Weinstock JV, eds. *Immunoregulation in Inflammatory Bowel Diseases – Current Understanding and Innovation.* Falk Symposium 153. 2007   ISBN-13 978-1-4020-5888-2

154. Adler G, Fiocchi C, Lazebnik LB, Vorobiev GI, eds. *Inflammatory Bowel Disease – Diagnostic and Therapeutic Strategies.* Falk Symposium 154. 2007
ISBN-13 978-1-4020-6115-8